Nasal Polyps: Epidemiology, Pathogenesis and Treatment

Nasal Polyps: Epidemiology, Pathogenesis and Treatment

Guy A. Settipane, M.D.

Valerie J. Lund, M.S., F.R.C.S.

Joel M. Bernstein, M.D., Ph.D.

Mirko Tos, M.D., Ph.D.

OceanSide Publications, Inc.

Providence, Rhode Island 1997

OceanSide Publications, Inc.

Library of Congress Catalog Card Number 96-070568

Published by OceanSide Publications, Inc., 95 Pitman Street, Providence, Rhode Island 02906

Printed in the United States of America
ISBN 0-936587-09-1

Contributors

Mark L. Benson, M.D. Clinical Instructor
Russell H. Morgan Department of
Radiology and Radiological Sciences
The Johns Hopkins Medical Institutions
Baltimore, Maryland 21287

John P. Bent, III, M.D.
Service Chief,Pediatric Otolaryngology
Children's Medical Center
Medical College of Georgia
Augusta, Georgia 30912-4060

Joel M. Bernstein, M.D., Ph.D.
Clinical Associate Professor
Departments of Otolaryngology and
Pediatrics, and Research Professor,
Department of Speech and
Communication Sciences
State University of New York at Buffalo
15 South Forest Road
Williamsville, New York 14221

David J. Brain, F.R.C.S.
Honorary Consultant Surgeon
Department of Otolaryngology and
Head and Neck Surgery
Queen Elizabeth Hospital
Birmingham, England UK

Peter M.G. Deane, M.D.
Clinical Assistant Professor
of Medicine and Emergency
Medicine
220 Alexander Street Suite 402
Rochester, New York 14607

Jerry Dolovich, M.D.
Professor, Department of Pediatrics
McMaster University
1200 Main Street West Room 3V41
Hamilton, Ontario, Canada L8N 3Z5

Adrian B. Drake-Lee, Ph.D., F.R.C.S.
Consultant ENT Surgeon
Queen Elizabeth Hospital
Edgbaston, Birmingham,
England B15 2TH

**Henrik B. Hellquist, M.D., Ph.D.,
F.C.A.P.**
Associate Professor,
Department of Pathology II
University Hospital
Linköping, Sweden

Hal M. Hoffman, M.D.
Department of Allergy & Immunology
University of California, San Diego
9500 Gilman Drive
La Jolla, California 92093-0635

Manel Jordana, M.D., Ph.D.
Associate Professor of Pathology
McMaster University
1200 Main Street West Room 4H21
Hamilton, Ontario, Canada L8N 3Z5

David W. Kennedy, M.D.
Professor and Chair Otorhinolaryngology:
Head and Neck Surgery
University of Pennsylvania Medical Center
Philadelphia, Pennsylvania

Frederick A. Kuhn, M.D.
Director, Georgia Rhinology and Sinus
Center
Georgia Ear Institute
4700 Waters Avenue
Savannah, Georgia 31414

Knud Larsen, M.D.
ENT Clinic
Jernbanegade 22
6700 Esbjere, Denmark

Torben Lildholdt, M.D., Ph.D.
Department of Otorhinolaryngology
Vejle Hospital,
DK-7100 Vejle, Denmark

**Valerie J. Lund, M.S., F.R.C.S.,
F.R.C.S.Ed.**
Professor in Rhinology
Honorary Consultant Surgeon
Professional Unit
The Institute of Laryngology & Otology
University College London
London, WCIX 8EE England UK

Ian S. Mackay, M.D., F.R.C.S.
Consultant ENT Surgeon
Charing Cross Hospital and
Royal Brompton Hospital
London, England UK

Niels Mygind, M.D.
Otopathological Laboratory,
Department of Otorhinolaryngology,
Rigshospitalet,
Copenhagen, Denmark

Patrick J. Oliverio, M.D.
Clinical Instructor
Russell H. Morgan Department of
Radiology and Radiological Sciences
The Johns Hopkins Medical Institutions
Baltimore, Maryland 21287

Maurice Roth, M.D.
Assistant Professor of Otolaryngology-
Head and Neck Surgery

Thomas Jefferson University
Philadelphia, Pennsylvania and
Lecturer, Department of Otolaryngology-
Head and Neck Surgery
University of Pennsylvania
Philadelphia, Pennsylvania

Robert H. Schwartz, M.D.
Professor of Pediatrics,
Director, Clinical Pediatric Allergy
Division of Immunology, Allergy and
Rheumatology
Department of Pediatrics
University of Rochester Medical Center
601 Elmwood Avenue
Rochester, New York

Guy A. Settipane, M.D.
Clinical Professor of Medicine
Brown University School of Medicine
Providence, Rhode Island

Russell A. Settipane, M.D.
Clinical Assistant Professor of Medicine
Brown University School of Medicine
Providence, Rhode Island

Heinz Stammberger, M.D.
Professor and Head
Department of General ORL
Head and Neck Surgery
University Medical School
Graz, Austria

Pontus Stierna, M.D., Ph.D.
Associate Professor, Department of
Otorhinolaryngology
Huddinge University Hospital
S-141 86 Huddinge, Sweden

Mirko Tos, M.D., Ph.D.
Professor and Chairman
Department of Otorhinolaryngology
Gentofte Hospital
University of Copenhagen
Hellerup, DK-2900 Denmark

Stephen I. Wasserman, M.D.
The Helen M. Ranney Professor and
Chairman, Department of Medicine
University of California, San Diego
402 Dickinson St. Suite 380
San Diego, California 92103

S. James Zinreich, M.D.
Associate Professor
Russell H. Morgan Department of
Radiology and Radiological Sciences
The Johns Hopkins Medical Institutions
Baltimore, Maryland 21287

Cover Photo: An endoscopic view of the nasal cavity, showing the middle turbinate with a small polyp in the anterior middle meatus. *(Courtesy of Valerie J. Lund, M.S., F.R.C.S., F.R.C.S. Ed. The Institute of Laryngology and Otology, University College London, London, England.)*

Foreword

Nasal polyposis is not a rare condition. Therefore this book, *Nasal Polyps: Epidemiology, Pathogenesis and Treatment,* which is the first book devoted entirely to the subject, is long overdue. The Editors have enlisted a stellar group of contributors whose knowledge and expertise are recognized internationally in laboratory research, clinical investigation or clinical practice. With their critical insights, the authors are able to provide in-depth presentations of the various facets of this illness. In a logical and systematic fashion, the authors cover the Historical Background, Epidemiology, Anatomy, Histopathology, Pathogenesis, Immunology, Pathophysiology, Clinical Relationships, Diagnosis and both Medical and Surgical Therapy.

Since the etiology of nasal polyps has not been defined, this condition presents a challenge to many clinicians. In addition, nasal polyps have been associated with conditions such as cystic fibrosis, aspirin sensitivity and allergic fungal sinusitis which are quite different in their pathogenesis and manifestations. The relationships of nasal polyps to inflammation via infection, allergy and other mechanisms are presented in a clear understandable manner. The same can be said for the chapter that discusses the management of polyps, both medical and surgical. Therefore, this book will be of interest to not only otorhinolaryngologists but also physicians interested in infectious disease, pediatrics, internal medicine, allergy and clinical immunology.

Philip Fireman, M.D.
Professor of Pediatrics and Medicine
University of Pittsburgh
School of Medicine

Preface

Rhinology is a diverse and expanding specialty, embracing basic science and many disciplines of medicine and surgery. Nowhere is this more apparent than in the study of nasal polyps, a common condition which produces chronic misery for sufferers, but which has proved tantalisingly difficult to manage and whose aetiology and pathophysiology has remained obscure. Happily, significant advances have been made in recent years and this book, the first entirely devoted to the subject, represents a distillation of that knowledge by some of the most prominent contributors in the field.

Clearly, this is a rapidly changing area but our contributors have responded to the challenge in record time and we thank them for their diligence and clarity of style.

*We wish to thank our publishing staff:
Cynthia Burke, Candace E. Crowshaw,
Michele A.L. Doherty, Carole Fico, and
Virginia Loiselle, for their help in
publishing this book.*

Contents

Chapter I

Introduction

Guy A. Settipane, M.D., Valerie J. Lund, M.S., F.R.C.S., Joel M. Bernstein, M.D., Ph.D.
and Mirko Tos, M.D., Ph.D.

Polypus—many footed.

The condition of nasal polyposis has been an enigma in the recorded history of mankind. It is found in a wide number of diseases and has varied histological components determined by the basic disease state. Thus it may represent a common pathological end point in a number of disease processes and offers a spectrum of severity ranging from discrete localized lesions to massive diffuse mucosal change producing significant facial deformity.

There has never been a comprehensive book on nasal polyps and as far as we know this is the first book devoted entirely to the subject. However, a considerable amount of research has been performed on the subject as evidenced by the mass of published work in the medical literature. In an attempt to render some order to the prolific data on this topic we have organized the book by including authors in various specialties. These contributors from medicine and surgery cover the field of medical history, basic science, histopathology, otorhinolaryngology, internal medicine, pediatrics, infectious diseases, allergy and clinical immunology. The list includes many of the foremost contributors in this field who have offered a distillation of their knowledge on the subject and in presenting this multi-disciplinary approach is very much in keeping with the philosophy of Dr. Cottle.

Chapter II
HISTORICAL BACKGROUND
David J. Brain

The history of nasal polyps goes back for a period of over 4,000 years to Ancient Egypt and this condition may, perhaps, be the earliest recorded disease in which we know the names of both the patient and the physician. Further

significant advances were made in Ancient Greece and Renaissance Europe but the real transformation of nasal polypectomy, from an extremely painful and potentially dangerous procedure, into a routine minor operation did not occur until the end of the 19th century.

Chapter III
EPIDEMIOLOGY OF NASAL POLYPS
Guy A. Settipane

Nasal polyps are found in 36% of patients with aspirin intolerance, 7% of those with asthma, 0.1% in children, and about 20% in those with cystic fibrosis. Other conditions associated with nasal polyps are Churg-Strauss Syndrome, allergic fungal sinusitis, and cilia dyskinetic syndrome, (Kartagener's) and Young Syndrome. Nasal polyps are statistically more common in non allergic asthma vs. allergic asthma (13% vs. 5%, P < 0.01). About 40% of patients with surgical polypectomy have recurrences. There appears to be a hereditary factor for developing nasal polyps. A classification system for staging nasal polyps is proposed in order to standardize treatment, consider differential diagnosis, and harvest meaningful comparative research information.

Chapter IV
ANATOMY OF NASAL POLYPS
Ian S. Mackay

The ciliated mucous membrane lining the nose is continuous with that of the paranasal sinuses. The latter develop embryologically as out pouchings from shallow grooves and furrows laterally to form the maxillary and ethmoidal sinuses, with the sphenoid sinus posteriorly and the frontal sinus superiorly. The nasal cavity is divided sagittally into left and right halves by the nasal septum. Above, the nose and paranasal sinuses are separated from the intracranial cavity by the roof of the ethmoids, sphenoids and cribriform plate while the orbital contents are divided from the ethmoids by the delicate lamina papyracea. The lateral wall of the nose is characterized by the superior, middle and inferior turbinates lateral to each of which is a corresponding meatus. The nasolacrimal duct drains tears from the lacrimal sac to the inferior meatus. The maxillary sinus drains via its ostium into the middle meatus which also drains the anterior ethmoid and frontal sinuses. This region, termed the ostiomeatal complex (OMC), is therefore of great importance as obstruction here will interfere with the drainage and aeration of the maxillary, anterior ethmoid and frontal sinuses. The posterior ethmoidal sinuses drain via the superior meatus. The spheno ethmoidal recess lies medial to the superior turbinate and is the location of the ostium of the sphenoid sinus.

Chapter V
HISTOPATHOLOGY
Henrik B. Hellquist

Sinonasal polyps are benign mucosal swellings that occur in four different histological patterns. The most common type is the oedematous, eosinophilic (so-called "allergic") nasal polyp, which constitutes 85–90% of nasal polyps. The oedematous polyp is morphologically characterized by oedema, goblet cell hyperplasia of the epithelium, thickening of the basement membrane, and of numerous leukocytes, predominantly eosinophils. The second histological type is a fibroinflammatory polyp characterized by chronic inflammation and metaplastic changes of the overlying epithelium. Another rare variant presents with pronounced hyperplasia of seromucinous glands but otherwise shows many similarities with the oedematous type of polyp. The fourth type is very rare and is a polyp with atypical stroma. This latter polyp calls for awareness and careful histological examination to avoid misdiagnosis of a neoplasm.

Chapter VI
CHEMICAL MEDIATORS IN POLYPS
Hal M. Hoffman and Stephen I. Wasserman

This chapter outlines the many chemical mediators of inflammation that have been studied in nasal polyps. The cell sources and actions of traditional as well as newer mediators are discussed. Results of research in this area are presented and implications for further study of nasal polyps and related disease states are postulated.

Chapter VII
EOSINOPHILS IN NASAL POLYPS
Manel Jordana and Jerry Dolovich

Nasal polyposis represents a paradigm of chronic airways inflammation. Eosinophils comprise the most prevalent inflammatory cell type in nasal polyp tissues except in those occurring in patients with Cystic Fibrosis and Kartagener Syndrome. These cells have a demonstrated ability to release mediators such as eosinophil peroxidase (EPO), eosinophil derived neurotoxin (EDN), eosinophil cationic protein (ECP) and other capable of causing cellular injury and tissue damage. In addition, it has become clear over the last few years that eosinophils and, specifically, eosinophils in nasal polyp tissues, can also synthesize and release a number of powerful regulatory molecules referred to as cytokines. Interestingly, some of these molecules such as GM-CSF, TNFα and IL-4 can, directly or indirectly, contribute to the further recruitment and activation of eosinophils. Others, such as TGFα and TGFβ can participate in the tissue structural abnormalities characteristic of nasal polyposis. This evidence establishes novel roles for eosinophils in the regulation of upper airways inflammation and, we suggest, provides the molecular basis for self-perpetuating eosinophilia.

Chapter VIII
THE PATHOGENESIS OF NASAL POLYPS
Adrian Drake-Lee

Pathogenesis has three stages, the evaluation of any underlying condition, understanding any factors in the genesis of tissue oedema and finally the symptoms that these reactions may cause. Nasal polyps occur almost solely in humans, more commonly in men and are found in all racial groups. Simple polyps may arise at any age after two and are usually due to cystic fibrosis in childhood. The mucosal changes may not be limited to the upper respiratory tract since patients may have co-existing asthma or other respiratory diseases. There is some evidence for a genetic predisposition and certain conditions such as immune deficiency, ciliary dyskinesia, Young's syndrome and aspirin hypersensitivity are associated with the condition. The origins of the tissue oedema may be explained at the cellular level: mast cells are degranulated with the resultant inflammatory mediators which attract eosinophils which in turn may damage tissue and perpetuate the changes. These reactions are exaggerated by the relatively poorly developed blood supply of the ethmoid sinuses. Finally, neurovascular reflexes and the complex anatomy of the ethmoid labyrinth can predispose to the persistence of oedema. Patients complain about nasal blockage, loss of sense of smell and also may suffer from attacks of sneezing, anterior rhinorrhea, pain and post nasal drainage.

Chapter IX
EARLY STAGE OF POLYP FORMATION
Mirko Tos

In 1977 Tos' group described the epithelial rupture theory on formation of nasal polyps. He postulated that polyp formation can start with a rupture of the epithelium caused by pressure from the edematous and infiltrated lamina propria. The lamina propria protrudes through the epithelial defect and the mucosa tends to cover it by migration of the epithelium from the edges of the defect. If the regeneration of the epithelium does not occur soon enough to cover the prolapse, or if the prolapse of the lamina propria continue to grow, the polyp will be formed and the vessel stalk established. During the early growth of the polyp some special long tubulus glands are found. These glands have a completely different structure, shape and size than the nasal seromucous glands and are a definitive proof that the polyp is not a prolapse of protrusion of the nasal or sinus mucosa. The polyp pathogenesis is divided into the following stages: 1) Epithelial damage, necrosis and rupture due to tissue pressure by inflammatory edema and infiltration of the cells of the nasal mucosa leading to a prolapse of the lamina propria. 2) Epithelialization of the prolapse. 3) Gland formation. 4) Enlargement due to gravity and elongation of the glands. 5) Changes of the epithelium and stroma of the well-developed polyp.

The first two stages are difficult to prove in the human nose, but experimentally we have been able to demonstrate, in three different models, including experimental acute otitis and long term tubal occlusion, that the epithelial necrosis in fact takes place during the infection. These experiments are briefly described.

Chapter X
BASIC SINUS IMAGING AND RADIOLOGICAL ASPECTS OF NASAL POLYPOSIS
Patrick J. Oliverio, Mark L. Benson
and S. James Zinreich

Coronal CT scanning is the imaging modality of choice in patients with sinus disease. CT scanning provides an initial screening of these patients and can display both anatomy and pathology both before and after surgery. CT is essential in surgical planning, and it provides an operative "roadmap". Close cooperation between the radiologist and otolaryngologist-head and neck surgeon allows for more accurate diagnosis and brings to light findings predisposing the patient to operative complications. When complications occur, the radiologist can provide assistance in evaluation using CT, MR, and nuclear medicine studies. Interactive image-guided, computer-assisted surgery now exists and holds great promise in objectively and directly integrating the imaging information with the endoscopic view and thus improve the accuracy and safety of the operative management of patients undergoing sinus surgery.

Chapter XI
THE IMMUNOHISTOPATHOLOGY AND PATHOPHYSIOLOGY OF NASAL POLYPS
Joel M. Bernstein

Bernstein reviews his data on nasal polyps and turbinates. Monoclonal antibodies were used to identify macrophages, lymphocytes and plasma cells. The remainder of the polyps and turbinates were treated with protease to achieve disaggregation of the epithelial cells. Transepithelial potential differences and resistance were measured daily. At the time of maximal transepithelial potential difference, the epithelial cells were mounted and modified in Ussing chambers and exposed to a sodium positive channel blocker (amiloride hydrochloride) and to selected chloride negative channel agonists (isoproterenol bitartrate and adenosine triphosphate). Middle turbinates and polyps were found to have more macrophages, lymphocytes, plasma cells, HLA-DR positive cells and eosinophils than the inferior turbinates. IgA represents the most common immunocyte present and is distributed primarily around the glands and in general outnumber IgG producing immunocytes 5–10 to 1. Epithelial cells obtained from polyps exhibited higher transepithelial potential differences and equivalent short circuit currents than turbinate cell cultures. The responses to amiloride, isoproterenol and adenosine triphosphate were also greater for polyp than for turbinate cultures. A theory for the pathogenesis of nasal polyps is proposed. Local release of inflammatory mediators could cause sodium absorption and chloride permeability to be higher in polyps than in turbinate epithelia. Increased sodium absorption is consistent with the hypothesis that epithelial fluid absorption contributes to the development of nasal polyps and is secondary to the increased recruitment of inflammatory cells which are present in nasal polyps. Finally, the differential diagnosis of unilateral and bilateral nasal masses is reviewed.

Chapter XII
THE CLINICAL RELATIONSHIP OF NASAL POLYPS TO ASTHMA
Knud Larsen

The clinical relationship of nasal polyps to asthma was reviewed by Knud Larsen of Denmark. From a meta-analysis on the clinical related literature on asthma and nasal polyps, it was found that patients with asthma had polyps in 7–15% of the time with the highest frequency in the age group above 50 years. Patients with nasal polyps had a diagnosis of asthma at an average of 29.9% in those referred to ENT-departments. Not all polyp patients had an associated lower airway disease, neither as manifest asthma, nor as hyper reactive airways as tested by methacholine challenge test. Asthma developed before the onset of polyps in an average of 69% of the series. Most patients showed improvement or at the least were unchanged in the control of their asthma after surgery. Bronchospasm during endonasal surgery was observed in less than 2%. Control of polyps and sinus disease showed a poorer outcome in patients with asthma, and this was even more pronounced in patients having ASA intolerance.

Chapter XIII
NASAL POLYPS AND
IMMUNOGLOBULIN E (IgE)
Guy A. Settipane

The association of nasal polyps to immunoglobulin E (IgE) or atopy is discussed by Guy A. Settipane. Nasal polyps are usually found in non allergic individuals. However, when nasal polyps and atopy occur together a special interaction exists. Total and specific immunoglobulin E (IgE) are found in significantly greater concentration in nasal polyp tissue than in serum and tonsil tissue. Patients with nasal polyps and allergies seem to have a greater recurrence rate after surgical polypectomy. Precipitating factors for recurrence are a specific pollen season in sensitive individuals, and upper respiratory infections. Nasal ciliary beat frequency is inhibited in patients with chronic sinusitis, allergic nasal reactions, and non specific nasal eosinophilia syndromes (NARES, BENARS). Nasal polyps are frequently associated with these conditions, which may predispose the nasal mucosa to infections and increased risk for developing nasal polyps. When nasal polyps and allergies occur together, it is important to treat the allergic condition. This takes the form of identifying the allergens, eliminating them from the environment (if possible), using antihistamines/decongestants, and nasal antiinflammatory drugs such as topical steroids. Hyposensitization may be considered in resistant cases.

Chapter XIV
NASAL POLYPS AND ASPIRIN INTOLERANCE
Guy A. Settipane and Russell A. Settipane

The relationship between nasal polyps and aspirin intolerance is discussed by Guy A. Settipane, and his son, Russell A. Settipane. The tetrad of aspirin intolerance (bronchospastic type), nasal polyps, asthma and chronic sinusitis is well established. However, nasal polyps and aspirin intolerance frequently occur alone. There are many similar characteristics between nasal polyps and aspirin intolerance. Both have an increased frequency with increased age, both are not mediated by IgE anti-

body, both are usually associated with eosinophilia, and both have a familial occurrence. Nasal polyps are most frequently found in association with non allergic asthma. The pathological mechanism of aspirin intolerance is through the inhibition of the cyclo-oxygenase pathway of arachidonic metabolism resulting in increased production of leukotriene, which can cause acute bronchospasm. Nasal polyps do not appear to be associated with this mechanism. However, the effect of the new antileukotriene drugs on nasal polyps has not been determined. Surgical removal of nasal polyps does not appear to cause or aggravate asthma. Surgical polypectomy in patients with aspirin intolerance is associated with a shorter interval of polyp recurrence than the interval of polyp recurrence in those without aspirin intolerance.

Chapter XV
NASAL POLYPS, RELATIONSHIP TO
INFECTION AND INFLAMMATION
Pontus L. E. Steirna

Since no single predisposing disease can account for the formation of nasal polyps in all patients, medical and surgical therapy has to be directed towards the inflammatory process and/or the underlying infection together with the development of local tissue pathology. Light and electron microscopical studies in experimental models have revealed that the initial polyp formation sequence involves multiple epithelial disruptions with proliferating granulation tissue where immature branching epithelium migrates to cover the mucosal defect. Other branches spread into the underlying connective tissue where intraepithelial microcavities with a differentiated epithelial lining separate the developing polyp body from the adjacent mucosa. Polyp formation and growth is thus activated and perpetuated by an integrated process of mucosal epithelium, matrix and inflammatory cells, which in turn may be initiated by both infectious and noninfectious inflammation. Glucocorticosteroids display a favorable therapeutic profile directly preventing both polyp formation and polyp growth but also by reducing local pathology and inflammatory exudate together with bacterial colonization. Steroids often combined with antibiotics or surgery aimed at specific events in polyp development have to be used in relation to disease progression and severity as well as differences in clinical behavior due to the multifactorial pathophysiological events of nasal polyposis.

Chapter XVI
ALLERGIC FUNGAL SINUSITIS
John P. Bent and Frederick A. Kuhn

It is estimated that 100% of patients with fungal sinusitis have associated nasal-sinus polyp disease. The four types of fungal sinusitis are discussed: acute/fulminant, chronic/ indolent, fungus ball and allergic fungal sinusitis. These can be further sub classified as invasive, non-invasive, acute and chronic. Surgical treatment initially results in dramatic improvement, and oral steroids help maintain postoperative success. However, recurrent disease eventually prevails, leaving a glaring need for improved medical treatment.

Chapter XVII
NASAL POLYPS IN CYSTIC FIBROSIS
Peter M.D. Deane and Robert H. Schwartz

Nasal polyps in cystic fibrosis are reviewed by Peter Deane and Robert Schwartz from the University of Rochester Medical Center. They state that about one third of children and almost one half of adults with this condition suffer from multiple, bilateral nasal polyps. These patients also suffer from chronic pansinusitis. The etiology of the polyps is believed to be related to the chronic sinus inflammation and excessive epithelial sodium and water reabsorption. The histology of the nasal polyps from CF patients differs significantly from those of non-CF allergic rhinitis patients, with less tissue eosinophils and more lymphocytes and plasma cells. Also, the basement membrane is not thickened. Treatment is based on degree of symptoms. Polyps may spontaneously regress. Smaller polyps may respond to topical nasal steroids. More significant and refractory polyps require surgery. Simple polypectomy is helpful but recurrence of the polyps is common.

Chapter XVIII
TREATMENT: MEDICAL MANAGEMENT
Niels Mygind and Torben Lildholdt

The objectives of medical management of nasal polyposis are (1) to eliminate nasal polyps and rhinitis symptoms, (2) to re-establish nasal breathing and olfaction, and (3) to prevent recurrence of nasal polyps. Whilst antibiotics are used for infectious complications of nasal polyposis, only glucocorticosteroids (steroids) have a proven effect on the symptoms and signs of nasal polyps. Topically applied steroid is the therapeutic modality which has been best studied in controlled trials. It reduces rhinitis symptoms, improves nasal breathing, reduces the size of polyps and the recurrence rate, but it has a negligible effect on the sense of smell and on any sinus pathology. Topical steroids can, as long-term therapy, be used alone in mild cases or combined with systemic steroids/surgery in severe cases. Systemic steroids, which are less well studied, have an effect on all types of symptoms and pathology, including the sense of smell. This type of treatment, which can serve as a "medical polypectomy", is usually used for short-

term improvement due to the risk of adverse effects. Individualized management of nasal polyposis may use long-term topical steroids, short-term systemic steroids, as well as surgery, in various combinations. Exactly how these therapies, which differ in their control of various symptoms, are optimally combined is not yet well established.

Chapter XIX
TREATMENT: SURGICAL TREATMENT-NASAL POLYPS
Valerie J. Lund

For most patients the management of nasal polyposis comprises a combination of medical and surgical therapies. Surgical intervention ranges from the most conservative intranasal polypectomy performed with a snare to radical external fronto-ethmo-sphenoidectomy. There is a significant paucity in the literature of well constructed trials considering the various surgical approaches and/or comparing them to medication, but of the operations available, a clearance performed under endoscopic control is felt by many surgeons to offer the best results in the long-term. However, even with the most meticulous surgery it is difficult to replace polypoid sinonasal mucosa with one of macroscopic normality by surgical interference. As a consequence, surgical success must be measured in subjective symptomatic improvement, objective measurement of clinical change, the duration of symptom-free interval and possible improvement of related disorders such as asthma.

Chapter XX
TREATMENT: RHINOSCOPIC SURGERY
Heinz Stammberger

Over the last two decades, a considerable change has taken place in the surgical approach to nasal polyposis. With the advent of the endoscope as a diagnostic tool, better visualization and the ability to "view around the corner" has enabled not only earlier detection, but less traumatic and more precise surgical treatment of diseases presenting with nasal polyps. The concept of Functional Endoscopic Sinus Surgery (FESS) offers individualized surgery according to the respective patient's disease. Routine radical surgical approaches can be avoided with good functional results. In a stepwise fashion, after exact diagnosis, diseased compartments of the ethmoids are approached and—depending on the extent of the disease—maxillary, frontal and sphenoid sinuses opened via their natural ostia. Care is taken not to denude bone, but leave peripheral mucosa in all operated cavities. Rarely, middle turbinates need to be resected. Patients with nasal polyposis histologically dominated by dense eosinophilic infiltration as present in Aspirin Intolerance, Allergic Fungal Sinusitis and many asthmatics, require a more aggressive approach and in many instances a combined therapy with corticosteroids. In these cases, extensive aftercare and follow-up is required by the physician and a good compliance by the patients to preserve the good postoperative results and to prevent regrowth of polyps. Massive scarring, postoperative osteoneogenesis and disease processes far laterally in the frontal and—rarely—the maxillary sinuses especially after previous external surgery, may present limitations to an exclusively endoscopic approach.

Chapter XXI
TREATMENT: OUTCOME AND COMPLICATIONS OF SURGICAL TREATMENT
Maurice Roth and David W. Kennedy

Until a cure is found for sino-nasal polyposis, surgical therapy will continue to play an important role in the overall management of this disorder. Overall results show that at least 85% of patients report marked improvement in nasal obstruction, congestion, and facial pain related to concurrent chronic sinusitis. Nasal drainage also improves in most cases. Improvement in associated asthma is less clear. Poorer prognosis is directly associated with greater extent of initial disease. Results are usually short term if patients do not receive concurrent medical therapy along with close observation. The use of the endoscope allows for greater precision in diagnosis and management and can be used as an effective tool when combined with medical therapy for the long term treatment of polyposis. There is no evidence that endoscopic sinus surgery has decreased the overall complication rate from surgical therapy although most major centers with good endoscopic experience report less than 1% risk of major complications. Avoidance of complications is best achieved through careful preoperative planning including comprehensive nasal endoscopy, computed tomography, and aggressive pre-operative medical management. Endoscopic surgical experience including the recognition and treatment of surgical complications is essential for all surgeons engaged in the treatment of sino-nasal polyposis.

Chapter II

Historical Background

David J. Brain, F.R.C.S.

ABSTRACT

The history of nasal polyps goes back for a period of over 4,000 years to Ancient Egypt and this condition may, perhaps, be the earliest recorded disease in which we know the names of both the patient and the physician. Further significant advances were made in Ancient Greece and Renaissance Europe but the real transformation of nasal polypectomy, from an extremely painful and potentially dangerous procedure, into a routine minor operation did not occur until the end of the 19th century.

The first medical practitioner whose name is known to us was an Egyptian rhinologist called Ni-Ankh Sekhmet (formerly incorrectly known as Sekhet' enanch). He was the Court Physician to King Sahura and his picture together with that of his wife were found on a slab in the tomb of the king together with a testimony of royal gratitude which states "he had made his nostrils well" (Fig. 2). This tablet had formerly been placed in an ante-room of the palace where it could be seen and read by all. We do not know the nature of the disease from which the king suffered but it seems more than likely that it was nasal polyposis. Pahor[1] has shown that the Egyptians were familiar with nasal polyps which they described as "grapes coming down from the nose". Treatment included medicaments containing alcohol and Pahor has postulated that some of the Egyptian surgical instruments may well have been used to remove polyps. At any rate, although the exact details are obscure, the history of nasal polyposis goes back nearly 5,000 years.

PATHOLOGY

Hippocrates thought that disease resulted from a disturbed equilibrium between the 4 "humours". When the humours were too thick it could result in the development of polyps. The underlying cause of this process was a constitutional factor. This theory was accepted by Roman authorities such as Galen, and did in fact linger on to much more recent times as shown by a case history recorded by Forestus[2] in 1591, who describes the remarkable case of a woman in whose nostrils had grown a huge polyp due to her carrying heavy weights on her head which forced the mucus down into the membranes of her nose. She was cured by ligation of the polyp and the application to its stump of vitriol but when she resumed her occupation it returned and was again cured in the same way.

Later, nasal polyps were regarded as neoplasms. Clinical observation revealed that certainly a small proportion were malignant, and it therefore seemed quite logical to believe that the majority were benign tumours. Thus we find in an early edition (1854) of Paget's "Surgical Pathology", that nasal polyps are classified as fibrocellular tumours. Shortly afterwards, the great Virchow (1863), considered the nasal polyp to be a myxoma. The dominant position of the neoplastic theory was not seriously challenged until 1882, when Zuckerkandl[3] published an important pathological study of this disease which he found to be very common, and present in every eighth routine autopsy. In all 39 of the post mortems showed evidence of nasal polyposis, the gradual removal of the bony parts, enabled the exact origin of the lesions to be located with precision. All arose from the middle meatus, and the most common site was around the edges of the hiatus semilunaris. Zuckerkandl drew attention to the striking conformity between the histological changes in nasal polypi, and in the maxillary mucosa, in "catarrhal inflammation", and he regarded these two processes as indentical. He considered that the oedematous mucosa hung downwards due to its weight, producing a kink of its blood supply, which in turn produced a further increase in the oedema.

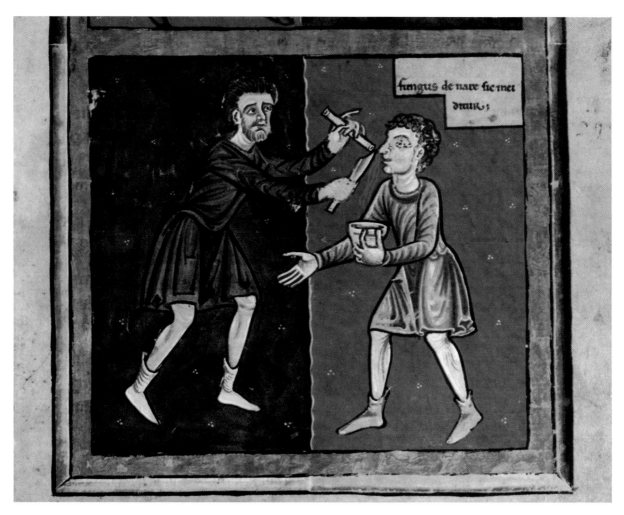

Figure 1. Nasal surgery in medieval times. 12th Century English Manuscript reproduced by kind permission of the Bodleian Library, Oxford. (MS Ashmole, 1462).

In 1885, Woakes[4] (Fig. 3) agreed that polypi were inflammatory lesions and stated that they were always caused by a "necrosing ethmoiditis". The logical therapeutic implication of this theory was to include routinely an ethmoidectomy in the treatment of nasal polyposis and this heralded an era of radical surgical treatment which was often performed through external incisions. Woakes pursued the propagation of his views with an evangelical zeal but the work of Hajek[5], Zuckerkandl[6], Heath[7], and others failed to confirm the presence of sinusitis in many cases of nasal polyposis, and indeed they challenged the existence of "necrosing ethmoiditis". Bacterial infection and sinusitis at best only provided an incomplete answer to the problem of nasal polyposis and an allergic cause for this disease was suggested by Bourgeois[8] in 1925.

The allergic theory has won wide recognition and has received much support, from among others, Hansel[9], Hirsch[10], Wiethe[11], Kern and Schenck[12] and Opheim[13].

MORBID ANATOMY

As we have seen, the Egyptians described nasal polypi as "grapes coming down from the nose". Celcus (A.D. 23–79) likened the polyp in appearance to the nipple of the female breast, whereas the great Persian physician, Avicenna (980–1037) considered that the polyp resembled the haemorrhoid.

Choanal polypi have been known for many years but the precise morbid anatomy of the antro-choanal polyp was first described by Lermoyez[14] in 1909.

SYSTEMIC DISEASES ASSOCIATED WITH NASAL POLYPS

1. Asthma

Voltolini[15] recorded a patient with asthma which was associated with nasal polyposis in 1872, many and similar cases were later recorded by Hanisch, Porter, Daly, Todd, Spencer, Mulhall, Joal and Jacquin. It was then postu-

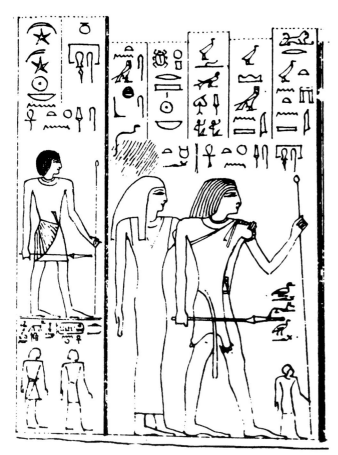

Figure 2. Ni-Ankh Sekhmet and wife, Vth Dynasty. (Courtesy of Mr. Ahmes Pahor).

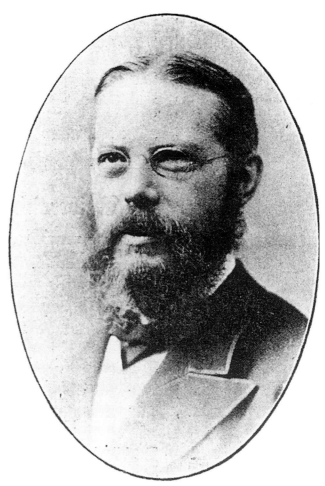

Figure 3. Edward Woakes. (Courtesy of Journal of Laryngology and Otology).

lated that the attacks of asthma were induced by nasal reflexes activated by the polypi. Later the frequent allergic causation of asthma was used as evidence that nasal polyposis was also allergic in origin.

2. Asthma, Aspirin intolerance and nasal polyposis

This well known syndrome was first described by Widal, Abrami, and Lermoyez[16] in 1922.

3. Cystic Fibrosis

The high incidence of nasal polyposis in children suffering from cystic fibrosis was recorded by Schwachman, Kylszycky, and Mueller[17] in 1961.

TREATMENT

Following the preliminary initial work which took place in Egypt and which has already been mentioned, the next major advance in the study and treatment of this disease occurred in Greece and is associated with the name of Hippocrates. This era of dramatic progress has been admirably reviewed by Baldewein[18] in his paper entitled

"Rhinology of Hippocrates". The treatment was tailored to fit each different type of polyp. When the lesions were soft and pedunculated, Hippocrates noted that they would move in and out during deep inspiration and expiration. These cases were suited to his sponge technique (Fig. 4–7) where a piece of sponge was cut to an appropriate size and shape and then tied to the ends of 3 or 4 strings. The other ends of the strings were inserted through the nose and into the pharynx using a slender soft tin or lead probe. Withdrawal of the strings through the mouth enabled firm traction to be applied which dragged the sponge through the nose, hopefully detaching and displacing the polyps on its way. With the more solid and firmer type of lesion, the principle of a snare was used. The loop of a sinew was adjusted around the polyp and the other end of the sinew was passed through the nose, into the pharynx and finally through the mouth where traction enabled the polyp to be removed. Hippocrates advised cautery as the treatment for the fleshy type of polyp. After all these operations he used the application

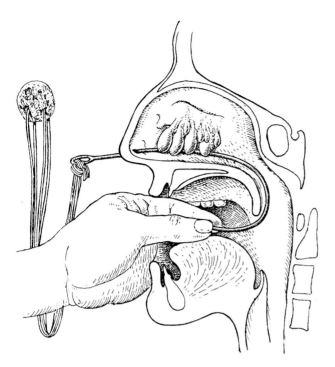

Figure 4. Hippocrates technique for nasal polypectomy.

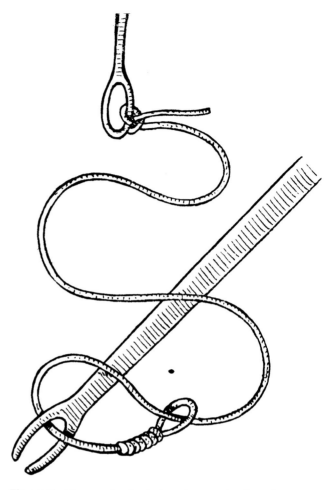

Figure 6. Hippocrates technique for nasal polypectomy.

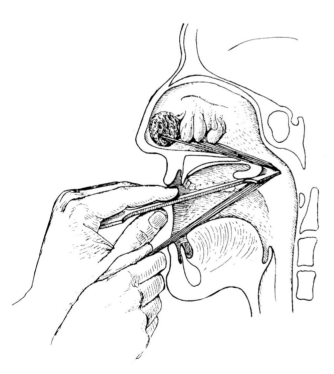

Figure 5. Hippocrates technique for nasal polypectomy.

This brilliant epoch of Greek medicine passed but although Greek culture was fading in the country of its birth, it was absorbed and further developed by Rome.

The Romans scorned to soil their hands in the practice of medicine, a calling only fit for slaves and foreigners, but they were interested in the subject and its knowledge was part of the broad educational background of every cultured Roman. One such example was Pliny the Elder (A.D. 23–79) who wrote a monumental natural history in 37 volumes[19] which included medicine and there was a very comprehensive pharmacopoeia which remained in use as late as the Middle Ages. Some of the medicaments were used to treat nasal polyps. Pliny was very critical of the medical profession in general, and he said "It is unfortunate that there is no law to punish ignorant physicians and that capital punishment is never inflicted on them. Yet they learn by our suffering and they experiment by putting us to death". Celcus was the author of another great encyclopaedia dealing with philosophy, military strategy, law, medicine and other subjects[20]. He also likened the nasal polyp in appearance to the nipple of the

of copperas powder and the insertion of stents in the nostrils which had been smeared with oil and honey. Certainly the work of Hippocrates is a major landmark in the history of this disease.

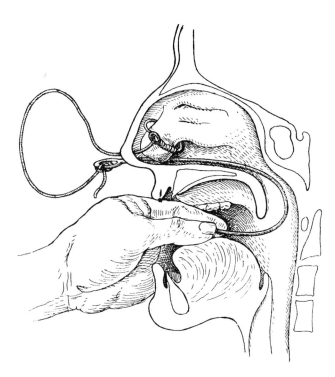

Figure 7. Hippocrates technique for nasal polypectomy.

the Arab surgeons and he was a strong advocate of the use of cautery. He also used to pull the nasal polyp forward with a hook, cut through the pedicle with scissors and then wash the nasal cavity with vinegar.

The next great advance of civilization occurred during the Renaissance, and this also included great progress in medicine. Gabriel Fallopius[21] (1522–62) combined the professorship of anatomy, surgery and botany at Padua (Fig. 8). Although now best known for his anatomical discoveries, he was also responsible for major advances in the treatment of nasal polyps. He did advocate the use of the ligature but found that in most cases the pedicle of the polyp was inaccessible and it was for this reason that he invented the snare. The tube was made of silver and the loop from harpsichord wire (Fig. 9). He used this instrument for the treatment also of rectal polyps. Some polyps were too hard to snare and for these Fallopius pulled down the lesion with forceps (Fig. 10) so that he could cut through the pedicle with a knife.

The 17th and 18th centuries were periods of consolidation rather than of major advance. Surgical education greatly expanded and several important textbooks were published at that time. Sir Percival Pott (Fig. 11)[22] clearly differentiated between malignant and benign polyps. He

female breast and used a sharp instrument like a spatula to cut through the pedicle of the polyp after which it was removed by hooks. Later, Galen advocated the local application of astringents to nasal polyps. Rome fell to the barbarians in 455 AD and this heralded a very bleak period lasting many centuries in Western Europe. Not only did medical progress come to a virtual halt but much of the existing knowledge was lost. Civilization persisted in the Byzantine Empire where Paulus Aegineta (607–690) practiced as the last civilised physician in the classical tradition. He wrote an encyclopedia called the Epitome and one of the 7 volumes was devoted to surgery. In it he describes a technique for removing nasal polyps which obviously owes much to Hippocrates, although a knotted string is used instead of a sponge. This book preserved and perpetuated the knowledge of Greek and Roman medicine. Throughout its history, the Byzantine Empire was in almost constant conflict with its Moslem neighbours to the East and the South. However, the Epitome became known to the Arabs who held it in high regard. The next great reservoir of medical knowledge was provided by the Arabs themselves who in addition to absorbing the earlier learning added much original work of their own. Their greatest contributions were, however, in the fields of pharmacology and ophthalmology rather than rhinology. The Arabs were not well versed in the art of surgery which was regarded as inferior to medicine and its practice relegated to craftsmen rather than scholars. Albucasis (936–1013) of Cordova was the greatest of

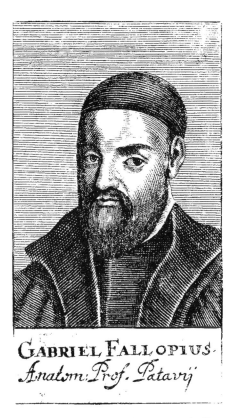

GABRIEL FALLOPIUS.
Anatom: Prof. Patavij

Figure 8. Gabriel Fallopius. (1523–1562) (Courtesy of Wellcome Institute Library, London). Engraving by anonymous artist, 17th Century.

11

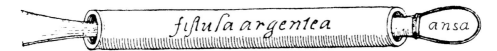

Figure 9. Nasal snare designed by Fallopius.

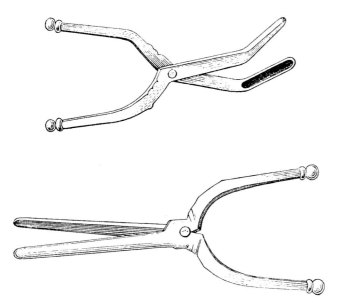

Figure 10. Nasal forceps designed by Fallopius.

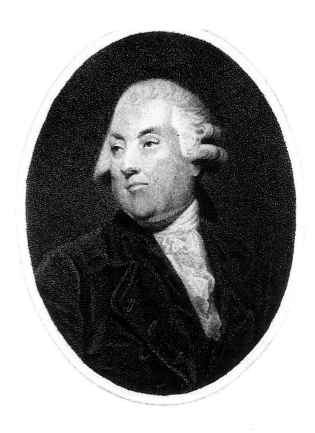

Figure 11. Sir Percival Pott. (1714–1788) (Courtesy of Wellcome Institute Library, London). Portrait by J. Heath, after Joshua Reynolds, published by J. Johnson, 1790.

recommended the use of the probe as a diagnostic tool. When the polyp was painful, red or dark purple in colour, hard, and found to be fixed when touched with the probe, it should be regarded as malignant and no attempt at treatment should be made. He did adopt a somewhat cautious attitude to benign polyps which he stated "to be most difficult totally and perfectly to eradicate, and most liable to reproduction". He also emphasizes the dangers of polypectomy, particularly haemorrhage which had been fatal on at least one occasion. This conservatism was probably tempered by the fact that Pott himself suffered from nasal polyposis. He noted that there was some variation in the size of the polyps which he attributed to climatic change. When the weather was moist, the polyps were in "a state of relaxation", and he then removed his own polyps using window forceps. He repeated the process until clearance had been achieved. His son-in-law, Sir James Earle, records that "Pott removed several from himself in front of a mirror . . . to some of them adhered a small portion of bone—sufficient proof that it required no small degree of fortitude and perseverance to perform the operation on his own person". Pott states that "of late years he had entirely got rid of them, but there had remained such a thickness of the whole membrane, that he continued totally to be deprived of the sense of smelling, a circumstance which he never much regret-

ted". Another of the major surgical textbooks written about that time was by Sir Charles Bell[23], who described a technique of snaring choanal polyps (Fig. 12) and also records a case report of a fatal complication following the operation where "There succeeded to the operation, pain in the face, headache and fever. On the 4th day, the patient became insensible and died on the 6th day". An autopsy showed that the cribriform plate had been perforated and that death was due to intracranial sepsis. Bell concluded "There is good reason for us avoiding violence with the forceps directed upwards in the nose". Sir Astley Cooper[24] (Fig. 13) endeavoured to identify the pedicle of polyp with a probe before removing it with forceps. At this time the use of forceps (Fig. 14 & 15) was very com-

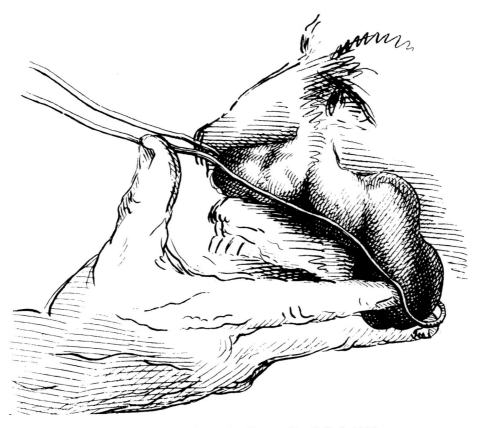

Figure 12. Taken from "A system of Operative Surgery" by C. Bell, 1807.

mon due to the simplicity and speed of the procedure but complications still frequently occurred. Michel[25] states "As a result of operations by others with forceps, I have seen luxation of the cartilaginous septum, fracture of the bones, removal of portions of the turbinated bones, circumstances which increase the suffering of patients, and render the operation quite horrible".

The operation was in fact unsatisfactory because it was always painful, and potentially dangerous because it almost completely lacked visual control by the surgeon. Further progress depended on developments in other fields which included adequate lighting and anterior rhinoscopy, anaesthesia (both general and topical) and an understanding of bacteriology which brought with it,

firstly, the antiseptic surgery of Lister and shortly afterwards aseptic surgery. All these advances occurred during the latter half of the 19th century.

Subsequently, the availability of electricity enabled the use of cautery to be simplified and made more controllable. Certainly Morell Mackenzie[26] regarded galvano cautery as the method of choice in 1884. Later, during this century, the cryosurgical probe and the laser have been used to destroy polyps. Radium has also been implanted in an effort to minimize the risk of recurrence of the disease after polypectomy and the endoscope has achieved great importance but this is all very recent history and in merging with the present, will be dealt with elsewhere in this book.

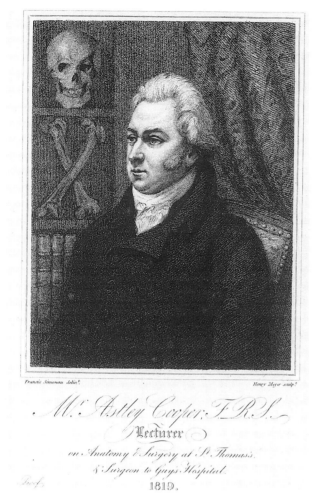

Figure 13. Sir Astley Paston Cooper. (Courtesy of Wellcome Institute Library, London). Engraving by H. Meyer, 1819 after F. Simoneau.

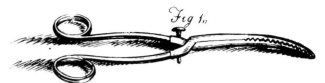

Figure 14. Nasal forceps. Early 19th Century. Taken from "A system of Operative Surgery" by C. Bell, 1807.

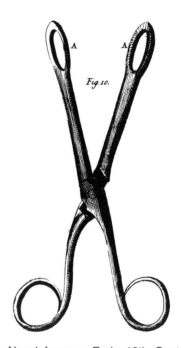

Figure 15. Nasal forceps. Early 19th Century. Taken from "A system of Operative Surgery" by C. Bell, 1807.

REFERENCES

1. Pahor A. L. Rhinology in Ancient Egypt. Paper read at the European Rhinological Meeting, Athens, 1986 F. med (BR), 94:203–5.

2. Forestus, 1591, quoted in History of Laryngology and Rhinology by J. Wright, Lea & Febiger, St. Louis, 1893, p. 165.

3. Zuckerkandl, E. Normale und pathologische Anatomie der Nasenhohle und ihrer pneumatischen Anhange. Vol. 2, Wein, Wilhelm Braumuller p. 222 (24 Tafeln).

4. Woakes E. The relation of Necrosing Ethnoiditis to Nasal Polypus. Brit Med J 50:701, 1885.

5. Hajek M. Ueber die pathologischen Veranderungen der Siebbein-Knochen im Gefolge der entzundlichen Schleimhauthypertrophie und der Nasenpolypen. Arch Laryng Rhinol 4:277, 1896.

6. Zuckerkandl E. A discussion on the aetiology of mucous polyp. Brit Med J 2:476, 1892.

7. Heath C. The surgery of the nose and accessory sinuses. Brit Med J 2:1282, 1892.

8. Bourgeois H. A propos d'un cas de coryza spasmodique. Progr. med. Paris, 95–96, 1925.

9. Hansel FK. Allergy of the nose and paranasal sinuses. A monograph on the subject of allergy as related to otolaryngology. St. Louis, C.V. Mosby Co. 1936, p. 820.

10. Hirsch O. Polypen und Allergie. Wein med Wehnschr 8:1461–2, 1931.

11. Wiethe C. Polyposis Nasi auf allergischer Grundlage. Monatschr Ohrenh 1932, 66:1378–82.

12. Kern RA, Schenck HP. Importance of allergy in etiology and treatment of nasal mucous polyps. J.A.M.A. 103: 1293–7, 1934.

13. Opheim O. Om allergiske neselidelser. Nord Med 16: 1607–19, 1938.

14. Lermoyez J. Ann d mal de l'oreille 1909, 35 Pt. I, p. 60 Kubo.

15. Voltolini H. Die Anwendung d GalvanoKaustik. Wien, 1872, p. 246.

16. Widal F, Abrami P, Lermoyez J. Anaphylaxie et idiosyncrasie. Presse Medicale 30:189–93, 1922.

17. Schwachman H, Kylszycky L. L., Mueller HD. Nasal polyposis in patients with cystic fibrosis. Amer J Dis Children 102:768–9, 1961.

18. Baldewain. Rhinology of Hippocrates. quoted in "History of Laryngology and Rhinology" by J. Wright, Lea & Febiger, St. Louis, 1893, pp. 57–59.

19. Pliny GPS. Historia Naturalis. ed. L. Jan and K. Mayhoff (Teubner 1892–1933).

20. Finlayson J. Celcus. Glas Med Jour 67:321, 1892.

21. Fallopius tractate, "De Tumoribus praeter Naturam" was first published in 1573 which was 11 years after his death in 1562.

22. Pott P. The Chirugical Works. London, Lowndes, 1753, Vol. 3, pp. 243–265.

23. Bell C. A System of Operative Surgery. London. Longman 1807, pp. 208–231.

24. Cooper A. Lectures on the Principles and Practice of Surgery. Westley, 1829, p. 425.

25. Michel F. Die Krankheiten der Nasenhohle. Berlin, 1876, p. 57.

26. McKenzie M. Manual of diseases of the throat and nose. London, Churchill, 1884, p. 380.

Chapter III

Epidemiology of Nasal Polyps

Guy A. Settipane, M.D.

ABSTRACT

Nasal polyps are found in 36% of patients with aspirin intolerance, 7% of those with asthma, 0.1% in children, and about 20% in those with cystic fibrosis. Other conditions associated with nasal polyps are Churg-Strauss Syndrome, allergic fungal sinusitis, and cilia dyskinetic syndrome, (Kartagener's) and Young Syndrome.

Nasal polyps are statistically more common in non allergic asthma vs. allergic asthma (13% vs 5%, P < 0.01). About 40% of patients with surgical polypectomy have recurrences. There appears to be a hereditary factor for developing nasal polyps.

A classification system for staging nasal polyps is proposed in order to standardize treatment, consider differential diagnosis, and harvest meaningful comparative research information.

Nasal polyps are found in many disease states (Table 1.) Indeed, it is unusual to find them alone, not associated with other diseases. Nasal polyps have a relatively moderate frequency in patients with nonallergic rhinitis but this is questionable since the presence of nasal polyps in the nasal cavity can by itself produce symptoms of nasal stuffiness and rhinorrhea due to irritation from the polyps. In allergic rhinitis the frequency of nasal polyps is quite low (1.5%).[1] Nasal polyps commonly are found in aspirin intolerant patients as manifested by acute bronchospasm and rhinorrhea within 3 hours of ingestion of aspirin. The urticaria type of aspirin intolerance is not associated with nasal polyps.

Characteristics of patients with nasal polyps are listed in Table 2. Polyps are equally divided between males and females and are most frequently found in patients with asthma.[1,2] Table 3 demonstrates that the type of asthma most commonly associated with nasal polyps is non allergic asthma. Nasal polyps are found in 13% of non allergic asthma and in only 5% of allergic asthma (P < 0.01). Some patients with nasal polyps do not have a history of asthma and have a negative pulmonary methacholine challenge test.[3,4] Therefore, not all patients with nasal polyps have an associated lower respiratory problem.[5]

The frequency of nasal polyps increases with age, reaching its peak in those individuals fifty years and older, Table 4. In asthmatic patients who are forty years or over, the frequency of nasal polyps is four times greater than asthmatics under forty (12.4% vs 3.1%, P < 0.01). In children, the frequency of nasal polyposis is extremely low, about 0.1%. Any child 16 years or younger with nasal polyps should be evaluated for cystic fibrosis.

Severe steroid-dependent asthmatics with aspirin intolerance have an even higher association with nasal polyps than other types of asthma. Slavin's group[6] reported on 33 patients with severe asthma and sinusitis. Fifteen of these patients were receiving corticosteroids: 10 received continuous corticosteroids and 5 required intermittent bursts. Of these 33 patients, 30 (90%) had a diagnosis of nasal polyps and 17 (52%) had aspirin intolerance. This data demonstrates that the nasal polyps as well as aspirin intolerance found in asthmatic patients usually indicate the presence of a severe asthmatic state.

The triad of nasal polyps, aspirin intolerance, and asthma was first described by Widal, Abrami, Lermoyez in 1922.[7] This association was later emphasized by Samter.[8] There seems to be a time sequence in developing this triad. When all three arms or components of this triad are present, asthma usually has occurred first followed by nasal polyps within the next 10 years[9,10] (Table 5). Aspirin intolerance usually occurs within one year of asthma onset. In many cases only two parts of the triad are present, such as asthma and aspirin intolerance.

There may be a hereditary factor for nasal polyps. A recent investigation of fifty patients with nasal polyps and

Table 1. Frequency of Nasal Polyps in Various Diseases

Diagnosis	Frequency (%)
Aspirin intolerance	36
Adult asthma	7
Intrinsic asthma	13
Atopic asthma	5
Chronic rhinosinusitis	2
Nonallergic rhinitis	5
Allergic rhinitis	1.5
Childhood asthma/rhinitis	0.1
Cystic fibrosis	20
Churg-Strauss syndrome (asthma, fever, eosinophilia vasculitis and granuloma)	50
Allergic fungal sinusitis	85
Kartagener's syndrome (bronchiectasis, sinusitis, situs inversus)	?
Young's syndrome (sinopulmonary disease, azoospermia)	?

Table 2. Nasal Polyps (211 Cases): Characteristics

Clinical Categories	No.	%
Males	106	50.2
Females	105	49.8
Asthma	149	70.6
Rhinitis (alone)	62	29.4
Positive allergy skin tests	117	55.5
Total aspirin intolerance	30	14.2
Subtypes of aspirin intolerance		
Bronchospasm	21	70.0
Urticaria	4	13.3
Both bronchospasm and urticaria	2	6.7
Rhinitis	3	10.0

Reprinted from Settipane GA, Chafee FH. Nasal polyps in asthma and rhinitis: a review of 6,037 patients. Allergy Clin Immunol 59:17–21, 1977.

Table 3. Nasal Polyps in Allergic and Nonallergic Asthma

	Total Patients	Polyps	%	p value
Nonallergic Asthma	511	64	13%	
				<0.01
Allergic Asthma	1,717	85	5%	
Total	2,228	149	6.7%	

28 matched controls reported that 14% of those with nasal polyps had a family history of nasal polyps compared with none in the control population.[11] Some patients had more than one immediate family member with nasal polyps, a finding which we also have observed[12] (Fig. 1) (Table 6). Lockey, et al.[13] reported on identical female twins, both of whom had asthma but only one had nasal polyps and aspirin intolerance. We studied male identical twins whose monozygotic nature was verified by typing 9 different blood factors.[14] Our twins were 36 years old when studied. Both twins had steroid-dependent asthma but only one twin had nasal polyps and aspirin intolerance. Our twins had the bronchospastic type of aspirin intolerance while one of Lockey's twins had both the bronchospastic and urticarial type of aspirin intolerance. These data are consistent with the theory that although there may be a genetic predisposition toward forming nasal polyps, local mucosal and environmental factors also play an important role. Some of these factors may be in the form of family spread infections.

Other disease states that are genetically transmitted may contribute to the development of nasal polyps, such as cystic fibrosis, Young's syndrome, and primary cilia dyskinesia.

It is important to describe the incidence of recurrence of nasal polyps after surgical polypectomy. We reviewed 167 patients with verified nasal polyps either by direct contact with the operating surgeon, or reviewing the pathologic reports. The recurrence rate was found to be 40%, (Table 7).[9,15] It was also noted that those patients with positive allergy skin tests had a higher frequency of multiple polypectomies than those with negative allergy skin tests[9]. This seems to indicate that although allergy is not a basic etiology in the pathogenesis of nasal polyps, it does increase the recurrence rate. The recurrence rate

Table 4. Frequency of Nasal Polyps in Various Age Groups
of Asthmatic Patients

Age When First Seen (yr)	No. with Asthma		No. with Nasal Polyps		%		p
10–19	491 ⎫		9 ⎫		1.8 ⎫		
20–29	465 ⎬ 1,374		18 ⎬ 43		3.9 ⎬ 3.1		
30–39	418 ⎭		16 ⎭		3.8 ⎭		<0.01*
40–49	410 ⎫ 854		41 ⎫ 106		10.0 ⎫ 12.4		
50 and over	444 ⎭		65 ⎭		14.6 ⎭		
Total	2,228		149		6.7		

*The difference between the 10–39-year-old group (43/1.374), 3.1%, compared to the 40-year-old and over group (106/854), 12.4%, is statistically significant.

Reprinted from Settipane GA, Chafee FH. Nasal polyps in asthma and rhinitis: a review of 6,037 patients. J Allergy Clin Immunol 59:17–21, 1977.

Table 5. Asthma with Nasal Polyps: Onset of Polyps versus Onset
of Asthma

Initial Diagnosis	Total Patients	%	Mean Time Interval between Diagnosis (yr)	Range of Time Interval (yr)
Polyps (first)	35	29.4	11.2	1–46
Asthma (first)	73	61.3	9.5	1–37
Both together	11	9.2	0	
Total	119			

*Aspirin sensitivity usually occurs within one year of asthma onset.

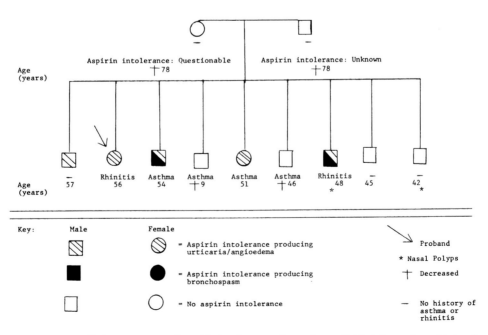

Figure 1. Familial occurrence of aspirin intolerance (based on reliable information obtained from the proband after repeated questioning of her relatives). Ref 12

19

Table 6. Nasal Polyps and Family History of Nasal Polyps

Patient #	Age	Sex	Asthma	Aspirin Intolerance	Family Members With Nasal Polyps
1	35	M	No	No	Father
2	50	M	No	No	Sister, Mother
3	56	M	Yes	No	Brother
4	56	M	No	No	2 Sisters
5	63	M	Yes	No	Father
6	69	F	No	No	3 Brothers
7	76	F	Yes	No	Brother

Table 7. 167 Patients with Verified Polyps and Polypectomies

Total Patients	No. of Polypectomies	No. of Patients	%
167	1 or more	143	86
143	2 or more	57	40
143	3 or more	34	24
143	4 or more	22	15
143	5 or more	17	12
143	6 or more	11	8

of nasal polyps also is aggravated by aspirin intolerance where the recurrence interval is shorter in intolerant individuals as compared to aspirin tolerant patients[16].

The method of treating nasal polyps obviously affects the recurrence rate. The mean interval of recurrence is six times shorter in patients treated with oral prednisone bursts compared to those treated by surgical polypectomy, Table 8[16]. Although surgical intervention is more traumatic than oral prednisone, it does produce longer intervals of remission than oral prednisone.

Other precipitating factors increasing the recurrence rate are upper respiratory infections and seasonal occurrence of pollens in sensitized individuals. These will be discussed in detail in Chapter XIII.

The frequency of nasal polyps occurring in the paranasal sinuses is unknown. It certainly occurs most of the time in allergic fungal sinusitis. In aggressive recurrent sino nasal polyposis, erosion of ethmoid bones and other sinus walls may occur.[17] This type of bone ero-

sion and expansion is called "Woakes Syndrome"[18] and may result in marked facial malformations "frog nose", and ptosis (Figs. 2A, 2B, 3)[15]. It is important to obtain paranasal sinus imaging, preferably CT scan, to complete the evaluation of nasal polyps.

Patients with cystic fibrosis have a high frequency of nasal polyps (20%). Children aged 16 or younger who have nasal polyps should always be evaluated for cystic fibrosis. Similarly, the polyps associated with the chronic dyskinetic cilia syndrome and Young's syndrome have the neutrophil as the predominant cell. Primary ciliary dyskinesia is classically manifested on Kartagener's syndrome, which is an uncommon genetic condition with an estimated incidence of 1 in 20,000 births[19,20]. It appears to be inherited as an autosomal recessive trait and is characterized by bronchiectasis, chronic sinusitis, and situs inversus (complete reversal of internal organs with heart on the right, liver on the left, etc.). Situs inversus is found in 50% of patients with this syndrome. The ciliary abnormality in these cases usually involves the entire body including the respiratory and genital tract. The disorder affects the cilia themselves with absence of the dynein arms leading to an incoordinated beat. Increased susceptibility to infection, often caused by Pseudomonas aeruginosa, is found in patients with both Kartagener's syndrome and cystic fibrosis[21].

Young's syndrome consists of recurrent respiratory diseases, azoospermia, and nasal polyposis. The respiratory disease consists of severe chronic sinusitis which may be associated with bronchiectasis[22,23]. These patients have normal sweat chloride values and pancreatic function and, therefore, do not have a variant of cystic

Table 8. Occurrence after surgical and medical polypectomy

type	total patients	polypectomies	mean interval (yrs)	range (yrs)
surgery	29	49	6.3	1–24
prednisone bursts	10	34	0.9	0.2–7

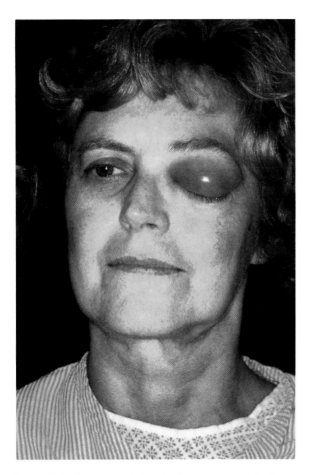

Figure 2A. Severe periorbital edema preoperatively.

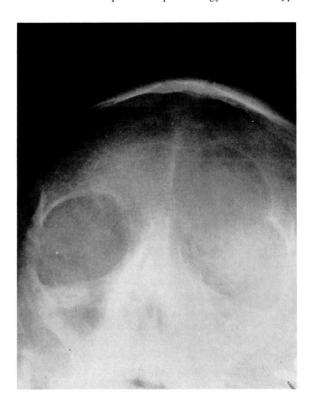

Figure 2B. Sinus films showing erosion of the orbital rim.

fibrosis. Cilia structures are normal in sperm tails taken from testicular biopsy specimens and in the cilia from tracheal biopsy specimens; and therefore, these patients do not have a chronic form of cilia syndrome. The azoospermia in Young's syndrome is due to a block in the epididymis that is distinguishable from the defect in the vas deferens associated with cystic fibrosis. However, spermatogenesis is normal. The prevalence of Young's syndrome is considerably higher than that of cystic fibrosis or Kartagener's syndrome. It is responsible for 7.4% of cases of male infertility. In Churg-Strauss Syndrome (allergic vasculitis), 50% of these patients have nasal polyps.[24]

Allergic fungal sinusitis is reportedly found in 6 to 7% of chronic sinusitis patients requiring surgery[25–28]. Practically all of these patients have associated polypoid changes in their sinuses. Classically, the inspissated sinus exudate is tan to gray-brown with a peanut butter-like consistency. Histologically, the exudate contain eosinophilia, basophilic mucin and Charcot-Leyden crystals. Hyphae are easily identified using a Gomori methenamine silver stain (GMS). The diagnosis of allergic fungal

sinusitis should be considered in any atopic patient with sinusitis and nasal polyposis who is unresponsive to conventional therapy. Besides the typical histological characteristics, the diagnostic criteria include culture identification, positive immediate skin test to fungus, positive serum precipitins, and elevated specific IgE and IgG antibodies. Allergic fungal sinusitis will be discussed in detail in Chapter XVI. Thus far, we have attempted to quantitate the nasal polyp problem and establish its frequency of association with other diseases. From this material it is apparent that nasal polyps may represent the tip of an iceberg where other diseases associated with polyps are the main underlying disease process.[28–32]

Table 9 represents a proposed working classification of nasal polyps. This proposed classification will be of help in the standardization of treatment, considering differential diagnosis, and comparing research data on nasal polyps.

One of the great difficulties in the treatment and research on nasal polyps is the lack of a uniform classification. Different types of nasal polyps may come from different origins and may require different treatment. In addition, research information may apply to one type of polyps and not to another. For these reasons it is important to have a standard clinical classification for staging nasal polyps. This standard classification should be simple enough to be activated at an outpatient facility using

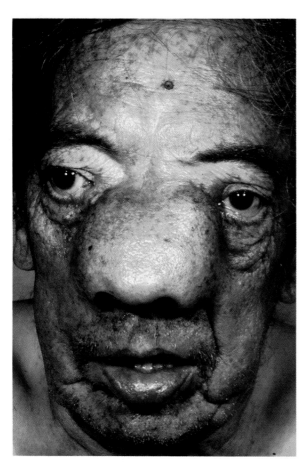

Figure 3. Massive hypertelorism ("frog nose") in a case of long standing nasal polyps. (*Photo courtesy of Valerie J. Lund, M.S., F.R.C.S. with kind permission of the Editor of The Journal of Laryngology and Otology*)

Table 9. Clinical Classification of Nasal Polyps

I. UNILATERAL
   A. Predominant Cell: Eosinophils
      1. See II.A
   B. Predominant Cells: Lymphocytes, Neutrophils, RBC
      1. Rule out neoplasm

II. BILATERAL
   A. Predominant Cell: Eosinophils
      1. Two or more of polyp tetrad (aspirin intolerance, asthma, sinusitis)
      2. Allergic rhinitis
      3. Allergic fungal sinusitis
      4. Churg Strauss Syndrome
   B. Predominant Cells: Lymphocytes, Neutrophils
      1. Cystic fibrosis
      2. Kartagener's syndrome
      3. Young's syndrome

III. MISCELLANEOUS-ADDITIONAL INFORMATION
   A. Recurrent (Number)
   B. Anatomical Origin
   C. Bone erosion
   D. Immunological abnormalities

Predominant cells determined by nasal scrapings. For histopathology classification see chapter v.

readily available procedures. These procedures should include physical examination with special visualization of the nose, by rhinoscopy/endoscopy which is very important. Other requirements are nasal scraping for identification of predominant cells such as eosinophils, lymphocytes, neutrophils, and red blood cells. (Figs. 4–6)[2] Over 80% of nasal polyps are of the eosinophilic type. Other characteristics of this classification may also include microbiology, CT scan, magnetic resonance imaging (MRI), and immunologic evaluation. Additional information might include the recurrent rate of the polyps, their anatomical origin, presence of bone erosion and immunological abnormalities.

Using this classification, a description of nasal polyps would be as follows: a polyp classified as IA would be a unilateral polyp with eosinophils as the predominating cell. Characteristics are usually the same as for bilateral nasal polyps with eosinophils covered in section II.A. A polyp characterized in Section. IB (unilateral, lympho-

cytes, neutrophils and red blood cells) would raise the suspicion of a neoplasm. II A. Polyp (bilateral with eosinophil) in an asthmatic patient would alert the physician of a probably coexisting aspirin intolerance and increased recurrency. Other conditions which should be considered in the II.A classification are allergic rhinitis, allergic fungal sinusitis, and Churg Strauss syndrome. Appropriate laboratory tests such as allergy skin tests, CT scan or MRI of the paranasal sinuses should be done. Allergic fungal sinusitis would require surgical debridement and appropriate fungal cultures, whereas Churg Strauss syndrome would require an evaluation for a multi system disease and a biopsy to confirm vasculitis.

The II.B classification would indicate the polyps are of an inflammatory origin with the predominant cells being lymphocytes and neutrophils. In this category the diagnoses to be considered are cilia dyskinetic syndromes (cystic fibrosis, Kartagener's syndrome) and Young's syndrome. In a child or young adult with a IIB classification, cystic fibrosis must be considered and the appropriate diagnostic test done forthwith (Chapter XVII). In addition, a IIB classification would need a chest x-ray to help rule out Kartagener's syndrome (Situs inversus).

The category III in this classification provides additional information. For example, are the polyps recurrent, choanal, located inside the sinuses, associated with

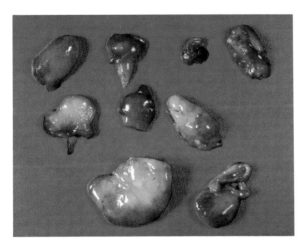

Figure 4. Gross photograph of multiple nasal polyps from a 64 year-old male.

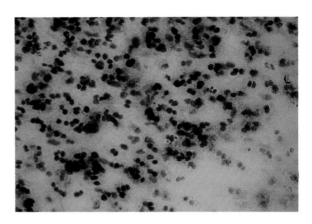

Figure 6. Smear of nasal secretions from a patient with nasal polyps reveals eosinophils.

bone erosion or associated with immunological abnormalities. Examples of using the supplement category III are as follows:

II A1 recurrent × 3 = would mean that the polyps are bilateral with the eosinophil as the predominant cell, associated with the aspirin intolerance syndrome and had recurred three times after appropriate treatment (either surgery or medical systemic corticosteroids)

II A2 = bilateral polyps associate with allergies (increased IgE)

II A3 bone erosion = bilateral polyps associated with allergic fungal sinusitis and bone erosion

II A4 Antrochoanal = bilateral polyps associated with Churg Strauss Syndrome and a polyp presenting in the nasopharynx with origin in the sinuses

II B1 = bilateral polyps in cystic fibrosis

II B2 = bilateral polyps with Kartagener's syndrome

II B3 = bilateral polyps with Young's syndrome

With classification, authors of research reports could describe precisely the type of polyp their data involves. Polyps arising from various sinuses or nasal meatuses have a different outcome and may deserve different types of treatment. A polyp that demonstrates bone erosion may be malignant or have the characteristics of Woakes' syndrome. Immunologic abnormalities such as IgA deficiency or immunosuppressive disease need to be diagnosed and treated appropriately. Polyps associated with aspirin intolerance have a high recurrence rate and may occur in individuals with severe asthma. Polyps associated with eosinophils would be more responsive to corticosteroids while those associated with neutrophils and lymphocytes may need antibiotics and additional evaluation for possible systemic diseases.

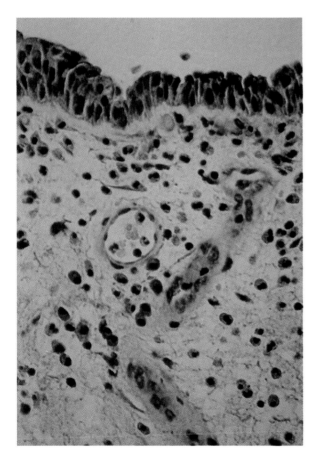

Figure 5. Nasal polyp (HE stain 400 × magnification): This high-power view shows orderly pseudo stratified columnar epithelium overlying an intact basement membrane. The stroma is edematous, vascular and contains eosinophils.

Editors of medical journals should require that authors precisely describe the characteristics of polyps in their data including information as indicated in this classification. It is apparent that different types of polyps may differ not only in treatment but also in prognosis and recurrence rate. Thus, a surgeon who describes a new procedure to prevent polyp recurrence may not have included the stubborn cases of Widal's syndrome (triad of aspirin intolerance) in their series. To organize medical knowledge, consider appropriate differential diagnosis, standardize treatment, and harvest meaningful comparative research information, a classification system for nasal polyps is needed. Such a classification system is proposed in Table 9.

REFERENCES

1. Settipane GA & Chafee FH. Nasal polyps in asthma and rhinitis: A review of 6,037 patients. J Allergy Clin Immunol: 59:17–21, 1977.
2. Settipane GA (Ed). In: Rhinitis, Second Edition, OceanSide Publications, Providence, 1992, pg 175, 176.
3. Downing ET, Braman S, Settipane GA. Bronchial reactivity in patients with nasal polyps before and after polypectomy. J Allergy Clin Immunol 69 (Part 2): 102, 1982.
4. Miles-Lawrence R, Kaplan M, Chang K. Methacholine sensitivity in nasal polyposis and the effects of polypectomy. J Allergy Clin Immunol 69 (Part 2): 102, 1982.
5. Settipane GA. Aspirin intolerance presenting as chronic rhinitis. RI Med J. 63:63–65, 1980.
6. Slavin RG, Linford P & Friedman WH. Sinusitis and bronchial asthma. J Allergy Clin Immunol: 69 (Part 2): 102, 1982.
7. Widal MF, Abrami P, Lermoyez J. Anaphylaxie et idiosyndraise. Presse Med 1922; 22:191.
8. Samter M, Beers RF. Concerning the nature of intolerance to aspirin. J Allergy 40: 281, 1967.
9. Settipane GA, Klein DE, Lekas, MD. Asthma and nasal polyps. In: Myers E, ed. New Dimensions in Otorhinolaryngology, Head and Neck Surgery. Amsterdam: Excerpta Medica, 1987, pp. 499–500.
10. Settipane GA. Nasal polyps: Epidemiology, pathology, immunology and treatment. Am J Rhinol 1: 119–126, 1987.
11. Greisner WA, Settipane GA. Hereditary factor for nasal polyps. J Allergy Clin Immunol. 95: No. 1 (Part 2), p 205, 1995.
12. Settipane GA, Pudupakkam RK. Aspirin intolerance. III. Sub-types, familial occurrence, and cross-reactivity with tartrazine. J. Allergy Clin Immunol 56:215–221, 1975.
13. Lockey RF, Rucknagel DL & Vanselow, NA. Familial occurrence of asthma, nasal polyps and aspirin intolerance. Ann Intern Med. 78:57, 1973.
14. Settipane GA. Benefit/Risk ratio of aspirin. NES Allergy Proceed: 2:96–102, 1981.
15. Settipane GA (ed). Rhinitis, First Edition, Providence: NER Allergy Proc, 1984, pg. 152.
16. Settipane GA, Klein DE, Settipane RJ. Nasal polyps, State of the art. Rhinol; 11:33–36 (Suppl.). 1991.
17. Parker GS, Tami TA, Wilson JF. Aggressive sino nasal polyposis. Ann J Rhinol: 2: 1–5, 1981.
18. Wentges RT, Woakes E. The history of eponym. J Laryngol Otol 86:501–512, 1972.
19. Atzellus BA. Disorders of ciliary motility. Hospital Practice 21: 73–80, 1986.
20. Rossman CM, Lee RM, Forrest JB & Newhouse MT. Nasal ciliary ultrastructure and function in patients with primary ciliary dyskinesia compared with that in normal subjects and in subjects with various respiratory diseases. Am Rev Respir Dis 129: 161–167, 1984.
21. MacKay DN. Antibiotic treatment of rhinitis and sinusitis. Am J Rhinol 1:83–85, 1987.
22. Schanker HM, Rajfer J & Saxon A. Recurrent respiratory disease, azoospermia, and nasal polyposis. Arch Intern Med 145:2201–2203, 1985.
23. Handelsman DJ, Conway AJ, Boylan LM & Turtle JR. Young's Syndrome. Obstructive azoospermia and chronic sinopulmonary infections. N Engl J Med 310:3–9, 1984.
24. Olsen Kdm Neel HB, DeRemee RA, Weiland LH. Nasal manifestations of allergic granulomatosis and angiitis (Churg-Strauss syndrome). Otolaryngol Head Neck Surg 88:85–89, 1990.
25. Schwietz LA, Gourley DS. Allergic fungal sinusitis. Allergy Proc 13:3–6, 1992.
26. Katzenstein AA, Sale SR, Greenberger PA: Allergic aspergillus sinusitis: A newly recognized form of sinusitis. J Allergy Clin Immunol 72:89–93, 1983.
27. Gourley DS, Whisman BA, Jorgensen NL, Martin ME, Redi MJ. Allergic Bipolaris sinusitis: clinical and immunopathologic characteristics. J Allergy Clin Immunol 85:583–591, 1990.
28. Bent JP III, Kuhn FA. Diagnosis of allergic fungal sinusitis. Otolaryngol HNS 111: 580–588, 1994.
29. Greenberger PA. Allergic fungal sinusitis in allergic bronchopulmonary aspergillosis ED Patterson, Greenberger, Roberts. OceanSide Publications, Providence, RI, 1995.
30. Rossman Cm, Lee RM, Forrest JB, Newhouse MT. Nasal ciliary ultrastructure and function in patients with primary ciliary dyskinesia compared with that in normal subjects and in subjects with various respiratory diseases. Am Rev Respir Dis 129: 161–167, 1984.
31. Oppenheimer EH, Rosenstein BJ. Differential pathology of nasal polyps in cystic fibrosis and atopy. Lab Invest 40:445–449, 1979.
32. Schanker HM, Raifer J, Saxon A. Recurrent respiratory disease, azoospermia, and nasal polyposis. Arch Intern Med 145:2201–2203, 1985.

Chapter IV

Anatomy of the Nose and Sinuses

Ian S. Mackay, M.D., F.R.C.S.

ABSTRACT

The ciliated mucous membrane lining the nose is continuous with that of the paranasal sinuses. The latter develop embryologically as out pouchings from shallow grooves and furrows laterally to form the maxillary and ethmoidal sinuses, with the sphenoid sinus posteriorly and the frontal sinus superiorly. The nasal cavity is divided sagitally into left and right halves by the nasal septum. Above, the nose and paranasal sinuses are separated from the intracranial cavity by the roof of the ethmoids, sphenoids and cribriform plate while the orbital contents are divided from the ethmoids by the delicate lamina papyracea. The lateral wall of the nose is characterised by the superior, middle and inferior turbinates lateral to each of which is a corresponding meatus. The nasolacrimal duct drains tears from the lacrimal sac to the inferior meatus. The maxillary sinus drains via its ostium into the middle meatus which also drains the anterior ethmoid and frontal sinuses. This region, termed the ostiomeatal complex (OMC), is therefore of great importance as obstruction here will interfere with the drainage and aeration of the maxillary, anterior ethmoid and frontal sinuses. The posterior ethmoidal sinuses drain via the superior meatus. The sphenoethmoidal recess lies medial to the superior turbinate and is the location of the ostium of the sphenoid sinus.

INTRODUCTION

Air entering the nose will first pass into the vestibule, a skin lined prechamber with hairs which filter out some of the larger particles. It then passes through a narrow 'nasal valve' where the upper lateral cartilages are overlapped by the lower lateral cartilages to form the narrowest part of the nasal airway.

The nasal cavity is divided in two by the nasal septum, the roof is the cribriform plate, separating it from the anterior cranial cavity while inferiorly the hard palate separates the nasal cavity from the oral cavity. The lateral wall is formed by horizontal projections, the inferior, middle and superior turbinates (or concha). Occasionally there may be a supreme turbinate. Below and lateral to each are found the inferior, middle and superior meatus. (Fig. 1)

The maxillary sinus, anterior ethmoidal and frontal sinuses **all** drain into the middle meatus via the **ostiomeatal complex.** This is formed by the slit-like ostium/ infundibulum of the maxillary sinus and the middle meatus being bounded by the middle turbinate medially, the inferior turbinate inferiorly and the orbital wall laterally. (Fig. 2 and 3) Inflammation and swelling in this region, whether it be due to allergy, infection, anatomical variants, polyps or any other cause, will result in obstruction of all three sinuses draining into this area.

Posteriorly the nose communicates with the nasopharynx via the posterior choanae. In children, this area may be obstructed by the lymphoid tissue of the adenoids, which usually atrophy away and it is rare to find any adenoidal tissue in adults. Rarely, a congenital abnormality results in choanal atresia, with the nasal airway ending as a blind cul-de-sac. If bilateral, this will be diagnosed at birth, as neonates are obligatory nose breathers and can not be suckled unless a nasal airway is established. Unilateral choanal atresia, may go undiagnosed for years and may not present until adult life.

EMBRYOLOGY

The maxillary sinus expands laterally as a shallow groove from the ethmoidal infundibulum in the fourth intrauterine month. It extends laterally to reach the lateral cartilaginous plate so that, at birth, there is a small sinus cavity with its lower border about 4mm above the nasal floor. Expansion and pneumatization continue until 8–9

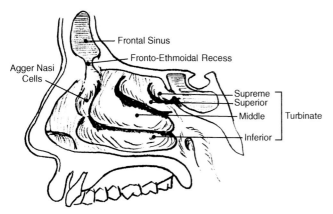

Figure 1. Lateral wall of the nose.

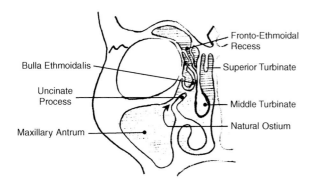

Figure 2. Coronal view of right side of nose.

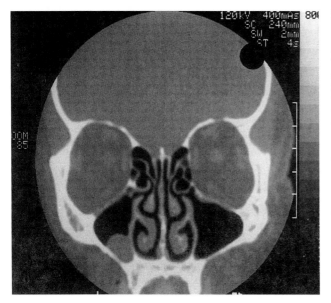

Figure 3. Coronal CT Scan

years of age when the floors of the sinus and nasal cavity are roughly equal and the sinus is $2 \times 2 \times 3$ cm in dimension. Growth continues at the rate of 2–3 mm/year until the adult stage is reached when the sinus floor is usually lower than the nasal cavity by 0.5–10mm.

The ethmoids arise from furrows between folds which develop on the lateral wall of the nose in the fourth intrauterine month. The cells and clefts are primarily evaginations of nasal mucosa which grow into the lateral ethmoidal masses and by further growth and resorption of bone, become established as the cellular labyrinth which is well-pneumatized at birth.

The frontal sinus is absent at birth and only develops between 6–12 years of age. It develops by:

1. Direct extension of the whole frontal recess
2. From one or more of the anterior ethmoid cells
3. Occasionally from the ventral extremity of the ethmoidal infundibulum.

The sphenoid is recognizable from the third intrauterine month as a cleft in the sphenoethmoidal recess. At birth it is approximately $0.5 \times 2 \times 2$ mm and becomes fully pneumatized at about the age of 8 years.

Children are potentially vulnerable to ethmoidal and maxillary sinusitis whereas sphenoiditis is very unlikely in young children and frontal sinusitis is rare before puberty.

ULTRASTRUCTURE

Nasal Epithelium

The nasal lining comprises a pseudostratified columnar ciliated mucous membrane which is in continuity with the paranasal sinuses and the pharynx. Anteriorly, the nasal vestibule is lined by skin. Superiorly, is the specialised olfactory mucosa innervated by the first cranial nerve.

The nasal epithelium comprises columnar ciliated cells, goblet cells and basal cells. Goblet cells produce mucus which forms a protective barrier over the nasal surface, important in filtration and host defence [as a source of lysosyme and lactoferrin]. Columnar cells possess superficial villous projections [microvilli] which greatly increase the epithelial surface area. Most columnar cells possess 50–100 mobile cilia which project into the overlying mucus. This "mucus blanket" has fluid [sol] and superficial gelatinous [gel] layers. The cilia will normally beat at 12–15 beats per second within the sol mucus phase which propels the thicker gel phase from anterior to the post-nasal space in approximately 10–20 minutes. Similarly, mucus from the sinuses drain via their respective ostia to join the main nasal mucus stream draining into the nasopharynx.

Nasal Submucosa

The nasal submucosa represents loose connective tissue containing blood vessels, submucosal glands and many different cell-types. The nasal mucosa is highly vascular. Blood may travel from the arterioles either directly via arteriovenous anastomoses, the venous system or alternatively via the extensive mucosal capillary network. Between the capillary system and the venules there is erectile tissue in the form of cavernous sinusoids which are normally constricted by ongoing sympathetic stimulation but dilate in the face of reduced sympathetic or increased parasympathetic activity. Engorgement of the sinusoids may result in marked mucosal swelling and nasal obstruction. Submucosal glands are either serous [opening predominantly anteriorly in the nasal cavity] or seromucous and are under parasympathetic nervous control via the seventh cranial [facial] and vidian nerves. Cell types within the nasal submucosa include macrophages, fibroblasts, lymphocytes and plasma cells. Neutrophils are occasionally present and increase with infections whereas eosinophils are characteristic of atopic allergic disease and some types of nonallergic diseases. Mast cells are of two types: mucosa mast cell with tryptase only [MC_T] and connective tissue mast cell with tryptase and chymase containing cells [MC_{TC}], present in roughly equal proportions. Mast cells and eosinophils are found in the nasal epithelium and MC_T mast cells and eosinophils migrate into the epithelium of hayfever sufferers during seasonal exposure to pollens.

NASAL MUCOCILIARY CLEARANCE (NMCC)

Congenital abnormalities of mucociliary clearance such as primary ciliary dyskinesia and Youngs syndrome are relatively rare but secondary defects due to the specific effects of bacteria such as *Streptococcus pneumoniae* and *Haemophilus influenzae* are common.[1,2] These bacteria are the commonest pathogens in both acute and chronic sinus infection but in the latter, a mixed growth is often found, which includes anaerobes.

PATHOPHYSIOLOGY

The importance of the middle meatus in the development of sinusitis was recognized by Caldwell a century ago and mucociliary mechanisms in this region were described by Hilding in the 1930s.[3] In 1978 Messerklinger[4] published in English an account of his *in vivo* endoscopic findings on patients and fresh cadavers using time-lapse photography. He noted that whenever two mucosal surfaces came into direct contact, localized disruption of the mucociliary clearance occurred, causing retention of secretions in the area of contact, preventing or slowing drainage, predisposing the patient to infection and leading to inflammation and oedema which could further increase contact leading to a vicious circle. Anatomically, areas of mucosal contact are most likely to occur in the narrow clefts of the middle meatus and ethmoids.

APPLIED ANATOMY

Inferior Meatus

The inferior meatus lies lateral to the inferior turbinate, below its attachment. It is the largest of the three meatuses, extending almost the entire length of the lateral wall of the nose. It is highest at the junction of the anterior and middle thirds, at the genu of the inferior turbinate. The nasolacrimal duct opens just anterior and inferior to this point. The bone is thinnest in the superior central portion of the meatus where it can easily be penetrated for lavage or fenestrated during inferior intranasal antrostomy.

The blood supply to the inferior meatus is derived from the lateral sphenopalatine artery, a terminal branch of the maxillary artery. It enters the nasal cavity through the sphenopalatine foramen beneath the horizontal attachment of the middle turbinate. The vessel supplying the inferior meatus enters posteriorly, and runs inferiorly and forwards between 4 and 5cm along the bony lateral wall, leaving the central portion of the meatus relatively avascular.

The anterior superior alveolar nerve is a branch of the infraorbital nerve and contributes to the superior dental plexus. It is related to the anterior attachment of the inferior turbinate where a branch is given to the mucosa of the lateral wall as high as the maxillary ostium. Damage to this nerve during anterior enlargement of an inferior meatal antrostomy may result in alteration in dental sensation. Paraesthesia can also result from direct damage to the infraorbital nerve during a Caldwell-Luc approach. The infraorbital canal represents a constant thinning of the bone in the orbital floor and may be dehiscent. The nerve may also be damaged as it leaves the infraorbital foramen to supply the soft tissue of the anterior cheek.

Middle Meatus

The configuration of the middle meatus is complex and subject to considerable variation. The middle turbinate provides the key to understanding the surgical anatomy. Anteriorly it is attached vertically to the skull base and posteriorly to the maxilla and lamina papyracea by a horizontal attachment. Joining the two is an oblique lamella of bone, the basal which divides the ethmoid complex into anterior and posterior ethmoidal cells.(Fig. 4)

Uncinate Process

The uncinate process is a thin crescent of ethmoid bone which attaches to the anterior edge of the maxillary hiatus but in life a variable area of the hiatus anterior and posterior to this attachment are filled with mucosa and membrane and are termed respectively the anterior and posterior fontanelles. (Fig. 5) It is in these natural areas of weakness that accessory ostia are found. The relationship of maxillary ostium to frontonasal recess

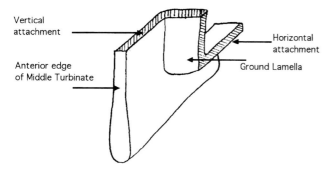

Figure 4. "Step-shaped" attachment of the left Middle turbinate. The ground lamella can be identified by passing an endoscope under the horizontal attachment posteriorly, advancing it anteriorly and superiorly. This area would normally be hidden by the bulla ethmoidalis and sinus lateralis when present.

will depend upon the superior attachment of the uncinate process. If the uncinate joins the lamina papyracea, a separate cul-de-sac results, the recessus terminalis. Adjacent to the uncinate and just anterior to the anterior attachment of the middle turbinate, the agger nasi area is found which is usually pneumatized. Anterior to the attachment of the uncinate process to the maxilla is the nasolacrimal duct, generally lying in thick bone but occasionally encroached upon by the agger nasi cells.

Ethmoidal Bulla

The ethmoidal bulla contains the anterior ethmoidal cells though can be poorly or completely unpneumatized in 8%[5]. The hiatus semilunaris is a two-dimensional space between the posterior edge of the uncinate process and the anterior face of the bulla. (Fig. 5) Passing through this boomerang shaped slit one enters the ethmoidal infundibulum, a funnel-shaped space leading to the maxillary ostium laterally and superiorly it will lead up to the frontal sinus or the recessus terminalis depending on its

superior attachment. Posteriorly, the bulla may fuse with the basal lamella of the middle turbinate or there may be a cleft, the sinus lateralis.(Fig. 6)

Frontal Recess

The term "frontal recess" is preferred to "frontonasal duct" as it is usually an hour-glass constriction rather than a tubular duct. It is found in the most anteriosuperior part of the middle meatus, often lying medial to the ostium of a suprabullar cell. However, accessory channels are found in 12% of the Caucasian population.[5]

The ethmoid bone is completed superiorly by the frontal bone which is generally thicker bone, resistant to disease and trauma. Where the frontal bone joins the ethmoid, particularly medially, the bone is thin and delicate which is further weakened by the passage of the anterior ethmoidal artery. It is at this point that the anterior cranial fossa may be easily breached. This vessel may also be damaged as it traverses the roof and lateral wall, from which it may retract, producing in the worst instance, a rapidly developing orbital haematoma. The posterior ethmoidal vessel by contrast is usually more protected, running within bone.

The level of the ethmoidal roof varies in 12% of the population between right and left, with the right side being more usually the lower [8%][6]. This may in part explain the tendency for the right side to be the site of iatrogenic CSF leaks.

Posterior Ethmoids

The posterior ethmoid cells are generally larger, pyramidal and few in number. They drain via the superior meatus. A supreme turbinate is discernible in two-thirds of subjects[7]. The sphenoethmoidal recess lies medial to the

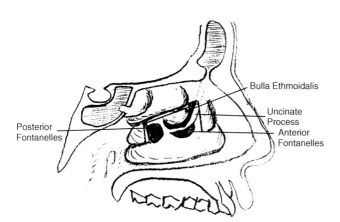

Figure 5. Lateral wall of nose with segment of Middle turbinate removed.

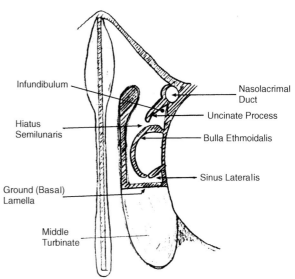

Figure 6. Axial section of right side of nose (after Stammberger).

superior turbinate and is the location of the ostium of the sphenoid sinus. The most posterior ethmoidal cell can extend lateral to the sphenoid, a variant described by Onodi[8]. The optic nerve is particularly vulnerable in such cells and even under normal circumstances has been estimated to be clinically dehiscent in 6% of the normal Caucasian population[5]. Ethmoidal cells may also pneumatize the floor of the orbit, forming Haller cells, which can encroach on the ethmoidal infundibulum[5]. This pneumatization can occur from the anterior system [70%] or posterior [30%].

Sphenoid Sinus

The ostium of the sphenoid sinus is usually located in the sphenoethmoidal recess and therefore lies medial to the superior (or supreme turbinate when present). It is intimately related to the optic nerve which can be seen in its bony canal superiorly with the internal carotid artery below. The bone overlying both can be extremely thin or dehiscent in 25% of the population.[5]

ANATOMIC VARIANTS

In the literature, a number of anatomical variants are cited as potentially predisposing to persistent infection. These include:

concha bullosa (pneumatised middle turbinate)

enlarged (or over pneumatized) ethmoidal bulla

everted uncinate process (or "double middle turbinate")

paradoxical middle turbinate (concave of normal convex curvature)

Haller cells (which lie between the uncinate process and orbital wall)

septal deflection (particularly where this impinges on the OMC)

One or more anatomical variants are found in 62% of patients with chronic rhinosinusitis and the incidence of some of these variants appears to be higher in patients than in control subjects[9]. However it does not necessarily follow that the anatomical variant per se is responsible for the sinus pathology. Surgery should only be advocated when the history, clinical findings and under-lying pathology have been considered and the anatomical variant, such as a concha bullosa, can be shown to be contributing to narrowing of the ostiomeatal complex.

A knowledge of the variable and intricate anatomy of the nasal cavity is useful to the understanding of the pathophysiology and medical treatment of nasal polyps. It is an essential prerequisite before embarking on surgical treatment with or without an endoscope.

FURTHER READING

J. Lang. Clinical Anatomy of the Nose, Nasal Cavity and Paranasal Sinuses 1989 Georg Thieme Verlag Stuttgart.

H. Stammberger. Functional Endoscopic Sinus Surgery 1991 B.C.Decker Philadelphia.

REFERENCES

1. Read R, Wilson R, Rutman A. et al, Interaction of non-typable *Haemophilus influenzae* with human respiratory mucosa in vitro. Journal of Infectious Disease, 1991 163: 549–558.
2. Feldman C, Read R, Rutman R et al. The interaction of Strepotococcus pneumonia with intact human respiratory mucosa in vitro. European Respiratory Journal, 5:576–583, 1992.
3. Hilding A C. Physiology of drainage of nasal mucous: experimental work on accessory sinuses. American Journal of Physiology. 100:644, 1932.
4. Messerklinger W. Endoscopy of the Nose. Baltimore: Urban & Schwarzenberg. 1978.
5. Stammberger H. Functional Endoscopic Sinus Surgery. Philadelphia: B C Decker. 1991.
6. Dessi P, Castro F, Triglia J M. et al. Difference in the height of the right and left ethmoid roofs: a possible risk factor for ethmoid surgery. Journal of Laryngology and Otology 1994. 108, 261–262.
7. Schaeffer J P. The Nose, Paranasal Sinuses, Nasolacrimal Passageways and Olfactory Organ in Man. Philadelphia: Blakiston, 1920.
8. Onodi A. Die Eroffnung der Kieferhohle im mittleren Nasengang. Arch Laryngol Rhinol 14:154–160, 1903.
9. Lloyd G A S, Lund V J and Scadding G K. Computerised tomography in the preoperative evaluation of functional endoscopic sinus surgery. Journal of Laryngology and Otology. 105:181–185, 1991.

Chapter V

Histopathology

Henrik B. Hellquist, M.D., Ph.D.

ABSTRACT

Sinonasal polyps are benign mucosal swellings that occur in four different histological patterns. The most common type is the oedematous, eosinophilic (so-called "allergic") nasal polyp, which constitutes 85–90% of nasal polyps. The oedematous polyp is morphologically characterized by oedema, goblet cell hyperplasia of the epithelium, thickening of the basement membrane, and of numerous leukocytes, predominantly eosinophils. The second histological type is a fibroinflammatory polyp characterized by chronic inflammation and metaplastic changes of the overlying epithelium. Another rare variant presents with pronounced hyperplasia of seromucinous glands but otherwise shows many similarities with the oedematous type of polyp. The fourth type is very rare and is a polyp with atypical stroma. This latter polyp calls for awareness and careful histological examination to avoid misdiagnosis of a neoplasm.

INTRODUCTION

Sinonasal polyps are swellings of the sinonasal mucosa which histologically can be composed of anything from an oedematous transformed mucosa to a neoplasm. In general terms, nasal polyps are non-neoplastic swellings that usually arise from the middle meatus and ethmoid sinuses and prolapse into the nasal cavity. Polyps may also arise from the maxillary sinuses and from the middle and superior turbinates. Support that nasal polyps can originate from the nasal mucosa was given in a study by Larsen and Tos, though this study could not preclude the presence of underlying ethmoid involvement[1]. The pathogenesis of nasal polyps is dealt with in other chapters of this book and here will only different histological features be described. Swelling and polyposis of the sinonasal mucosa constitute a clinical problem rather than a histological one. Numerous studies have been performed concerning polyposis, particularly concerning the etiology, clinical behaviour, and treatment policies,[2,3,4] but few studies have paid attention to differences in histological appearance and to any possible implication that this might have. It is the author's belief that the common grouping of polyps into allergic and nonallergic polyp is inappropriate, particularly as polyps are produced in many different pathological conditions, both benign and malignant. Histological investigation is essential for accurate diagnosis and the most important differential diagnoses will be discussed towards the end of this chapter.

SINONASAL MUCOSA

Most polyps arise in the middle meatus and ethmoidal region, particularly from the mucosa of the middle concha, and the ethmoidal air cells which may be filled with polyps. The sinonasal tract (apart from the vestibulem and the area of olfactory epithelium) is lined by an ordinary respiratory tract epithelium, i.e. a pseudostratified, ciliated columnar cell epithelium with interspersed goblet cells and scattered areas of metaplastic squamous cell epithelium. The normal sinonasal respiratory epithelium always shows areas of squamous metaplasia but also cuboidal metaplasia (Fig. 1). The normal gradual metaplastic transformations have been studied and described in detail[5]. These metaplastic changes of epithelium may thus also be present in the epithelium of a polyp. In fact, on rare occasions areas with dysplastic changes can be seen in the overlying epithelium of a polyp. The mucosa contains a variable amount of vessels, nerves and seromucinous glands. The seromucinous glands are more frequent in the mucosa of the turbinates than elsewhere in the nasal cavity (Fig. 2).

The epithelium of the nasal cavity is still called by many the Schneiderian membrane. Schneider (1660) described the histological features of the nasal mucosa and

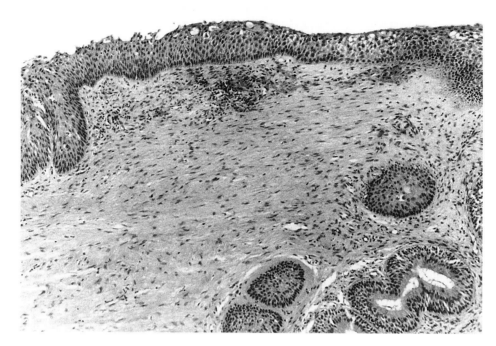

Figure 1. Photomicrograph of nasal mucosa with extensive squamous metaplasia. Squamous metaplasia is also present in three seromucinous glands (H & E, × 100).

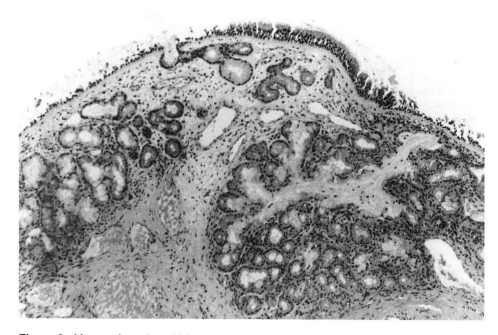

Figure 2. Mucosa from the middle turbinate lined with respiratory epithelium which shows some goblet cell hyperplasia (left). Note the abundance of seromucinous glands (H & E, ×50).

disproved the contemporary theory that nasal secretion was produced by the pituitary gland. Histologically the Schneiderian membrane is an ordinary pseudostratified, columnar and ciliated respiratory epithelium. The term "transitional cell epithelium," on the other hand, is a misnomer, as transitional cell epithelium is found in the urogenital tract, and not in the sinonasal tract. Similarly, the so-called transitional cell papilloma (carcinoma) should correctly be termed columnar (cylindrical) cell papilloma (carcinoma)[6].

The normal surface epithelium in the paranasal sinuses differs somewhat when compared with that of the nasal cavity. The surface lining of the paranasal sinuses is thinner, less specialized and contains fewer cilia and goblet cells than that of the nasal cavity[7]. Moreover, there are less seromucinous glands in the lamina propria of the sinuses than in that of the nasal cavity. These circumstances probably contribute to the lower resistance to infection of the sinuses compared to that of the nasal cavity.

GROSS APPEARANCE

Sinonasal polyps are usually soft, lobular and mobile swellings. They usually have a smooth and shiny surface with a bluish-grey or pink translucent appearance. The cut surface is moist and pale but appears more pink or red if the polyp is more vascular. The polyp often has an elongated stalk, which may be accentuated by pulling during the surgical removal. The gross appearance is not as opaque as that of the sinonasal inverted papilloma, nor does it have the corrugated or pitted surface of an inverted papilloma. Polyp size varies considerably, usually being 2–3 cm in diameter. However, often they are larger, multiple and bilateral, and may lead to visible broadening of the external nose[8]. The antrochoanal polyp, which is a separate entity originating from the mucosa of the maxillary sinus, usually in children, is often of considerable size. Due to its size the antrochoanal polyp bulges backwards into the nasopharynx via the posterior choana.

HISTOLOGICAL STRUCTURE

Four histologically different types of sinonasal polyps can be recognized. This subdivision may seem academic but it is sometimes essential due to the differential diagnosis of neoplastic disease. The so-called allergic, oedematous and eosinophilic polyp is the commonest type, followed in frequency by the polyp that histologically is characterized by chronic inflammation. The third type of polyp has many features in common with the eodematous polyp but furthermore shows hyperplasia of seromucinous glands. This latter type can be misdiagnosed as an adenoma. The rare nasal polyp with stromal atypia constitutes the fourth variant[9]. Combinations of these histological patterns may occasionally be present within a

single polyp, and also different polyps in patients with multiple polyps may display different histological subtypes. Possible etiologies of the different histological types of polyps, and their association with allergy, asthma, etc, will not be commented upon here as they are dealt with in other chapters of this book.

Oedematous, Eosinophilic (So-called "Allergic") Polyp

The oedematous polyp is by far the most common and constituted 86% a series of 107 polyps[10]. The histological hallmarks comprise I) oedematous stroma (Fig 3), II) hyperplasia, often pronounced, of goblet cells in the overlying respiratory epithelium (Fig 4), III) numerous eosinophils and mast cells in the stroma (Fig 4 a & 5) and IV) a thickened, slightly hyalinized basement membrane separating the oedematous stroma and the epithelium (Fig. 3). The stroma shows a sparse amount of fibroblasts whilst there are numerous inflammatory cells. The oedematous stroma is partly filled with fluid creating pseudocystic spaces (Fig. 3 b). The inflammatory infiltrate can be very pronounced, however, commonly there is a moderate amount (Fig. 4a). The oedematous polyp is often bilateral.

Chronic Inflammatory Polyp (Fibroinflammatory Polyp)

The lack of stromal oedema and goblet cell hyperplasia are the most striking features of this type of polyp. Goblet cells are present but the epithelium is devoid of goblet cell hyperplasia. The epithelium frequently shows squamous and cuboidal metaplasia. There may be a thickening of the basement membrane though not as pronounced as in the oedematous type of polyp. The inflammatory infiltrate is often intense but lymphocytes predominate, although intermixed with eosinophils. The stroma contains numerous fibroblasts and fibrosis is not exceedingly rare. In many "fibroinflammatory" polyps there is a slight hyperplasia of seromucinous glands, and dilated vessels can often be seen (Fig. 6). This type represents less than 10% (8.4%) of sinonasal polyps[10].

Polyp with Hyperplasia of Seromucinous Glands

This type of polyp is characterized by numerous seromucinous glands, often in a rather loose, oedematous stroma. It has several features in common with the oedematous polyp. The abundance of glands and ductal structures are the distinguishing histological features. The hyperplasia of the glandular elements may mimic a benign glandular neoplasm, and the author believes that many cases described in the literature as tubulocystic adenoma[11] represented a hyperplastic reaction in a polyp rather than a true neoplastic lesion. The polyp is composed of numerous glands where the cells are cylindrical

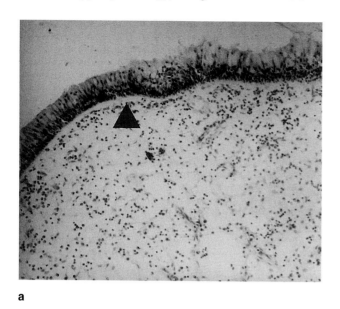

a

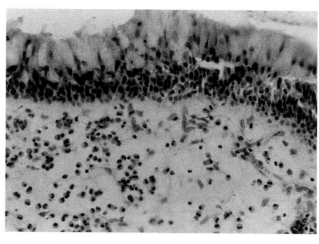

a

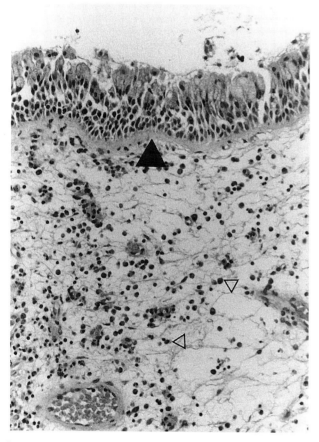

b

b

Figure 4. a) Photomicrograph showing the pronounced hyperplasia of goblet cells in the respiratory epithelium. The majority of the inflammatory cells in the loose, oedematous stroma are eosinophils (H & E, ×250). **b)** A polyp where parts of the respiratory epithelium is almost entirely replaced by goblet cells (H & E, ×100).

Figure 3. a) Oedematous, eosinophilic polyp. Note the abundance of inflammatory cells, most of which are eosinophils and mast cells. There is a thickening of the basement membrane (arrow) (H & E, ×100). **b)** Another oedematous polyp with goblet cell hyperplasia, thickening of the basement membrane (thick arrow), and the loose stroma contains pseudocystic spaces filled with fluid (empty arrows) (H & E, × 200).

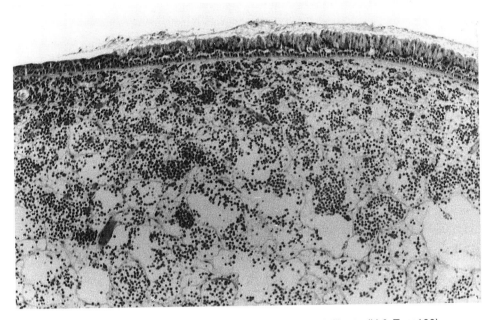

Figure 5. An oedematous polyp with intense inflammatory infiltrate (H & E, ×100).

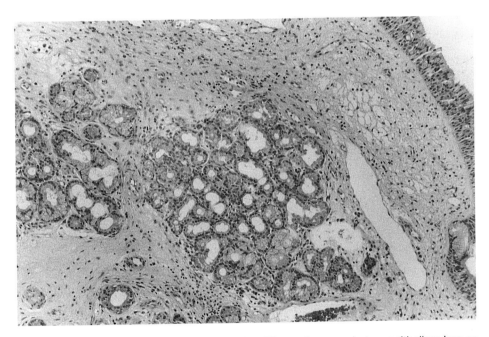

Figure 6. A chronic inflammatory type of polyp. The surface respiratory epithelium has areas with cuboidal metaplasia but no goblet cell hyperplasia. The basement membrane does not show any pronounced hyalinization. The stroma consists of connective tissue with some dilated vessels and a moderate amount of lymphocytes. There are more seromucinous glands than found in the oedematous type of polyp (H & E, ×100).

with the nuclei eccentrically placed towards the basal part of the cells. The glands are frequently in connection with the overlying epithelium and display no atypia. Moreover, in contrast to glandular tumours, the glands are separated from each other and seldom lying neck-to-neck as usually seen in tumours (Fig. 7). This type of polyp is rare and constitutes less than 5% of sinonasal polyps[10].

Polyp with Stromal Atypia

This very rare sinonasal polyp has a distinct histological appearance and can easily be mistaken for a neoplasm if not familiar with its existence and its histological features. Macroscopically it may have the same appearance as any other polyp but histologically it is characterized by stromal cells that are bizarre and "atypical" (Fig. 8). The cells tend to be stellate and hyperchromatic, but may also be more irregular and plump with vesicular cytoplasm. Usually only certain areas of the polyp will show these "atypical" cells, which represent reactive fibroblasts (Fig. 8b). Occasionally the entire polyp consists of atypical stromal elements. The lack of mitoses is the main feature to distinguish a polyp with atypical stroma from

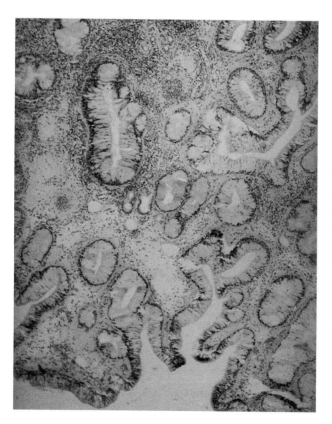

Figure 7. Nasal polyp with hyperplasia of seromucinous glands. Note that the glands are lacking atypia and rarely arranged neck-to-neck. There is no atypia (H & E, ×100).

a neoplasm. Furthermore, there are no cytoplasmic cross-striations and the glycogen content is minimal in these bizarre cells. Immunostaining in any case of polyp with bizarre fibroblast-like cells will be of great help to rule out malignant melanoma, neurogenic sarcoma, etc. Only one of the 107 polyps reported by Davidsson and Hellquist represented a polyp with atypical stroma[10].

CELLULAR ELEMENTS

The cellular infiltrate is composed of leukocytes, of which eosinophils predominate, mast cells and lymphocytes. Nasal polyps in patients with cystic fibrosis contain more mast cells than non-cystic fibrosis polyps, and eosinophils are rarely seen in cystic fibrosis nasal polyps[12]. Investigation of subsets of lymphocytes in nasal polyps indicate that T lymphocytes predominate over B cells, and that there are more T suppressor (CD8+) than T helper (CD4+) cells[4]. Interestingly, IgE-producing mast cells are rarely found in polyps of patients with nasal allergy[4]. In contrast, the amount of histamine, which is mainly found in mast cells, has been found to be less in aspirin-induced asthma-related polyps than in allergy-related polyps[13]. The exact composition of the cellular infiltrate in histologically different polyps in patients with and without allergy or allergy-like conditions, remains to be clarified. The migration of eosinophils and other inflammatory cells into the stroma of the polyps is not only dependent on attractant factors, eg. the chemokine RANTES. The upregulation of certain endothelial adhesion molecules on the vessel endothelium in the polyps is also of great importance. For example, the eosinophilic adhesion to nasal polyp endothelium is P-Selectin dependent whereas the vascular cell adhesion molecule 1 (VCAM-1) is not upregulated[14]. Also the transepithelial ion transport differs in polyp-derived epithelium compared to turbinate-derived epithelium[15,16]. The mechanisms of ion transport and the role of chemokines, proinflammatory cytokines and adhesion molecules in the recruitment of the cellular elements, call for further studies to enlighten our understanding of the pathogenesis, and to improve treatment strategies of sinonasal polyposis.

NECESSITY OF HISTOLOGICAL EXAMINATION OF POLYPS

The vast majority of clinically typical sinonasal polyp are histologically benign polyps with an appearance as described above. On rare occasions, however, both benign and malignant neoplasms may have a very similar macroscopical appearance to a polyp, and histological examination of all sinonasal polyps is therefore necessary. Histologically the bizarre cells in atypical nasal polyps may give the impression of embryonal rhabdomyosarcoma. The absence of mitotic activity, and the

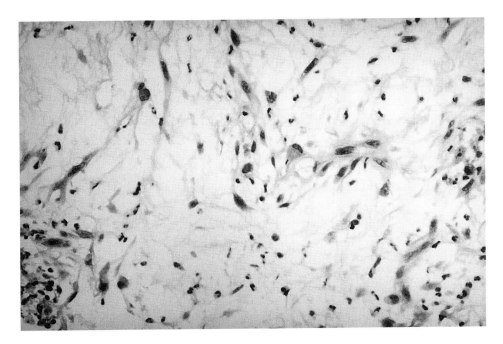

a

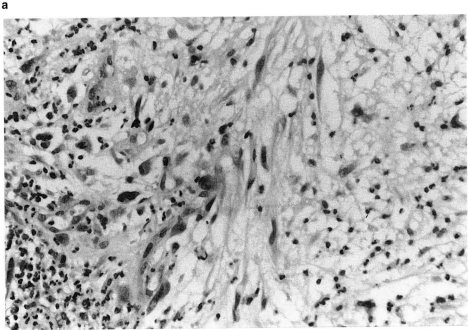

a

Figure 8. a) Photomicrograph of a polyp with atypical stroma. The stroma is rather oedematous with inflammatory cells but there are numerous bizarre, partly stellate-shaped cells. The nuclei of these "atypical" cells often tend to be hyperchromatic. Note the absence of mitosis (H & E, ×440). **b)** Another case of a polyp with atypical stroma. The atypical cells are seen in the center of the picture whilst there is a pronounced inflammation (left) and also oedema (right) (H & E, ×440).

minimal amount (if any) of cross striations, and of glycogen, constitute the main features to distinguish a polyp with atypical stroma from an embryonal rhabdomyosarcoma. An immunostaining with desmin may be helpful. In cases of amelanotic malignant melanoma (primary and metastatic) immunostaining for S-100, cytokeratin and HMB-45 can be of great help (Fig 9). Furthermore, adult muscle cells may occasionally be seen in polyps and care has to be taken not to misdiagnose such a lesion as teratocarcinoma.

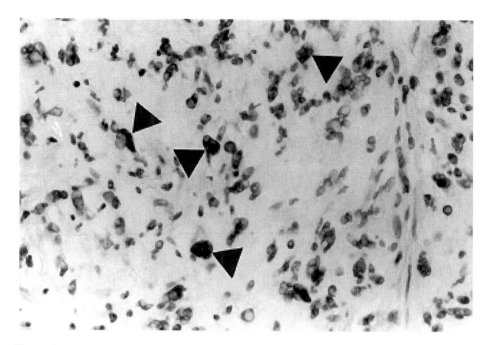

Figure 9. A unilateral nasal polyp which histologically has features compatible with a polyp with atypical stroma. An immunostaining was performed and most cells showed strong positivity for both S-100 and HMB-45 (arrows). After further clinical examination the primary malignant melanoma was found on the skin of the back (ABC, HMB-45, ×440).

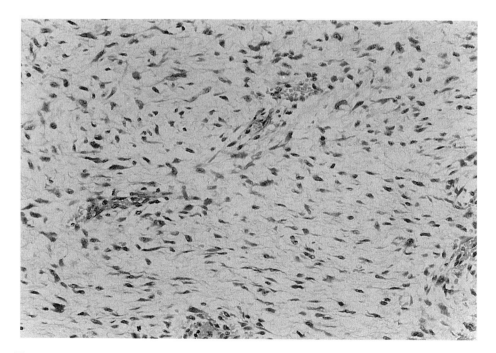

Figure 10. Photomicrograph of a nasal polyp which is a neurilemoma. The typical features are not obvious and only after examination (immunostaining included) of several blocks typical areas of both Antoni A and B were observed (H & E, ×200).

Fibromatosis (neurofibromatosis, aggressive fibromatosis as well as infantil fibromatosis) and neurilemoma are examples of benign tumours or tumour-like conditions which macroscopically may mimic a sinonasal polyp of the fibroinflammatory type. Careful histologic examination of several blocks is often necessary to reveal the true nature of fibromatosis, or of neurilemoma with palisading of cells (Fig 10).

The examples given in Figures 9 and 10 illustrate two cases that the author has experienced, and exemplify the necessity to examine all sinonasal polyps, irrespective of their gross appearance.

REFERENCES

1. Larsen PL, Tos M. Origin of nasal polyps. Laryngoscope 101: 305–312, 1991.

2. Braun JJ, Haas, F, Conraux C. La polypose nasosinusienne Epidémiologie et clinicque sur 350 cas. Traitement et résultats avec un recul supérieur à 5 ans sur 93 cas. Ann Oto-Laryngol (Paris) 109: 189–199, 1992.

3. Stoop AE, van der Heijden HAMD, Biewenga J, van der Baan S. Clinical aspects and distribution of immunologically active cells in the nasal mucosa of patients with nasal polyps after endoscopic sinus surgery and treatment with topical corticosteroids. Eur Arch Otorhinolaryngol 249: 313–317, 1992.

4. Liu C-M, Shun C-T, Hsu M-M. Lymphocyte subsets and antigen-specific IgE antibody in nasal polyps. Ann Allergy 72: 19–24, 1994.

5. Boysen M. The surface structure of the human nasal mucosa. Ciliated and metaplastic epithelium in normal individuals. A correlated study by scanning/transmission electron and light microscopy. Virchows Arch (B) 40: 279–294, 1982.

6. Shanmugaratnam K, Barnes L, Cardesa A et al. Histological Typing of Tumours of the Upper Respiratory Tract and Ear. World Health Organization International Classification of Tumours, 2nd Ed., Springer-Verlag, Berlin, Heidelberg, New York, 1991.

7. Tos M, Mogensen C. Mucus production in chronic maxillary sinusitis. A quantitative histopathological study. Acta Otolaryngol (Stockh) 97: 151–159, 1984.

8. Hellquist HB. Allergy and allergy-like conditions. In: Pathology of the nose and paranasal sinuses. Butterworths, London, 1990, pp. 24–32.

9. Compagno J, Hyams VJ. Nasal polyposis with atypical stroma. Arch Pathol Lab Med 100: 224–226, 1976.

10. Davidsson Å, Hellquist HB. The so-called 'allergic' nasal polyp. ORL J Relat Spec 55: 30–35, 1993.

11. Friedmann I, Osborn DA. Tumours of mucosal glands. In: Pathology of Granulomas and Neoplasms of the Nose and Paranasal Sinuses. Churchill Livingstone, Edinburgh, 1982, pp. 133–161.

12. Henderson WR Jr, Chi EY. Degranulation of cystic fibrosis nasal polyp mast cells. J Pathol 166: 395–404, 1992.

13. Ogino S, Abe Y, Irifune M et al. Histamine metabolism in nasal polyps. Ann Otol Rhinol Laryngol 102: 152–156, 1993.

14. Symon FA, Walsh GM, Watson SR, Wardlaw AJ. Eosinophilic adhesion to nasal polyp endothelium is P-Selectin-dependent. J Exp Med 180: 371–376, 1994.

15. Bernstein JM, Cropp GA, Nathanson I, Yankaskas JR. Bioelectric properties of cultured nasal polyp and turbinate epithelial cells. Am J Rhinol 4: 45–49, 1990.

16. Bernstein JM, Yankaskas JR. Increased ion transport in cultured nasal polyp epithelial cells. Arch Otolaryngol Head Neck Surg 120: 993–996, 1994.

Chemical Mediators in Polyps

Hal M. Hoffman, M.D., and Stephen I. Wasserman, M.D.

ABSTRACT

This chapter outlines the many chemical mediators of inflammation that have been studied in nasal polyps. The cell sources and actions of traditional as well as newer mediators are discussed. Results of research in this area are presented and implications for further study of nasal polyps and related disease states are postulated.

INTRODUCTION

Nasal polyps are the end result of an inflammatory process which is associated with various disease states, implying a multiplicity of etiologies and responsible mediators. The ready availability of nasal polyp tissue and the development of improved techniques for identifying chemical mediators has led to a proliferation of informative research into this fascinating disorder. This chapter will discuss the mediators and the cell sources implicated in the development of nasal polyps.

For this discussion a chemical mediator is defined as a molecule formed by one cell which has the ability to effect changes in other responding cells. Mediators may be peptides, proteins, amines, or lipids. In an effort to simplify the classification of the mediators, this chapter will organize mediators according to chemical family within the broader headings of traditional or new mediators.

MEDIATOR ACTIONS

The first mediators described had primarily local tissue effects such as vasoactive or spasmogenic actions. Several mediators share these actions including histamine, platelet activating factor (PAF), prostaglandins, leukotrienes, norepinephrine, neuropeptide Y (NPY), substance-P, and vasoactive intestinal peptide (VIP). Other mediators such as transforming growth factor (TGF), tumor necrosis factor

(TNF) and VIP can change the composition of extracellular matrix in a tissue. Preformed granular proteins and enzymes can cause tissue destruction as well. (Table 1)

All inflammatory processes involve the control of cell migration. Several mediators have been found to directly attract leukocytes such as high molecular weight-neutrophil chemotactic factor (HMW-NCF), histamine, prostaglandins, leukotrienes, PAF, interleukin-5 (IL-5) and a family of molecules termed chemokines. The discovery of adhesion molecules (i.e. selectins, integrins) on the cell surface has revealed another mechanism influencing the migration of inflammatory leukocytes to specific areas. Adhesion molecule expression is influenced by IL-1, IL-4, IL-6, TNF, as well as by some of the vasoactive or spasmogenic molecules, providing an indirect effect on leukocyte migration. (Table 2)

The ability to stimulate cell growth, differentiation, and proliferation via TGF, the colony stimulating factors, insulin-like growth factor (IGF), TNF, and several interleukins also is relevant to development and maintenance of inflammatory processes. Generally, the production or release of chemical mediators is initiated by activation of the cells that produce them. This activation may in turn be initiated or modulated by other chemical mediators. Mediators implicated in cell activation include several interleukins, vasoactive intestinal peptide, and adhesion molecules.

SOURCES OF MEDIATORS

The traditional mediator producing cells in the upper and lower respiratory tract have been mast cells, basophils, eosinophils, macrophages, and neutrophils. As a better understanding of immunologic cellular communication was achieved, attention focused on the role of T lymphocytes in orchestrating the inflammatory process. This occurs through production of cytokines which direct

Table 1 Local Tissue Effects

Mediator	Cell Sources	Action
Preformed		
Histamine	Mast Cells	Vasodilation
	Basophils	Smooth Muscle Contraction or Dilation
		Increase in Vascular Permeability
Proteases	Mast Cells	Tissue Destruction/Repair
	Neutrophils	Extracellular Matrix Remodeling
Granular Proteins	Eosinophils	Tissue Destruction
Generated		
Platelet	Mast Cells	Smooth Muscle Contraction
Activating	Neutrophils	Vasoconstriction
Factor (PAF)	Eosinophils	Increase in Vascular Permeability
	Monocytes	
Prostaglandins*	Mast Cells	Vasodilation
(PG)		Smooth Muscle Contraction
		Increase in Vascular Permeability
Leukotrienes*	Mast Cells	Smooth Muscle Contraction or Dilation
(LT)	Basophils	Vasoconstriction
	Eosinophils	Increase in Vascular Permeability
	Neutrophils	
	Monocytes	
Neurotransmitters		
Norepinephrine	Autonomic Nerves	Vasoconstriction
Neuropeptide Y	Autonomic Nerves	Vasoconstriction
Substance P	Sensory Nerves	Vasodilation
		Smooth Muscle Contraction
		Increase in Vascular Permeability
Vasoactive	Autonomic Nerves	Vasodilation
Intestinal		Cystic Degeneration of Glands
Peptide (VIP)		
Cytokines		
Transforming	Eosinophils	Extracellular Matrix Production
Growth Factor		Angiogenesis
(TGF)		
Tumor Necrosis	Eosinophils	Extracellular Matrix Degradation
Factor (TNF)	Mast Cells	Angiogenesis

*action varies with subtype

proliferation, activation, and localization of other mediator producing cells.

More recently attention has been directed at the microenvironment as a source of mediators, especially growth factors. Epithelial cells, endothelial cells and fibroblasts not only serve as structural framework for these tissues but also play a part in the cellular intercommunication through their production of mediators[1]. Their cell surface adhesion molecules also play a special role in directing inflammatory cell migration and activation. Finally, the extracellular matrix has also been implicated in this complex communication web[2].

SPECIFIC MEDIATORS STUDIED IN NASAL POLYPS

Traditional Mediators

Histamine

Histamine is released primarily by mast cells (but also basophils) after IgE mediated activation or activation by histamine releasing factors. Histamine is found in mast cells of nasal polyp tissue especially in the apex of the polyp[3], and is higher in patients with allergy and chronic sinusitis than in those with aspirin intolerance, whose levels are normal[4,5]. This histamine can be released, in vitro,

Table 2. Cell migration

Direct Effect	Indirect Effect (via adhesion molecule expression)

High Molecular Weight-
   Neutrophil Chemotactic Factor
   (HMW-NCF)
	Transforming Growth Factor (TGF)
	Tumor Necrosis Factor (TNF)

Histamine	Interleukin-1 (IL-1)
Prostaglandins (PG)	Interleukin-4 (IL-4)
Leukotrienes (LT)	Interleukin-6 (IL-6)
Platelet Activating Factor (PAF)	Macrophage Inflammatory Protein (MIP-1α)
Interleukin-5 (IL-5)	
Interleukin-8 (IL-8)	
Macrophage Inflammatory Protein (MIP-1α)	

by allergen in allergic individuals or, from non-allergic individuals, after in vitro sensitization with IgE[6]. Histamine content in nasal polyp fluid varies widely (20 to 1000 times that of serum) but does not correlate with skin test positivity[7], with IgE levels[8], or with presence of asthma or allergic rhinitis[7].

The three histamine degradative enzymes, histidine decarboxylase, histaminase, and histamine-N-methyl transferase (HMT) are present in nasal polyps. The latter predominates and is higher in polyps from aspirin sensitive patients, perhaps explaining the lower histamine content in polyps from these patients[5].

The increase in histamine which mediates the formation of polyps is thought to occur by one or both of two possible mechanisms: first, insufficient blood supply to the ethmoid sinus inhibits local degradative enzymes, causing increased histamine, with resulting edema and polyp formation[7]; alternatively, histamine is released by allergy or other stimuli[3].

Arachidonic Acid Metabolites
Arachidonic acid is the precursor of a family of chemical mediators. Two main pathways exist: the cyclooxygenase pathway producing prostaglandins, thromboxanes, and prostacyclin and the lipoxygenase pathway synthesizing hydroxyeicosatetraenoic acids (HETE), cystinyl-leukotrienes (LT), and lipoxins (LX). (Fig. 1)

The predominant arachidonic acid metabolite in nasal polyps is 15-HETE[9], found at levels 30 times that of normal or chronically inflamed nasal mucosa[10]. 5-HETE, 12-HETE and 15-HETE are produced when polyp tissue is stimulated[11]. All of the cystinyl-leukotrienes have been found in nasal polyp tissue[12], with LTE$_4$ more frequently identified in nasal lavage[11]. Both LTB$_4$ and LTC$_4$ have been found in higher concentration in polyps[9], and the level of LTB$_4$ is much higher in polyps from allergic than non-allergic patients[13]. LTC$_4$ and LTD$_4$ predominate in patients with aspirin sensitive asthma[14] and in chronic

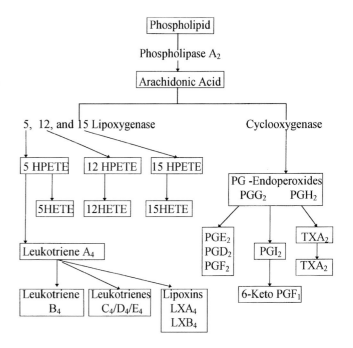

Figure 1. Arachidonic Acid Pathway.

allergic patients after aspirin challenge[15]. LTC$_4$ and LTD$_4$ are also produced upon addition of ragweed antigen to polyps from ragweed sensitive patients and from non-allergic patients passively sensitized with ragweed sensitive serum[6]. Nasal polyp tissue can also convert exogenous LTA$_4$ to lipoxins LXA$_4$ and LXB$_4$[16].

Nasal polyps contain detectable levels of prostaglandins D$_2$[15], E$_2$, and F$_{2\alpha}$[17] with PGE$_2$ predominating[14], especially in allergic patients[9]. Polyp tissue from aspirin sensitive patients has lower amounts of prostaglandins[14] and demonstrates inhibited prostaglandin release and biosynthesis following aspirin challenge[18]. Thromboxane B$_2$ and 6 keto-PGF$_{1\alpha}$ can also be identified in nasal polyp tissue[9,14].

15-HETE[10] and LTB$_4$[11] may be important chemotactic mediators in polyp development. In aspirin sensitivity nasal polyp development probably reflects increased synthesis of lipoxygenase products[18]. Others feel aspirin sensitive patients are hyperresponsive to leukotrienes[15].

Preformed Granular Proteins and Enzymes

Several important lysosomal proteases are released by inflammatory cells. These include collagenase, elastase, the thiol proteases cathepsin B and L, as well as the neutral proteases tryptase and chymase. Fibroblasts cultured from nasal polyp tissue produce collagenase, and production is augmented by the addition of extracts of secretions from patients with clinical sinusitis[19]. Neutrophil elastase is present occasionally in nasal polyp tissue[20], but is more prominent in nasal secretions[21]. Cathepsin B is the predominant thiol protease in nasal polyp tissue[21].

Tryptase and chymase are found in mast cells and differentiate mucosal mast cells which have tryptase only (MC$_T$) from connective tissue mast cells which have both chymase and tryptase (MC$_{CT}$). A significantly higher content of chymase and tryptase is found in nasal polyp stromal mast cells than in epithelial mast cells of the same tissue[22,23].

While the specific actions of each enzyme in nasal tissue are uncertain, processes such as allergy or chronic infection which are associated with polyp formation may release enzymes which directly induce polyps or may consume or overwhelm protease inhibitors leading to chronic inflammation[21] and tissue destruction[24] resulting in polyp growth[25].

The nonenzymatic, preformed granular proteins of eosinophils, eosinophil cationic protein (ECP) and major basic protein (MBP), have been localized in nasal polyp tissue by immunoelectron microscopy[26]. Both stored (EG1) and secretory (EG2) types of ECP, have been found in greater amounts in nasal polyp tissue than in nasal mucosal tissue[27]. Nasal lavage from patients with nasal polyps contain more ECP than fluid from patients without polyps, but levels do not change with seasonal allergen exposure[28]. MBP has also been found in mast cells in nasal polyps suggesting that mast cells may sequester this mediator[29]. The amount of MBP present in tissue has been correlated with amount of epithelial damage[20], which confirms the in vitro effect of MBP on respiratory epithelium. Taken together this data suggests that the eosinophils and mast cells present in nasal polyp tissue are important in the development of the tissue changes seen in nasal polyps.

New Mediators

Interleukins

Interleukins (IL) are a family of mediators released by a number of inflammatory and noninflammatory cells. In nasal polyps IL-1 (α and β) are found primarily in monocytes and to a lesser extent in polymorphonuclear cells[30].

IL-1β levels in monocytes are related directly to the weight of nasal polyp tissue[31]. The finding that nasal polyp mast cells are IL-2 receptor positive suggests the involvement of IL-2 in nasal polyps. CD4+ lymphocytes noted near these mast cells may be the source of the IL-2[32].

Polyp tissue from patients with chronic sinusitis has a higher number of IL-3 mRNA positive cells than normal controls. These cells were always found in the subepithelial region. A correlation exists between activated (EG2+) eosinophils and cells expressing IL-3, but not IL-5, mRNA. A higher density of IL-5 positive cells are found in nasal polyps from skin test positive patients[33]. IL-4 has been localized in eosinophils in nasal polyps[34] and the chemokine IL-8 has also been found in polyp mucosa[35]. In vitro nasal epithelial cells, in some conditions, can release IL-6[36], while T lymphocyte clones from polyp tissue stimulated with PHA can generate IL-4[37].

The above evidence suggests several interleukins may participate in the development of nasal polyps. IL-1β from monocytes may activate lymphocytes, which in turn release IL-2. IL-3 from inflammatory or stromal cells may participate in the later stages of polyp development by attracting and activating eosinophils. Finally, IL-6 may modulate monocyte and macrophage behavior[36]. Convincing roles for IL-4 and IL-5 have not yet been identified, but their importance in IgE synthesis, and eosinophil migration and activation suggests an important role in allergic polyposis.

Growth Factors

Several growth factors appear to be involved in the pathogenesis of polyps. Transforming growth factor (TGF) α and β_1 are expressed by the majority of eosinophils in nasal polyp tissue[38]. TGFβ_1 can be found throughout nasal polyp tissue by immunohistochemical and mRNA staining[39] in both eosinophils and extracellular matrix[40]. Insulin-like growth factor-I (IGF-I) is present in high concentrations in all polyp tissue in epithelial cells, activated macrophages, vascular endothelial cells, and lymphocytes, but is absent from areas of necrosis and is low in normal mucosa[41].

Certain hematopoietic growth factors, or colony stimulating factors (CSF's) have been found to be important in proliferation and differentiation of granulocyte precursors. They are classified by the cells they stimulate (i.e. macrophages (M-CSF), granulocytes (G-CSF), and both granulocyte and macrophages (GM-CSF)[39]. They are released from macrophages and lymphocytes, as well as from epithelial cells, endothelial cells, eosinophils, and fibroblasts in nasal polyp tissue. These findings suggest that the factors direct in-situ hematopoiesis or maintain and activate infiltrating inflammatory leukocytes[42].

GM-CSF appears to be the primary growth factor in nasal polyps. A larger proportion of cells in nasal polyp subepithelium stain with antibody to this factor than do cells in normal nasal mucosa[43]. GM-CSF mRNA was detected in polyp and nasal tissue from allergic but not normal individuals[44]. The number of GM-CSF staining cells correlates strongly with the number of activated (EG2+) eosinophils[33]. Interestingly, 30% of eosinophils in nasal polyp tissue express GM-CSF, and GM-CSF has also been detected in supernatants of nasal polyp tissue by ELISA[44].

Cell lines derived from nasal polyp tissue have been used to investigate the importance to the CSF's. Fibroblast and epithelial cells cultured from polyp tissue produce significant levels of all three CSFs in their supernatants[39,45], although M-CSF may not be present in all epithelial cultures[36]. More CSF's, and specifically 2–3 times more GM-CSF, is produced in fibroblasts and epithelial cells from polyp tissue than from inferior turbinate tissue[45,43,36].

Conditioned media from nasal polyp derived cell lines has been used to determine the specific actions of these growth factors. Epithelial cells from nasal polyp tissue survive and proliferate better than normal tissue in vitro[46]. The conditioned media from nasal polyp cells induces differentiation of monocytic[36] and neutrophilic cells to a much greater degree than media from allergic and normal nasal tissue; an effect inhibited by antibody to GM-CSF[45]. This media also stimulates growth of basophil/mast cell and eosinophil colonies from peripheral blood progenitors[47], an effect increased by addition of T lymphocytes from atopic individuals[48]. Supernatants of epithelial cells and fibroblasts increase eosinophil survival and activation[39], and this effect is abrogated by antibody to GM-CSF or by dexamethasone[49].

Interferons

Interferons which have been primarily implicated in protection from viral infection may also be important in nasal polyps. T lymphocyte clones from nasal polyp tissue make significant amounts of interferon-τ when stimulated with PHA. The same result was obtained with mononuclear cells in bulk culture stimulated with PHA and IL-2. This finding, together with low IL-4 production in these T cell clones, suggests a predominant TH1 pattern of inflammation[37].

Other Mediators

Several other mediators have been identified in nasal polyps. Platelet activating factor (PAF), a lipid mediator, is present in all polyps, and is increased by addition of PAF precursors, calcium ionophore, or anti-IgE[50]. High molecular weight neutrophil chemotactic factor (HMW-NCF) is released into the supernatant of antigen stimulated nasal polyp tissue[51]. Tumor necrosis factor-α (TNF-α) is present in most nasal polyp tissue, and localized to eosinophils[52]. Nasal polyp eosinophils are also positive for macrophage inflammatory protein-1α (MIP-1α), an important chemokine and T-lymphocyte chemo-

attractant[53]. A role for each of these mediators can be postulated, but none has been unequivocally defined.

Adhesion Molecules

Adhesion molecules are membrane proteins which effect cell to cell interaction. They have been grouped into families: selectins, integrins, addressins, and the immunoglobulin supergene family. In nasal polyp endothelial tissue intracellular adhesion molecule (ICAM-1), E-selectin, P-selectin, and possibly vascular cell adhesion molecule (VCAM-1) are expressed. These adhesion molecules may play a role in the migration of inflammatory cells into nasal polyps, as antibody to P-selectin completely inhibits eosinophil adhesion to polyp epithelium but antibodies to several other adhesion molecules have no effect. Antibody to the adhesion molecule Mac-1 also partially inhibits eosinophil adhesion suggesting the involvement of this integrin[54]. Additionally, cell interactions can be modulated by upregulating the adhesion molecules on the surface of the cell or by altering the molecules affinity, as is seen with the effect of IL-1 on CD11b expression in eosinophils[55].

Neurotransmitters

Neurotransmitters, released from autonomic and sensory nerves, have potent effects on the immune system and upper respiratory glands. Norepinephrine, a biogenic amine, has been found in nasal polyp tissue, primarily around blood vessels at the polyp base[3]. Vasoactive Intestinal Peptide (VIP), neuropeptide Y (NPY)[56], and substance P[57] have been localized by immunohistochemistry in nasal polyp tissue. NPY is found predominantly around thick walled vessels, whereas VIP is found in close proximity to the submucosa[56]. These neuropeptides may contribute to nasal polyp development by mediating tissue edema, inflammation, and cystic degeneration of glands.

CONCLUSION

Nasal polyps can be seen in a variety of disease states including allergy, infection, aspirin sensitivity, and cystic fibrosis, strongly suggesting the presence of multiple pathways leading to a final common end point.

The mediators released from eosinophils and mast cells appear to be important in the development of all nasal polyps, regardless of the associated disease process. However, individual mediators appear to assume different roles in different clinical situations. Histamine and prostaglandin levels are lower in patients with aspirin sensitivity, while LTC$_4$ and LTD$_4$ amounts are elevated in polyps from these patients. Also the presence of preformed granular proteins and lysosomal enzymes does not change in different disease states but the selective release of these mediators may be important in the final stages of polyp development.

Interleukins, cytokines and growth factors can logically be thought to be involved in the orchestration and perpetuation of the events leading to polyp development. Lymphocytes, monocytes, neutrophils, epithelial cells, fibroblasts, mast cells and eosinophils use these signals to communicate with each other and to alter adhesion molecule expression. Taken together, mediators of sufficient biological potency and diversity are present in nasal polyps tissue to explain their genesis and perpetuation. It is now essential to tease apart the relative importance of the various mediators in each of the different clinical situations in which nasal polyps occur.

BIBLIOGRAPHY

1. M. Jordana, C. Vancheri, T. Ohtoshi, D. Harnish, J. Gauldie, J. Dolovich, J. Denburg. Hemopoietic Function of the Microenvironment in Chronic Airway Inflammation. Agents Actions Supplement, 28, 85–95, 1989.

2. C. Nathan, M. Sporn. Cytokines in Context. The Journal of Cell Biology, 113, 5, 981–986, 1991.

3. R.M. Bumsted, T. El-Ackad, J. Montgomery Smith, M.J. Brody. Histamine, Norepinephrine and Serotonin Content of Nasal Polyps. The Laryngoscope, 89, 832–843, 1979.

4. W.G. Hosemann, H.W. Baenkler, F. Gunther. ASA-induced Release of Histamine from Nasal Mucous Membranes in Analgesic Intolerance and Polyposis Nasi. Rhinology, 28, 231–238, 1990.

5. S. Ogino, Y. Abe, M. Irifune, T. Harada, T. Matsunaga, I. Imamura, H. Fukui. Histamine Metabolism in Nasal Polyps. Ann Otol Rhinol Laryngol. 102, 152–156, 1993.

6. M. Kaliner, S. Wasserman, K. Frank Austen. Immunologic Release of Chemical Mediators from Human Nasal Polyps. N Engl J Med, 289 (6), 277–281, 1973.

7. A.B. Drake-Lee, R. Bickerton, P. McLaughlan. Free Histamine in Nasal Polyp Fluid. Rhinology, 22, 133–138, 1984.

8. A.B. Drake-Lee, P. McLaughlan. Clinical Symptoms, Free Histamine and IgE in Patients with Nasal Polyposis. Int. Archs Allergy appl. Immun, 69, 268–271, 1982.

9. T.T.K. Jung, S.K. Juhn, D. Hwang, R. Stewart. Prostaglandins, Leukotrienes, and other Arachidonic Acid Metabolites in Nasal Polyps and Nasal Mucosa. Laryngoscope, 97, 184–189, 1987.

10. D.M. Smith, J.M. Gerrard, J.G. White. Comparison of Arachidonic Acid Metabolism in Nasal Polyps and Eosinophils. Int. Archs Allergy appl. Immun, 82, 83–88, 1987.

11. H. Salari, P. Borgeat, S. Steffenrud, J. Richard, P.M. Bedard, J. Hebert, G. Pelletier. Immunological and Non-immunological Release of Leukotrienes and Histamine from Human Nasal Polyps. Clin. exp. Immunol, 63, 711–717, 1986.

12. R.J. Shaw, A. Drake-Lee, P. Fitzharris, O. Cromwell, A.B. Kay. Leukotrienes in Nasal Hypersensitivity and Polyposis. Thorax, 40, 215–216, 1985.

13. S. Ogino, M. Irifune, T. Harada, H. Kikumori, T. Matsunaga. Arachidonic Acid Metabolites in Human Nasal Polyps. Acta Otolaryngol (Stockh), Suppl. 501, 85–87, 1993.

14. T. Yamashita, H. Tsuji, N. Maeda, K. Tomoda, T. Kumazawa. Etiology of Nasal Polyps Associated with Aspirin-sensitive Asthma. Rhinology, Suppl. 8, 15–24, 1989.

15. M.L. Kowalski, M. Sliwinska-Kowalska, Y. Igarashi, M.V. White, B. Wojciechowska, P. Brayton, H. Kaulbach, J. Rozniecki, M.A. Kaliner. Nasal Secretions in Response to Acetylsalicylic Acid. J Allergy Clin Immunol, 91, 580–598, 1993.

16. J.A. Lindgren, C. Edentus, M. Kumlin, B. Dahlen, A. Anggard. Conversion of Leukotriene A_4 to Lipoxins by Human Nasal Polyps and Bronchial Tissue. Advances in Prostaglandin, Thromboxane, and Leukotriene Research, 21, 89–92, 1990.

17. D.M. Smith, J.M. Gerrard, S.K. Juhn, J.G. White. Arachidonic Acid Metabolism in Nasal Polyps and Allergic Inflammation. Minnesota Medicine, 64(10), 605–610, 1981.

18. S. Nigam, G. Kunkel, D. Herold, F.E. Baumer, L. Jusuf. Nasal Polyps and their Content of Arachidonic Acid Metabolites. NER Allergy Proc. 7(2), 109–112, 1986.

19. T. Matsuzaki. A Study on Collagenase Production of Nasal Polyp-derived Fibroblasts Stimulated by Nasal Secretions of Chronic Sinusitis. Journal of Oto-Rhino-laryngological Society of Japan, 92(4), 617–628, 1989.

20. T. Fujisawa, G.M. Kephart, B.H. Gray, G.J. Gleich. The Neutrophil and Chronic Allergic Inflammation: Immunochemical Localization of Neutrophil Elastase. Am Rev Respir Dis, 141, 689–697, 1990.

21. Y. Hamaguchi, M. Taya, H. Suzumura, Y. Sakakura. Lysosomal Proteases and Protease Inhibitors in Nasal Allergy and Non-atopic Sinusitis. Am J Otolaryngol, 11, 37–43, 1990.

22. S. Finotto, J. Dolovich, J.A. Denburg, M. Jordana, J.S. Marshall. Functional Heterogeneity of Mast Cells Isolated from Different Microenvironments within Nasal Polyp Tissue. Clin Exp Immunol, 95, 343–350, 1994.

23. S. Kawabori, J.A. Denburg, L.B. Schwartz, A.A. Irani, D. Wong, G. Jordana, S. Evans, J. Dolovich. Histochemical and Immunohistochemical Characteristics of Mast Cells in Nasal Polyps. Am. J. Respir. Cell Mol. Biol., 6, 37–43, 1992.

24. Y. Hamaguchi, M. Ohi, Y. Sakakura, Y. Miyoshi. Significance of Lysosomal Protease; Cathepsins B and H in Maxillary Mucosa and Nasal Polyp with Non-atopic Chronic Inflammation. Rhinology, 24, 187–194, 1986.

25. T. Kosugi, T. Morimitsu, O. Matsuo, H. Mihara. A Protease-Antiprotease System in Antrochoanal Polyp. Arch. Otorhinolaryngol, 225, 97–102, 1979.

26. M. Peters, M. Rodriguez, G.J. Gleich. Localization of Human Eosinophil Granule Major Basic Protein, Eosinophil Cationic Protein, and Eosinophil-derived Neurotoxin by Immunoelectron Microscopy. Laboratory Investigation, 54(6), 656, 1986.

27. A.E. Stoop, H.A.M.D. van der Heijden, J. Biewenga, S. van der Baan. Eosinophils in Nasal Polyps and Nasal Mucosa: An Immunohistochemical Study. J Allergy Clin Immunol, 91, 616–622, 1993.

28. P.K. Keith, M. Conway, S. Evans, D.A. Wong, G. Jordana, D. Pengelly, J. Dolovich. Nasal Polyps: Effects of Seasonal Allergen Exposure. J Allergy Clin Immunol, 93, 567–574, 1994.

29. J.H. Butterfield, D. Weiler, E.A. Peterson, G.J. Gleich, K.M. Leiferman. Sequestration of Eosinophil Major Basic Protein in Human Mast Cells. Laboratory Investigation, 62(1), 77, 1990.

30. Y. Liu, Y. Hamaguchi, M. Taya, Y. Sakakura. Quantification of Interleukin-1 in Nasal Polyps from Patients with Chronic Sinusitis. Eur Arch Otorhinolaryngol, 250, 123–125, 1993.

31. Y. Hamaguchi, H. Suzumura, S. Arima, Y. Sakakura. Quantitation and Immunocytological Identification of Interleukin-1 in Nasal Polyps from Patients with Chronic Sinusitis. Int Arch Allergy Immunol, 104, 155–159, 1994.

32. L.M. Larocca, N. Maggiano, A. Capelli, P. Bevilacqua, P. Ruscito, M. Maurizi, P. Bellioni. Immunopathology of Nasal Polyps: An Immunohistochemical Approach. Annals of Allergy, 63, 508–512, 1989.

33. D.L. Hamilos, D.Y.M. Leung, R. Wood, A. Meyers, J.K. Stephens, J. Barkans, Q. Meng, L. Cunningham, D.K. Bean, A.B. Kay, Q. Hamid. Chronic Hyperplastic Sinusitis: Association of Tissue Eosinophilia with mRNA Expression of Granulocyte-Macrophage Colony-Stimulating Factor and Interleukin-3. J Allergy Clin Immunol, 92, 39–48, 1993.

34. M. Nonaka, R. Nonaka, K. Woolley, E. Adelroth, K. Miura, P. O'Byrne, J. Dolovich, M. Jordana. Localization of Interleukin-4 in Eosinophils in Nasal Polyps and Asthmatic Bronchial Mucosa. Journal of Allergy and Clin Immunology, 95(1), 220, 1995.

35. T. Norlander, K.M. Westrin, P. Stierna. Inflammatory Response of the Sinus and Nasal Mucosa During Sinusitis: Implications for Research and Therapy. Acta Otolaryngol (Stockh), Supp. 515, 38–44, 1994.

36. T. Ohtoshi, C. Vancheri, G. Cox, J. Gauldie, J. Dolovich, J.A. Denburg, M. Jordana. Monocyte-Macrophage Differentiation Induced by Human Upper Airway Epithelial Cells. Am. J. Respir. Cell Mol. Biol., 4, 255–263, 1991.

37. C.H. Miller, D.R. Pudiak, F. Hatem, R.J. Looney. Accumulation of Interferon Gamma-producing TH1 Helper T Cells in Nasal Polyps. Otolaryngol Head Neck Surg, 111, 51–58, 1994.

38. A. Elovic, D.T.W. Wong, P.F. Weller, K. Matossian, S.J. Galli. Expression of Transforming Growth Factor—α and β_1 mRNA and Product by Eosinophils in Nasal Polyps. J Allergy Clin Immunol, 93, 864–869, 1994.

39. J. Gauldie, G. Cox, M. Jordana, I. Ohno, H. Kirpalani. Growth and Colony-stimulating Factors Mediate Eosinophil Fibroblast Interactions in Chronic Airway Inflammation. Annals New York Academy of Sciences, 725, 83–90, 1994.

40. I. Ohno, R.G. Lea, K.C. Flanders, D.A. Clark, D. Banwatt, J. Dolovich, J. Denburg, C.B. Harley, J. Gauldie, M. Jordana. Eosinophils in Chronically Inflamed Human Upper Airway Tissues Express Transforming Growth Factor β_1 Gene (TGFβ_1). J. Clin. Invest., 89, 1662–1668, 1992.

41. B. Petruson, H.A. Hansson, K. Petruson. Insulin-like Growth Factor I Is a Possible Pathogenic Mechanism in Nasal Polyps. Acta Otolaryngol (Stockh), 106, 156–160, 1988.

42. J.A. Denburg, J. Gauldie, J. Dolovich, T. Ohtoshi, G. Cox, M. Jordana. Structural Cell-derived Cytokines in Allergic Inflammation. Int Arch Allergy Appl Immunol, 94, 127–132, 1991.

43. I. Ohno, G. Cox, R. Lea, J. Dolovich, D. Clark, J. Gauldie, M. Jordana. Synthesis and Localisation of GM-CSF in Human Airway Tissues. Am Rev Resp Dis, 143(supp), A201, 1991.

44. I. Ohno, R. Lea, S. Finotto, J. Marshall, J. Denburg, J. Dolovich, J. Gauldie, M. Jordana. Granulocyte/Macrophage Colony-stimulating Factor (GM-CSF) Gene Expression by Eosinophils in Nasal Polyposis. Am. J. Respir. Cell Mol. Biol. 5, 505–510, 1991.

45. C. Vancheri, T. Ohtoshi, G. Cox, A. Xaubet, J.S. Abrams, J. Gauldie, J. Dolovich, J. Denburg, M. Jordana. Neutrophilic Differentiation Induced by Human Upper Airway Fibroblast-derived Granulocyte/Macrophage Colony-stimulating Factor (GM-CSF). Am. J. Respir. Cell, Mol. Biol., 4, 11–17, 1991.

46. H. Otsuka, J. Dolovich, M. Richardson, J. Bienenstock, J.A. Denburg. Metachromatic Cell Progenitors and Specific Growth and Differentiation Factors in Human Nasal Mucosa and Polyps. Am Rev Resp Dis, 136, 710–717, 1987.

47. J.A. Denburg, H. Otsuka, M. Ohnisi, J. Ruhno, J. Bienenstock, J. Dolovich. Contribution of Basophil/Mast Cell and Eosinophil Growth and Differentiation to the Allergic Tissue Inflammatory Response. Int. Archs Allergy appl. Immun., 82, 321–326, 1987.

48. M. Ohnishi, J. Ruhno, J. Bienenstock, R. Milner, J. Dolovich, J.A. Denburg. Human Nasal Polyp Epithelial Basophil/Mast Cell and Eosinophil Colony-stimulating Activity: The Effect is T-Cell-dependent. Am Rev Respir Dis, 138, 560–564, 1988.

49. A. Xaubet, J. Mullol, E. Lopez, J. Roca-Ferrer, M. Rozman, T. Carrion, J.M. Fabra, C. Picado. Comparison of the Role of Nasal Polyp and Normal Nasal Mucosa Epithelial Cells on in vitro Eosinophil Survival. Mediation by GM-CSF and Inhibition by Dexamethasone. Clinical and Experimental Allergy, 24, 307–317, 1994.

50. M. Furukawa, T. Yamashita, T. Kumazawa, K. Satouchi, K. Saito. Evidence of Platelet-Activating Factor in Nasal Polyps. ORL, 54, 29–32, 1992.

51. T. Nagakura, T. Onda, K. Akimoto, H. Nagakura, K. Tanaka, K. Ohno, T. Sudo, Y. Iikura. Release of High Molecular Weight-Neutrophil Chemotactic Activity from Human Tissues, Cells and Secretion. Int Arch Allergy Appl Immunol, 88, 187–190, 1989.

52. S. Finotto, I. Ohno, J.S. Marshall, J. Gauldie, J.A. Denburg, J. Dolovich, D.A. Clark, M. Jordana. TNF-α Production by Eosinophils in Upper Airways Inflammation (Nasal Polyposis). Journal of Immunology, 153, 2278–2284, 1994.

53. J.J. Costa, K. Matossian, M.B. Resnick, W.J. Beil, D.T.W. Wong, J.R. Gordon, A.M. Dvorak, P.F. Weller, S.J. Galli. Human Eosinophils Can Express the Cytokines Tumor Necrosis Factor-$\propto$ and Macrophage Inflammatory protein-1$\propto$. J. Clin. Invest., 91, 2673–2684, 1993.

54. F.A. Symon, G.M. Walsh, S.R. Watson, A.J. Wardlaw. Eosinophil Adhesion to Nasal Polyp Endothelium is P-Selectin-dependent. J. Exp. Med., 180, 371–376, 1994.

55. C. Walker, S. Rihs, R.K. Braun, S. Betz, P.L.B. Bruijnzeel. Increased Expression of CD11b and Functional Changes in Eosinophils after Migration across Endothelial Cell Monolayers. The Journal of Immunology, 150, 4061–4071, 1993.

56. S.Y. Fang, C.L. Shen, M. Ohyama. Presence of Neuropeptides in Human Nasal Polyps. Acta Otolaryngol (Stockh), 114, 324–328, 1994.

57. F. Beatrice, P. Aluffi, F. Bottomicca, L. Perlasco, A. Sartoris. Nasal Polyps and Substance P: A Preliminary Report. Acta Otorhinolaryngologica Italica, 41, 35–39, 1994.

Chapter VII

Eosinophils in Nasal Polyps

Manel Jordana, M.D., Ph.D., and Jerry Dolovich, M.D.

ABSTRACT

Nasal polyposis represents a paradigm of chronic airways inflammation. Eosinophils comprise the most prevalent inflammatory cell type in nasal polyp tissues except in those occurring in patients with Cystic Fibrosis and Kartagener Syndrome. These cells have a demonstrated ability to release mediators such as eosinophil peroxidase, eosinophil derived neurotoxin, eosinophil cationic protein and others capable of causing cellular injury and tissue damage. In addition, it has become clear over the last few years that eosinophils and, specifically, eosinophils in nasal polyp tissues, can also synthesize and release a number of powerful regulatory molecules referred to as cytokines. Interestingly, some of these molecules such as GM-CSF, TNFα and IL-4 can, directly or indirectly, contribute to the further recruitment and activation of eosinophils. Others, such as TGFα and TGFβ can participate in the tissue structural abnormalities characteristic of nasal polyposis. This evidence establishes novel roles for eosinophils in the regulation of upper airways inflammation and, we suggest, provides the molecular basis for self-perpetuating eosinophilia.

INTRODUCTION

Eosinophils are associated and, in fact, represent the most abundant inflammatory cell type in a number of diseases of the airways including *asthma, allergic rhinitis and nasal polyposis*. The contribution of these cells to the pathogenesis of these diseases has been long recognized primarily based upon their ability to release mediators such as EPO [eosinophil peroxidase], MBP [major basic protein], ECP [eosinophil cationic protein], EDN [eosinophil derived neurotoxin] and other substances with a well established capacity to cause cellular injury[1-3]. However, it has become apparent particu-

larly over the last five years that eosinophils possess a number of additional abilities. Probably one of the most important among them is the synthesis of powerful regulatory molecules, *cytokines*. These hormone-like messengers are relatively small molecules the source of which was originally thought to be restricted to the traditional immune-inflammatory cells such as lymphocytes and macrophages. This evidence undoubtedly suggests novel roles for eosinophils in the regulation of mucosal inflammation.

EOSINOPHILIC INFLAMMATION: GENERAL CONCEPTS

During the last decade there has been considerable progress in our understanding of the cellular and molecular regulation of airways inflammation. Much of this progress has focused on the events that *initiate* this reaction. At the cellular level, there is general agreement that both *lymphocytes and mast cells* play central roles in the initiation of airways inflammatory responses where eosinophils are the prevalent infiltrating leukocytes. There is also recognition that the accumulation of eosinophils into a tissue site involves a number of events including differentiation of bone marrow progenitors into functionally mature cells, adhesion to, and migration through the endothelium and, within the tissue, chemotaxis and activation[4]. In addition to these, modulation of survival is increasingly perceived as an important event in tissue eosinophilia. Eosinophils are relatively short-lived cells with an average half life in circulation of approximately 48h. Eosinophil death is a programmed event referred to as *apoptosis* which, in contrast to *necrosis,* describe "death from within" and requires activation of endogenous biochemical processes. Thus, it has been postulated that changes in the tissue microenvironment conducive to inhibition of apoptosis, i.e. promotion of survival, may contribute to the *sustained accumulation* of eosinophils in the tissue.

At the molecular level, the development of inflammation involves dozens, perhaps hundreds, of mediators. However, cytokines comprise in all likelihood a family of such pro-inflammatory mediators with central regulatory functions. Yet, given the polyfunctionality and the redundancy observed for many cytokines, it is highly unlikely in our view that a single cytokine will be found to play a critical [irreplaceable] role in tissue eosinophilia. Rather, we suggest that this process is controlled by a *network of cytokines* regulating specific events with probably distinct significances in different compartments [bone marrow, peripheral blood and tissue]. Granulocyte-macrophage colony-stimulating factor [GM-CSF], interleukin-3 [IL-3] and interleukin-5 [IL-5] are three cytokines with substantive overlapping activities on eosinophils. They all probably play significant roles in the differentiation of progenitors to mature eosinophils as well as in the promotion of survival and activation of mature eosinophils. Tumor necrosis factor α [TNFα] may be involved in tissue eosinophilia via its ability to stimulate tissue structural cells [fibroblasts, epithelial and endothelial cells] to synthesize cytokines including GM-CSF, as well as through its capacity to upregulate VCAM-1 [vascular cell adhesion molecule 1] on endothelial cells, a surface molecule important for the adhesion of eosinophils to the endothelium. In this later regard, interleukin 4 [IL-4] has been shown to have similar effects which are synergistic with TNFα. Another cytokine probably involved in eosinophil recruitment is RANTES [*r*egulated upon *a*ctivation, *n*ormal *T* cell expressed and *s*ecreted], a member of an increasing family called chemokines. This molecule, initially identified in T cells and, subsequently, on fibroblasts, epithelial and endothelial cells[5–8], has been shown to be chemotactic for memory T lymphocytes and monocytes[9]. In addition, this cytokine has strong eosinophil chemotactic and activating effects[10–11]. It needs to be recognized that the suggested contribution of these cytokines to human disease is based on either *in vitro* experimentation or *in vivo* descriptive studies. However, recent information in mouse models of airways eosinophilic inflammation as well as in transgenic mouse models strongly suggests significant functions for at least GM-CSF, IL-4, IL-5 and TNFα in the initiating events leading to tissue eosinophilia[12–15].

CHRONIC INFLAMMATION: THE NASAL POLYP PARADIGM

Asthma and nasal polyposis are both chronic inflammatory diseases and, unfortunately, much less is known about the mechanisms that *perpetuate,* as opposed to initiate, the inflammatory response. Indeed, paraphrasing Charles E. Reed, it is an enigma the apparent self-perpetuating mechanism operating in eosinophilic inflammation that once established tends to continue indefinitely[16]. Part of the difficulty to gain insight into this process is that, regarding human studies, tissues especially from asthmatics can only be obtained, in the vast majority of instances, from patients with mild disease. With respect to animal studies, the type of inflammation that can be generated in experimental models of airways inflammation is of a self-limiting nature. In this context, we view nasal polyps not only as an opportunity to obtain relatively abundant amounts of human inflamed tissue but also as a paradigm of chronic and severe eosinophilic airways inflammation.

We suggest that nasal polyps, with the exception of those occurring in patients with Cystic Fibrosis and Kartagener Syndrome where neutrophils are the prevalent infiltrating granulocytes[17], represent a model of *chronic eosinophilic inflammation.* Indeed, even though there is substantial heterogeneity in the histological presentation of nasal polyps[18,19], eosinophils are consistently present in significant numbers. In two different studies where we have quantified the eosinophil content in series of 10 and 12 consecutive nasal polyp tissues, we established that approximately 20% of *all cells* in the tissue were eosinophils[20,21]. In a previous study, we had determined that approximately three quarters of all eosinophils in the tissue stained positive for EG2[22], thus suggesting activation. Regarding other cell types, mast cells represent approximately 2% of all cells in nasal polyp tissues which is about twice the density observed in the normal nasal mucosa[18]. In contrast to these findings, we did not find statistically significant differences in the density of lymphocytes between nasal polyp and normal nasal mucosa tissues, and only a very small proportion of lymphocytes expressed CD25 [interleukin 2 receptor] used in this study as an indication of cell activation[22].

Peripheral blood eosinophilia is observed, with the exceptions noted above, in most patients with nasal polyposis. Moreover, the extent of this eosinophilia correlates with the likelihood of polyp recurrence[23]. On the other hand, peripheral blood eosinophilia does not assure the development of nasal polyps, or any other inflammatory disease of the airways. Hence, we hypothesize that disease expression requires the presence of two critical signals. A first signal, of a systemic nature either originating or having an important impact in the bone marrow, which determines *peripheral blood eosinophilia.* However, the establishment of *tissue eosinophilia* requires a second signal which likely originates at the tissue site. Admittedly, each of these signals may be a single distinct entity or, more likely, a set of molecules. Recent data indicating that tissue eosinophils have themselves the ability to synthesize a number of cytokines which directly or indirectly promote eosinophil survival and activation suggest that autocrine/paracrine mechanisms involving eosinophils may be an important component underlying the perpetuation of tissue eosinophilia.

SYNTHESIS OF REGULATORY MOLECULES BY EOSINOPHILS

GM-CSF is a heavily glycosylated protein with a molecular weight of 15-30 kDa[24]. GM-CSF acts in a species-specific manner and interacts with a cell membrane receptor of 45 kDa[25]. This cytokine was initially identified from lymphocytes although it is now clear that a number of additional cell types such as macrophages and structural cells [fibroblasts, endothelial and endothelial cells] are able to produce, the latter upon stimulation by IL-1 and TNFα particularly, GM-CSF[26–28]. GM-CSF was named from its ability to induce stem cell differentiation to granulocytes and macrophage/monocytes. However, it has also become apparent that this cytokine modulates numerous biologic activities on mature hemopoietic cells including increased survival and activation of lymphocytes and monocyte/macrophages[29–31]. Clearly, eosinophils are a target for GM-CSF upregulating activities such as survival, leukotriene production and parasite killing in vitro[32,28]. Of more interest is the demonstration that peripheral blood eosinophils are capable of producing GM-CSF protein under various conditions of stimulation in vitro[33,34]. In addition, we have shown that eosinophils in nasal polyp tissues express mRNA for GM-CSF[35]. Subsequently, we examined highly enriched populations of eosinophils directly isolated from nasal polyp tissues and detected significant levels of GM-CSF in the supernatant of these cells cultured without any stimulation. Moreover, the spontaneous survival of these cells ex vivo was, compared to that of peripheral blood eosinophils, markedly enhanced[20–21].

IL-3 and IL-5 have also been shown to enhance survival and induce activation of eosinophils[36,37], and it is clear that under appropriate conditions of stimulation, peripheral blood eosinophils produce these cytokines in vitro[33,38]. However, whether these cytokines are also involved in regulatory loops in the tissue remains to be elucidated. To our knowledge, there are no data examining expression of mRNA and immunoreactivity for these cytokines in nasal polyp tissues, although such evidence is available in the bronchial tissue of patients with asthma[39–40].

TNFα is a multifunctional cytokine with a broad array of pro-inflammatory effects[41]. TNFα was initially identified by its cytotoxic and cytostatic activities in vitro against tumor but not normal cell lines[42]. It is now known that TNFα stimulates most structural cell types to release other cytokines including GM-CSF[27] thus contributing to the amplification of the inflammatory response in general

and, indirectly enhancing eosinophil survival in particular. In addition, TNFα has also been shown to rapidly increase transcription of the VCAM-1 gene as well as protein expression on endothelial cells, hence promoting selective lymphocyte and eosinophil adhesion to the endothelium[43,44]. On eosinophils, TNFα stimulates the production of oxygen metabolites thus providing an additional mechanism of toxic cell injury[45]. Human peripheral blood eosinophils release TNFα under appropriate conditions of stimulation in vitro[34]. Moreover, we and others have demonstrated by means of in situ hybridization and immunohistochemistry, TNFα expression in nasal polyp tissues[46,47]. We showed that most cells expressing TNFα mRNA were eosinophils. Different cells types, especially mononuclear cells, expressed immunoreactive TNFα; a proportion of cells positively stained were eosinophils, and some could easily be detected in the epithelium. Therefore, TFNα could be involved in the pathogenesis of nasal polyposis through a number of direct and indirect mechanisms including promotion of eosinophil recruitment, enhancement of eosinophil survival and induction of eosinophil toxicity.

IL-4 is a 20 kDa glycoprotein which is a multifunctional cytokine considered to play an important role in allergic disease. In this regard, it has been shown that isotype switching of B cells to IgE synthesis is under the control of IL-4[48]. Also, transgenic mice overexpressing IL-4 develop high levels of circulating IgE as well as severe conjunctivitis characterized by mononuclear, mast cell and eosinophilic infiltration[49]. In addition, IL-4 has also been shown capable of upregulating VCAM-1 on endothelial cells[50]. It is of interest to note that this effect is, in contrast to that induced by TNFα, relatively modest and of relatively slow appearance. However, the combination of both cytokines leads to a prolonged and synergistic upregulation of VCAM-1[44]. While T-lymphocytes of the T_{H2} subset have been considered the primary source of IL-4[51], there is now evidence that human mast cells and basophils are also capable of producing this cytokine in vitro[52,53]. Furthermore, Bradding et al. have recently shown that the mast cell may be a primary source of immunoreactive IL-4 in allergic rhinitis as well as in bronchial tissues from patients with mild asthma[54,55]. We have recently performed a quantitative and comparative immunohistochemical study examining IL-4 expression in bronchial tissues from patients with very mild asthma and nasal polyposis tissues with the following key findings[56]. Firstly, the density of eosinophils in nasal polyp tissues was about 17 times greater than in asthmatic tissues, thus verifying the severe nature of the inflammatory response in the former. Secondly, the density of cells exhibiting IL-4 immunoreactivity was about three times greater in nasal polyp tissues compared to asthmatic tissues. Thirdly, using a double labelling technique with FITC we determined that the majority of cells expressing IL-4 immunoreactivity in the asthmatic tissues were not eosinophils, in agreement with the data by Bradding et al. In contrast, approximately 90% of the cells expressing IL-4 immunoreactivity in nasal polyp tissues were eosinophils. In this study, we also document IL-4 mRNA expression by Northern blot analysis in peripheral blood eosinophils as well as the ability of these cells to release IL-4 protein particularly upon stimulation with IgA immunecomplexes. The precise role of IL-4 in the pathogenesis of nasal polyposis in particular and of chronic inflammation in general remains to be determined, but this role may be completely independent of IgE regulation.

CD40 is a 45-50 kDa transmembrane glycoprotein originally identified in B cells, some B cells malignancies and carcinoma cell lines. More recently, CD40 expression has also been recognized in other cell types including follicular dendritic cells, thymic epithelial cells, monocytes and endothelial cells[57,58]. CD40 is a member of the nerve growth factor/TNF receptor superfamily. CD40 signalling can be initiated by crosslinking CD40 with anti-CD40 monoclonal antibodies or by direct interaction with CD40 ligand [CD40L], also referred to as gp39, which is expressed by CD4+ T cells[59] and, as recently shown, by human mast cells and basophils[60]. It is clear that this receptor/ligand interaction is, in the presence of IL-4 as a coactivation signal, of key importance in the switching of B cells to an IgE phenotype. However, it is also increasingly apparent that this receptor/ligand interaction may be involved in a number of potentially important activities. For example, receptor crosslinking in CD40 expressing monocytes or thymic epithelial cells results in the release of a number of pro-inflammatory cytokines including GM-CSF[61,62]. On endothelial cells, soluble gp39 induces the expression of E-selection as well as ICAM-1[58], thus participating in the recruitment of leukocytes into the tissue. We have recently demonstrated that peripheral blood eosinophils from allergic subjects express the CD40 mRNA by Northern blot analysis as well as CD40 immunoreactivity. Such expression is functional as crosslinking of CD40 leads to markedly increased eosinophil survival which is fully inhibited by incubating the eosinophils with an anti-GM-CSF antibody. Furthermore, CD40 mRNA is strongly expressed in nasal polyp tissues but not in the normal mucosa. Finally, we have observed by immunohistochemistry that a substantial proportion of cells expressing CD40 immunoreactivity in the tissue are eosinophils[63]. These findings suggest previously unrecognized interactions between eosinophils and cells expressing CD40L [gp39] such as T-lymphocytes and mast cells.

Transforming growth factor β [TGFβ] refers to a family of cytokines identified for their ability to induce transfor-

mation of cells to anchorage-independent growth. There are five known subtypes, but only three are known to be present in mammalian tissue and, of these, TGFβ$_1$ is the most prominent. This molecule is a protein of 25 kDa made up of two identical chains linked by disulfide bonds[64]. TGFβ is normally secreted as an inactive precursor that requires either acid treatment or enzymatic action for activation although in some instances such as with monocytes and neutrophils, it may be released in active form[65]. We and others have demonstrated strong mRNA TGFβ expression in nasal polyposis tissues and, by means of in situ hybridization and immunohistochemistry, expression of message and protein by eosinophils in such tissues[66,67]. Of the many effects demonstrated for TGFβ in primarily in vitro systems[64,68,69], there are at least three that may potentially play a role in nasal polyposis. First, this cytokine can directly affect gene expression of extracellular matrix molecules in fibroblasts, inducing collagen synthesis and collagenase inhibition, thus leading to increased collagen deposition. Second, TGFβ can promote chemotaxis and stimulate proliferation of fibroblasts either directly or indirectly through the induction of other growth factor such as PDGF [platelet-derived growth factor]. Third, TGFβ is a well known immunosuppressor capable of inhibiting T cell proliferation, generation of cytotoxicity, suppression of natural and lymphokine-activated killing by large granular lymphocytes and T lymphocyte adhesion to endothelium[64,70,71]. It is tempting to suggest that the relative lack of lymphocyte activity that we have observed in nasal polyp tissues may in fact be the result of active suppression mediated by TGFβ.

It has been recently shown that TGFβ inhibits the survival enhancing effects of the hemopoietins GM-CSF, IL-3 and IL-5 on eosinophils in vitro, thus inducing apoptosis[72]. That eosinophils synthesize a cytokine which induces their own death is intriguing. As suggested by Alam et al.[72], TGFβ may have a homeostatic function to prevent an excessive expansion of eosinophils. However, the finding that eosinophils make TGFβ in nasal polyp tissues, where they survive rather than die, suggests a dysfunction of this regulatory mechanism. Whether this is related to changes in the TGFβ receptor precluding an appropriate response to this cytokine or, simply, because the hemopoietin content in the tissue microenvironment overrides the apoptotic effect of TGFβ is unknown at present.

Transforming growth factor α [TGFα] is a peptide initially identified in malignant epithelial tumors, and it has been suggested that this cytokine may contribute to the transformed phenotype through autocrine mechanisms[73]. More recently, TGFα has also been shown to be expressed in certain normal tissues and cell types[74] suggesting a role in repair and remodeling processes. Wong et al. demonstrated mRNA expression and immunoreactivity in peripheral blood eosinophils from a patient with hypereosinophilic syndrome[75]. These researchers subsequently demonstrated similar findings in eosinophils in nasal polyp tissues[76]. The proportion of eosinophils expressing TGFα in these tissues was substantial. Indeed, 40–80% of the eosinophils expressed TGFα mRNA, and 20–60% expressed immunoreactive TGFα. As suggested by Elovic et al.[76], TGFα might reasonably be involved in the expansion of the polyp stroma through its angiogenic effects, and it might also contribute to the epithelial hyperplasia and squamous metaplasia often observed in nasal polyposis.

In this section, we have highlighted those molecules with powerful regulatory activities for which there is evidence of expression, both at the mRNA and protein levels, in nasal polyp tissues. However, peripheral blood eosinophils can also produce other cytokines such as IL-1, IL-6 and IL-8[77–79]. To our knowledge, whether eosinophils in nasal polyp tissues express these cytokines is not known. Similarly, the role of these cytokines in the pathogenesis of eosinophilic airways inflammation remains to be elucidated. Nevertheless, these findings further strengthen the view of eosinophils as cells with considerable effector capabilities.

DISCUSSION

By design, inflammation is a physiological response, essential for survival. But this reaction must be self-limited to remain within the homeostatic range, for granulocytes are equipped to destroy, not cells or tissues, but foreign biological agents such as parasites and bacteria. Consequently, a failure to terminate this response in a timely fashion will result in chronic inflammation, tissue damage and ensuing alterations in organ function. It is likely that apoptosis is a significant built-in terminating mechanism as, indeed, both eosinophils and neutrophils are scheduled to die shortly after exiting the bone marrow.

Against this background, the nasal polyp tissue presents itself as a highly *anti-apoptotic microenvironment*. Taking GM-CSF as a benchmark, this cytokine is highly expressed in nasal polyps tissues, being produced by a variety of cell types. TNFα might contribute to the supply of GM-CSF through its effects on structural cells GM-CSF synthesis. Moreover, a great proportion of eosinophils which comprise a large cell compartment [1 of every 5 cells] in these tissues express both GM-CSF and TNFα. Plausibly, the continuing exposure to these cytokines at such close range may significantly contribute to the prolonged survival of eosinophils in an activated state. Also, the potential availability of IL-5 and, perhaps, IL-3 in the nasal polyp tissue, as it has been shown in asthmatic tissue, would further enrich this anti-apoptotic microenvironment. On these grounds only, it is hard not to imagine the nasal polyp microenvironment as a paradise for eosinophil welfare. The release of TNFα and IL-4, on the other hand, might be an internal [independent of antigen exposure] mechanism of eosinophil recruitment through their effects on integrin upregulation on endothelial cells. And the presence of TGFβ in the tissue, part of it produced by eosinophils, might further skew the nature of inflammation by suppressing certain elements, i.e. lymphocytes, with likely critical roles in the initial development of the inflammatory process. While we do *not* think that the type of inflammation ongoing in nasal polyposis is fundamentally different than that in asthma or allergic rhinitis, we also think that the nasal polyp tissue uniquely portrays a scenario where *eosinophilia leads to further eosinophilia*.

We can only speculate with respect to the mechanisms mediating this apparently ever-expanding, and purposeless, tissue eosinophilia. Two studies reported over 20 years ago acquire now a new perspective. Donovan et al. documented that IgG, IgA and IgM were all present in nasal polyp fluid in considerable quantities, and that they were likely produced locally[80], and Brandtzaeg et al. carried out immunofluorescence studies demonstrating IgA plasma cells primarily in proximity to glandular areas and secretory ducts and IgG producing cells particularly in the stroma between the glands and the surface area[81]. The renewed interest on these findings stems from the recent evidence that eosinophils express the Fc receptors for IgG, IgA and IgE[82–84] and that these immunoglobulins, including secretory IgA, are all capable of triggering eosinophil degranulation[85–87]. Furthermore, these immunoglobulins, particularly secretory IgA, stimulate eosinophil synthesis of IL-5[38] and IL-4[56] as well as upregulation of the CD40 surface molecule, crosslinking of which will lead to eosinophil GM-CSF synthesis and release[63]. This may provide the framework for ongoing eosinophil activation as well as production of cytokines which, directly or indirectly, support further eosinophilia.

Regardless of the mechanisms involved in this process of self-perpetuating tissue eosinophilia, a practical implication of the findings supporting its existence may be to encourage early and aggressive anti-inflammatory treatment of airways eosinophilic inflammation, before autocrine/paracrine loops of stimulation leading to chronic disease and potentially irreversible structural alterations are established.

ACKNOWLEDGEMENTS

Work from our laboratory cited in this manuscript has been carried out with grants from the Medical Research Council [Canada] to M. J. and J. D. and from Astra

Canada. M. J. is a Career Scientist of the Ontario Ministry of Health. We are grateful to Dr. Xing Zhou MD, PhD for his critical review of the manuscript. The secretarial assistance of Mary Kiriakopoulos is gratefully appreciated.

REFERENCES

1. Gleich G J, and Adolphson C R. The eosinophil leukocyte: structure and function. Adv Immunol 1986; 39:177.

2. Weller P F. Eosinophils: structure and function. Current Opinion in Immunology 1994; 6:85.

3. Venge P, Dahl R, Fredens K, and Peterson C G B. Epithelial injury by human eosinophils. Am Rev Respir Dis 1988; 138:S54.

4. Resnick M B, and Weller P F. Mechanisms of eosinophil recruitment. Am J Resp Cell Mol Biol 1993; 8:349.

5. Schall T J, Jongstra J, Dyer B J, et al. A human T cell specific molecule is a member of a new gene family. J Immunol 1988; 141:1018.

6. Rathanswami P, Hachicha M, Sadich M, et al. Expression of the cytokine RANTES in human rheumatoid synovial fibroblasts. J Biol Chem 1993; 268:5834.

7. Herger P, Wolf G, Meyers C, et al. Isolation and characterization of cDNA from renal tubular epithelium encoding murine RANTES. Kidney Int 1992; 41:220.

8. Stellato C, Beck L A, Klunk D A, Schall T J, Ono S J, and Schleimer R P. Differential regulation by glucocorticoids [GC] of RANTES production in human epithelial and endothelial cells. J Allergy Clin Immunol 1995; 95:A634.

9. Schall T J, Bacon K, Toy K J, and Goeddel D V. Selective attraction of monocytes and T lymphocytes of the memory phenotype by the cytokine RANTES. Nature 1990; 347:669.

10. Rot A, Krieger M, Brunner T, Bischoff S C, Schall T J, and Dahinden C A. RANTES and macrophage inflammatory protein 1α induce the migration and activation of normal human eosinophil granulocytes. J Exp Med 1992; 176:1489.

11. Alam R, Stafford S, Forsythe P, Harrison, R, Faubion D, Lett-Brown M A, and Grant J A. RANTES is a chemotactic and activating factor for human eosinophils. J Immunol 1993; 150:3442.

12. Nakajima H, Iwamoto I, Tomoe S, Matsumura R, Tomioka H, Takatsu K, and Yoshida S. CD4+ T-lymphocytes and interleukin 5 mediate antigen-induced eosinophil infiltration into the mouse trachea. Am Rev Respir Dis 1992; 146:374.

13. Lukacs N W, Strieter R M, Chensue S W, and Kunkel S L. Interleukin 4-dependent pulmonary eosinophil infiltration in a murine model of asthma. Am J Respir Cell Mol Biol 1994; 10:526.

14. Kung T T, Stelts D, Zurcher J, Garlisi C G, Falcone A, Umland S P, Egan R W, Kreutner W, and Chapman R W. Cytokine profile of the pulmonary eosinophilia in allergic mice. Am J Respir Crit Care Med 1995; 151 [Part 2]:A220.

15. Brusselle G, Kips J, Joos G, Bluethmann, and Pauwels R. Allergen-induced airway inflammation and bronchial responsiveness in wild-type and interleukin-4 deficient mice. Am J Respir Cell Mol Biol 1995; 12:254.

16. Reed C E. Eosinophils in asthma. Part 1. History and histogenesis. In: Eosinophils, Biological and Clinical Aspects. Makin S and Fukuda T, eds. CRC Press, Boca Raton, FL, p325.

17. Settipane G A. Nasal polyps. Immunol Allergy Clin North Am 1987; 7:105.

18. Kakoi H, Hiraide F. A histological study of formation and growth of nasal polyps. Acta Otolaryngol [Stockh] 1987; 103:137.

19. Cauna N, Hinderer K H, Manzetti G W, and Swanson E W. Fine structure of nasal polyps. Ann Otol 1972; 81:41.

20. Ramis I, Finotto S, Dolovich J, Marshall J S, and Jordana M. Increased survival of nasal polyp eosinophils. Immunol. Let. 1995; 45:219.

21. Nonaka R, Takanashi S, Nonaka M, Dolovich J, and Jordana M. Effect of budesonide on the survival of eosinophils from both peripheral blood and nasal polyp tissues. J Allergy Clin Immunol 1994; 93:A324.

22. Kanai N, Denburg J A, Jordana M, and Dolovich J. Nasal polyp inflammation. Effect of topical nasal steroid. Am J Respir Crit Care Med 1994; 150:1094.

23. Wong D, Jordana G, Denburg J A, and Dolovich J. Blood eosinophilia and nasal polyps. Am J Rhinol 1992; 25:195.

24. Wong G G, Witek J S, Temple P A, et al. Human GM-CSF: molecular cloning of the complementary DNA and purification of the natural and recombinant proteins. Science 1985; 228:810.

25. Gearing D P, King J A, Gough N M, and Nicola N A. Expression cloning of a receptor for human granulocyte-macrophage colony-stimulating factor. EMBO J 1989; 8:3667.

26. Zucali J R, Dinarello C A, Oblon D J, Gross M A, Anderson L, and Weiner R S. Interleukin 1 stimulates fibroblasts to produce granulocyte-macrophage colony-stimulating factor activity and prostaglandin E_2. J Clin Invest 1986; 177:1857.

27. Broudy V C, Kaushansky K, Segal G M, Harlan J M and Adamson J W. Tumor necrosis factor α stimulates human endothelial cells to produce granulocyte-macrophage colony-stimulating factor. Proc Natl Acad Sci USA 1987; 83:7467.

28. Cox G, Ohtoshi T, Vancheri C, Gauldie J, Denburg J A, Dolovich J, and Jordana M. Promotion of eosinophil survival by human bronchial epithelial cells and its modulation by steroids. Am J Respir Cell Mol Biol 1991; 4:525.

29. Agro A, Jordana M, Chan K H, Cox G, Richards C, Stepien H, and Stanisz A M. Synoviocyte derived granulocyte macrophage colony stimulating factor mediates the survival of human lymphocytes. J Rheumatol 1992; 19:1065.

30. Smith P D, Lamerson C L, Wong H L, Wahl L M, and Wahl S M. Granulocyte-macrophage colony-stimulating factor stimulates human monocyte accessory cell function. J Immunol 1990; 144:3829.

31. Chen B D M, Clark C R, and Chou T. Granulocyte-macrophage colony-stimulating factor stimulates monocyte and tissue macrophage proliferation and enhances their responsiveness to macrophage colony-stimulating factor. Blood 1988; 71:997.

32. Rothenberg M A, Owen W F, Silberstein D S, Soberman R J, Austen K F and Stevens R L. Eosinophils cocultured with endothelial cells have increased survival and functional properties. Science 1987; 237:645.

33. Kita H, Ohnishi T, Okubo Y, Weiler D, Abrams J S, and Gleich G J. Granulocyte-macrophage colony-stimulating factor and interleukin 3 release from human peripheral blood eosinophils and neutrophils. J Exp Med 1991; 174:745.

34. Takanashi S, Nonaka R, Xing Z, O'Byrne P, Dolovich J, and Jordana M. Interleukin 10 inhibits lipopolysaccharide-induced survival and cytokine production by human peripheral blood eosinophils. J Exp Med 1994; 180:711.

35. Ohno I, Lea R G, Finotto S, Marshall J S, Denburg J A, Dolovich J, Gauldie J, and Jordana M. Granulocyte-macrophage colony-stimulating factor [GM-CSF] gene expression by eosinophils in nasal polyposis. Am J Respir Cell Mol Biol 1991; 5:505.

36. Rothenberg M E, Owen W F, Silbertstein D S, Woods J, Soberman R J, Austen K F, and Stevens R L. Human eosinophils have prolonged survival, enhanced functional properties, and become hypodense when exposed to human interleukin 3. J Clin Invest 1988; 81:1986.

37. Yamaguchi Y, Suda T, Ohta S, Tominaga K, Miura Y, and Kasahara T. Analysis of the survival of mature human eosinophils: Interleukin-5 prevents apoptosis in mature human eosinophils. Blood 1991; 78:2542.

38. Dubucquoi S, Desreumaux P, Janin A, Klein O, Goldman M, Tavernier J, Capron A, and Capron M. Interleukin 5 synthesis by eosinophils: association with granules and immunoglobulin-dependent secretion. J Exp Med 1994; 179:703.

39. Broide D H, Paine M M, and Firestein G S. Eosinophils express interleukin 5 and granulocyte-macrophage colony-stimulating factor mRNA at sites of allergic inflammation in asthmatics. J Clin Invest 1992; 90:1414.

40. Robinson D S, Hamid Q, Ying S, Tsicopoulos A, Barkans J, Bentley A M, Corrigan C, Durham S R, and Kay A B. Predominant T_{H2}-like bronchoalveolar T-lymphocyte population in atopic asthma. N Eng J Med 1992; 326:298.

41. Tracey K J, Vlassara H, and Cerami A. Cachectin/TNF. Lancet 1989; i:1122–6.

42. Sugarman B J, Aggarwal B B, Hass P E, Figari I S, Palladino M A, and Sheppard M M. Recombinant human tumor necrosis factor-α: effects of proliferation of normal and transformed cells in vitro. Science 1985; 230:943.

43. Briscoe D M, Cotran R S, and Pober J S. Effects of tumor necrosis factor, lipopolysaccharide and IL-4 on the expression of vascular cell adhesion molecule-1 in vivo. Correlation with CD3⁺ T cell infiltration. J Immunol 1992; 149:2954.

44. Iademarco M F, Barks J L, and Dean D C. Regulation of vascular cell adhesion molecule-1 expression by IL-4 and TNF-α in cultured endothelial cells. J Clin Invest 1994; 95:264.

45. Slungaard A, Vercellotti G M, Walker G, Nelson R D, and Jacob H S. Tumor necrosis factor/cachectin stimulates eosinophil oxidant production and toxicity toward human endothelium. J Exp Med 1990; 171:2025.

46. Finotto S, Ohno I, Marshall J S, Gauldie J, Denburg J A, Dolovich J, Clark D A, and Jordana M. TNFα production by eosinophils in upper airways inflammation [nasal polyposis]. J Immunol 1994; 153:2278.

47. Costa J J, Matossian K, Resnick M B, Beil W J, Wong D T W, Gordon J R, Dvorak A M, Weller P F, and Galli S J. Human eosinophils can express the cytokines tumor necrosis factor α and macrophage inflammatory protein-1α. J Clin Invest 1993; 91:2673.

48. Coffman R L, Ohara J, Bond M W, Carty J, Zlotnik E, and Paul W E. B-cell stimulatory factor-1 enhances the IgE response of lipopolysaccharide activated B cells. J Immunol 1986; 136:4538.

49. Tepper R I, Levinson D A, Stranger B Z, Campos-Torres J, Abbas A K, and Leder P. IL-4 induces allergic-like inflammatory disease and alters T-cell development in transgenic mice. Cell 1990; 62:457.

50. Schleimer R P, Sterbinsky S A, Kaiser J, Bickel C A, Klunk D A, Tomioka K, Newman W, Luscinkas F W, Gimbrone M A, McIntyre B W, and Bochner B S. IL-4 induces adherence of human eosinophils and basophils but not neutrophils to endothelium. Association with expression of VCAM-1. J Immunol 1991; 148:1086.

51. Le Gros G, Ben-Sasson S Z, Sedaer R, Finkelman F D, and Paul W E. Generation of interleukin 4 [IL-4]-producing cells in vivo and in vitro: IL-2 and IL-4 are required for the in vitro generation of IL-4 producing cells. J Exp Med 1990; 173:921.

52. Bradding P, Feather, Howarth P H, Mueller R, Roberts J A, Britten K, Bews J P A, Hunt T C, Okayama Y, Heusser C H, Bullock G R, Church M K, and Holgate S T. Interleukin 4 is localized to and released by human mast cells. J Exp Med 1992; 176:1381.

53. MacGlashan D Jr, White J M, Huang S, Ono S J, Schroeder J T, and Lichtenstein L M. Secretion of IL-4 from human basophils. J Immunol 1994; 152:3006.

54. Bradding P, Feather I H, Wilson S, Bardin P G, Heusser C H, Holgate S T, and Howarth H. Immunolocalization of cytokines in the nasal mucosa of normal and perennial rhinitic subjects. J Immunol 1993; 151:3853.

55. Bradding P, Roberts J A, Britten K M, Montefort S, Djukanovic R, Mueller R, Heusser C H, Howarth P H, and Holgate S T. Interleukin-4, -5, -6 and tumor necrosis factor α in normal and asthmatic airways: evidence for the human mast cell as a source of these cytokines. Am J Respir Cell Mol Biol 1994; 10:471.

56. Nonaka M, Nonaka R, Woolley K, Adelroth E, Miura K, Okhawara Y, Glibetic M, Nakano K, O'Byrne P, Dolovich J, and Jordana M. Distinct immunohistochemcial localization of interleukin 4 [IL-4] in human inflamed airways tissues: nasal polyposis and asthma. IL-4 is localized to eosinophils in vivo and released by peripheral blood eosinophils. J Immunol 1995 [September].

57. Noelle R J. Introduction: CD40, its ligand and immunity. Seminars in Immunology 1994; 6:257.

58. Hollenbaugh D, Mischel-Petty N, Edwards C P, Simon J C, Denfeld R W, Kiener P A, and Aruffo A. Expression of functional CD40 by vascular endothelial cells. J Exp Med 1995; 182:33.

59. Hollenbaugh D, Grosmaire L S, Kullas C D, Chalupny N J, Braesch-Andersen S, Noelle R J, Stamenkovic I, Ledbetter J A, and Aruffo A. The human T cell antigen gp39, a member of the TNF gene family, is a ligand for the CD40

receptor: expression of a soluble form of gp39 with B cell co-stimulatory activity. The EMBO J 1992; 11:4313.

60. Gauchat J F, Henchoz S, Mazzed G, Aubry J P, Brunner T, Blasey H, Life P, Talabot D, Flores-Romo L, Thompson J, Kishi K, Butterfield J, Dahinden C, and Bonnefoy J Y. Induction of human IgE synthesis in B cells by mast cells and basophils. Nature 1993; 365:340.

61. Galy A H M, and Spits H. CD40 is functionally expressed on human thymic epithelial cells. J Immunol 1992; 149:775.

62. Alderson M R, Armitage R J, Tough T W, Strockbine L, Fanslow W C, and Spriggs M K. CD40 expression by human monocytes: regulation by cytokines and activation of monocytes by the ligand for CD40. J Exp Med 1993; 178:669.

63. Ohkawara Y, Xing Z, Glibetic M, Dolovich J, and Jordana M. Expression of CD40 by human eosinophils and functional consequences of its activation. Am J Respir Crit Care Med 1995; 151 [Part 1]:A240.

64. Roberts A B, and Sporn M B. The transforming growth factors β. In: Sporn M B, Roberts A B, eds. Handbook of Experimental Pharmacology, Vol 95/I, Peptide Growth Factors and Their Receptors. New York. Springer-Verlag, 1990:419.

65. Grotendorst G R, Smale G, and Pencev D. Production of transforming growth factor β by human peripheral blood monocytes and neutrophils. J Cell Physiol 1989; 140:396.

66. Ohno I, Lea R G., Flanders K C, Clark D A, Banwatt D, Dolovich J, Denburg J A, Harley C B, Gauldie J, and Jordana M. Eosinophils in chronically inflamed human upper airway tissues express transforming growth factor β_1 gene. J Clin Invest 1991; 89:1662.

67. Wong D T W, Elovic A, Matossian K, Nagura N, McBride J and Chou J R. Eosinophils from patients with blood eosinophilia express transforming growth factor β_1. Blood 1991; 78:2702.

68. Border W A, and Ruoslahti E. Transforming growth factor-β in disease: the dark side of tissue repair. J Clin Invest 1992; 90:1.

69. McCartney-Francis N, and Wahl S M. TGFβ: a matter of life and death. J Leuk Biol 1994; 55:401.

70. Espevik T, Figari I S, Shalaby M R, et al. Inhibition of cytokine production by cyclosporin A and transforming growth factor β. J Exp Med 1987; 166:571.

71. Ranges G E, Figari I S, Espevik T, and Palladino M A. Inhibition of cytokine T cell development by transforming growth factor β and reversal by tumor necrosis factor α. J Exp Med 1987; 166:991.

72. Alam R, Forsythe P, Stafford S, Fukuda S. Transforming growth factor β abrogates the effects of hematopoietins on eosinophils and induces their apoptosis. J Exp Med 1994; 179:1041.

73. Derynck R, Goeddel D V, Ulrich A, Gutterman J U, Williams R D, Bringman T S, and Berger W H. Synthesis of messenger RNAs for transforming growth factor-α and β and the epidermal growth factor-receptor by human tumors. Cancer Res 1987; 47:707.

74. Derynck R. Transforming growth factor-α. Cell 1988; 54:593.

75. Wong D T W, Weller P F, Galli S J, Elovic A, Rand T H, Gallagher G T, Chiang T, Chou M Y, Matossian K, McBride J, Todd R. Human eosinophils express transforming growth factor α. J Exp Med 1990; 172:673.

76. Elovic A, Wong D T W, Weller P F, Matossian K, and Galli S J. Expression of transforming growth factors-α and β_1 messenger RNA and product by eosinophils in nasal polyps. J Allergy Clin Immunol 1994; 93:864.

77. Del Pozo V, De Andres B, Martin E, Maruri N, Zubeldia J M, Palomino P, and Lahoz C. Murine eosinophils and IL-1: αIL-1 mRNA detection by in situ hybridization. Production and release of IL-1 from peritoneal eosinophils. J Immunol 1990; 144:3117.

78. Hamid Q, Barkans J, Meng Q, Ying S, Abrams J S, Kay A B, and Moqbel R. Human eosinophils synthesize and secrete interleukin-6 in vitro. Blood 1992; 80:1496.

79. Braun R K, Francini M, Erard F, Rhis S, De Vries I J M, Blaser K, Hansel T T, and Walker C. Human peripheral blood eosinophils produce and release interleukin-8 on stimulation with calcium ionophore. Eur J Immunol 1993; 23:956.

80. Donovan R, Johansson S G O, Bennich H, and Soothill J F. Immunoglobulins in nasal polyp fluid. Int Arch Allergy 1970; 37:154.

81. Brandtzaeg P, Fjellanger I, and Gjeruldsen S T. Localization of immunoglobulins in human nasal mucosa. Immunochemistry 1967; 4:57.

82. Looney R J, Ryan D H, Takahashi K, Fleit H B, Cohen H J, Abraham G N, and Anderson C L. Identification of a second class of IgG Fc receptors on human neutrophils. A 40 kilodalton molecule also found on eosinophils. J Exp Med 1986; 163:826.

83. Monteiro R C, Hostoffer R W, Cooper M D, Bonner J R, Gartland G L, and Kubagawa H. Definition of immunoglobulin A receptors on eosinophils and their enhanced expression in allergic individuals. J Clin Invest 1993; 92:1681.

84. Gounni A S, Lamkhlioued B, Ochiai K, Tanaka Y, Delaporte E., Capron A, Kinet J P, and Capron M. High-affinity IgE receptor on eosinophils is involved in defence against parasites. Nature [Lond.] 1994; 367:183.

85. Abu-Ghazaleh R I, Fujisawa T, Mestecky J, Kyle R A, and Gleich G J. IgA-induced eosinophil degranulation. J Immunol 1989; 142:2393.

86. Khalife J, Capron M, Cesbron J Y, Tai P C, Taelman H, Prin L, and Capron A. Role of specific IgE antibodies in peroxidase [EPO] release from human eosinophils. J Immunol 1986; 137:1659.

87. Kaneko M, Swanson M C, Gleich G J, and Kita H. Allergen-specific IgGa and IgG3 through Fc$_\gamma$RII induce eosinophil degranulation. J Clin Invest 1995; 95:2813.

Chapter VIII

The Pathogenesis of Nasal Polyps

Adrian Drake-Lee, Ph.D., F.R.C.S.

ABSTRACT

Pathogenesis has three stages, the evaluation of any underlying condition, understanding any factors in the genesis of tissue oedema and finally the symptoms that these reactions may cause. Nasal polyps occur almost solely in human, more commonly in men and are found in all racial group. Simple polyps may arise at any age after two and are usually due to cystic fibrosis in childhood. The mucosal changes may not be limited to the upper respiratory tract since patients may have co-existing asthma or other respiratory diseases. There is some evidence for a genetic predisposition and certain conditions such as immune deficiency, ciliary dyskineisia, Young's syndrome and aspirin hypersensitivity are associated with the condition. The origins of the tissue oedema may be explained at the cellular level: mast cells are degranulated with the resultant inflammatory mediators which attract eosinophils which in turn may damage tissue and perpetuate the changes. These reactions are exaggerated by the relatively poorly developed blood supply of the ethmoid sinuses. Finally, neurovascular reflexes and the complex anatomy of the ethmoid labyrinth can predispose to the persistence of oedema. Patients complain about nasal blockage, loss of sense of smell and also may suffer from attacks of sneezing, anterior rhinorrhoea, pain and post nasal drainage.

INTRODUCTION

The pathogenesis of a condition is the origins, development and resultant effects of a disease. The term "polyp" comes from the Greek and means many footed (poly-pous). Unfortunately there has been much debate recently on the exact nature of a nasal polyp. Some workers differentiate a simple polyp from polyposis. Similarly some authors debate to what extent ethmoid disease is a pre-polypoidal condition. Established benign, mucous or simple nasal polyps are an easily recognisable clinical condition.

Clinically, polyps are pale bags of oedematous tissue which arise most commonly from the middle meatus and are relatively insensitive. The pale colour is due to the poor blood supply but in the presence of repeated trauma and inflammation they may become reddened. They are commonly bilateral and, when unilateral, require histological examination to exclude the transitional cell papilloma (syn Ringert's tumor, inverted papilloma) or malignancy.

A problem occurs with this definition because a physical finding is classified as a disease. The correct question should be, 'what is the clinical condition giving rise to polyps?' Part of the clinical puzzle, then, is the evaluation of any underlying disease.

Pathogenesis has three stages, the evaluation of any underlying condition, understanding any factors in the genesis of tissue oedema and finally the symptoms that these reactions may cause. The origins of the tissue oedema may be explained at the cellular level. Finally, neurovascular reflexes and the complex anatomy of the ethmoid labyrinth can predispose to the persistance of oedema. (Table 1)

Simple polyps may arise at any age after two. If seen before this, a menigocoele or encaphelocoele should be excluded. It is unusual for simple nasal polyps to arise before 10 years and so may be the presenting complaint of cystic fibrosis[1]. They occur more commonly in men and are found in all racial group. Chimpanzees are the only animal to have nasal polyps[2,3].

Although polyps are a disease of the ethmoid sinuses, the mucosal changes frequently extend further in the nose and into the other paranasal sinuses. The maxillary

Table 1. The Pathogenesis of Nasal Polyps

Genetic predisposition
Mucosal reactions
   Allergic inflammation
   Infection
   Non allergic infection
      Trigger cell
         Mast cell
         Eosinophil
         Lymphocyte
         Macrophage
      Inflammatory mediators
   Mucus glands
   Alteration in the connective tissue
Anatomical abnormality
   The general anatomy of the ethmoid labyrinth
   The junction of the ethmoid sinuses and the nasal
     cavity
   The Bernoulli phenomenon
Neurovascular changes
   The relative paucity of the sinus vascularity
   Loss of autonomic control

sinuses are affected more commonly than the frontal and sphenoid sinuses. The mucosal changes may not be limited to the upper respiratory tract since patients may have co-existing asthma or other respiratory diseases.

All polypoidal conditions were initially grouped together until histological classification helped to differentiate them from the neoplastic conditions when it was recognised that they were an inflammatory condition[4]. The histological changes in the sinuses are the same as those in polyps, demonstrating the oedema and eosinophilia. The condition is prone to recurrence.

GENETIC PREDISPOSITION

Moloney and Oliver looked at the HLA classification of 29 patients with nasal polyps and found that there was a higher incidence of A1/B8 in patients with nasal polyps, asthma and aspirin hypersensitivity[5].

Several members of a family may be affected with nasal polyps but there is little evidence for a genetic basis for this. Some evidence to support a genetic predisposition comes from the development of polyps in identical twins[6].

Cystic fibrosis (CF) is an autosomal recessive disease which is associated with a gene defect on the seventh chromosome but it is not know which phenotype is associated with nasal polyps. CF gene probes have been used in seven patients with nasal polyps but without CF[7]. G551D mutation was found to be higher than expected in this small report. Further studies are required. (See Chapter XVII.)

CONDITIONS FOUND WITH AN INCREASED INCIDENCE OF NASAL POLYPS

Asthma and nasal polyps

The association of nasal polyps and asthma has long been recognised[8]. Their review of several studies has shown that 20–40% of patients with polyps have coexisting asthma and it appears that a similar proportion of adults with asthma have nasal polyps (Table 2).

Late onset asthma is associated with nasal polyps[9]. The incidence of childhood asthma is about 5% of the population and it was 3.5% in a study of cases with nasal polyps[10]. Asthma usually developed around the onset of nasal polyps with over half getting either polyps or asthma within five years of each other. Surgery has little effect on asthma, if anything patients notice a subjective improvement in their asthma[11]. It has been suggested that patients with asthma may be a distinct subgroup within the disease because proportionately a greater number of patients with asthma and polyps are women whereas polyps usually occur more frequently in males.

Aspirin Hypersensitivity

Patients with aspirin hypersensitivity, asthma and nasal polyps are a well recognized subgroup[12] which occurs in up to 8% of patients with nasal polyps. The mechanism for both aspirin hypersensitivity and asthma is unclear, but it is not an allergic reaction and there is some suggestion that there is an alteration in prostaglandin synthesis[13].

Cystic Fibrosis

Cystic fibrosis is a multisystemic disease affecting the exocrine glands which is an autosomal recessive disease occurring in 1 in 2000 live births. The abnormality lies in the seventh chromosome in three quarters of the cases. The exocrine glands are unable to produce dilute sweat and values of above 60 mEq of sodium on 2 consecutive tests are diagnostic.

Transepithelial electrolyte transport controls the quantity and composition of the respiratory tract fluid and so is important in mucociliary clearance. (See Chapter XI.)

Table 2. Diseases Associated With the Development of Nasal Polyps

Cystic fibrosis

Young's syndrome

Immune deficiency, both congenital and acquired

Ciliary dyskinesia

Late onset asthma

Aspirin hypersensitivity

Cystic fibrosis epithelia have defective electrolytic transport especially of the chloride ion. This results in the airway secretions being thick and dehydrated.

The disease produces gastrointestinal and respiratory symptoms. The gastrointestinal symptoms may present at birth with failure of the neonate to pass meconium ileus or subsequently failure to thrive. Conversely some children have little in the way of gastrointestinal symptoms and present with recurrent respiratory tract infections, which may result in severe lung damage produced by persistent colonisation by staphylococci and pseudomonas.

Although the pathological changes in the sinuses were first described in detail by Bodian in 1952[14], the first description of polyps was made by Lurie in 1957[15]. The true incidence is uncertain and reports have varied from 3 to 48%. A study that compared polyp patients with a control group found that there was no greater incidence of allergic diseases and positive skin tests in the polyp patients[16].

Occasionally, the nasal symptoms may occur first but usually the other manifestations occur first[16]. Males predominate with a ratio of 5 to 1 which appears to be real, even though cystic fibrosis is slightly more common in males.

Other Respiratory Diseases

While the deficit in cystic fibrosis is in the function of the exocrine glands, hyperviscous mucus found in Young's syndrome can also predispose to polyp formation. Other abnormalities in the respiratory mucosa such as primary ciliary dyskinesia (Immotile cilial syndrome, Kartagener's syndrome) may eventually result in polyp formation. These two conditions are very rare causes of polyps in adults and often follow a long period of respiratory illness in childhood. Immune deficiencies, both congenital and acquired, can predispose to polyp development.

MUCOSAL REACTIONS

Different theories have been put forward to explain the pathogenesis of nasal polyps. Although a single aetiology would be attractive, this is unlikely. There are a variety of levels in the mucosa where alterations may occur but the important consideration to bear in mind is that the reactions and compounds measured or described may well occur because the tissue is respiratory mucosa and they may not be due to disease at all.

Nasal polyp tissue continues to behave like normal respiratory mucosa in some respects and it is able to produce immunoglobulins from the plasma cells present.

Histological examination has demonstrated that polyps are mainly oedema[17] and the extracellular oedema is easy to extract and has been analyzed in different studies[4,18,19]. After they are removed, polyps may be coarsely minced and centrifuged and the resulting oedema is collected and analyzed. Matched serum may be taken at the same time. Berdal injected polyp fluid subcutaneously and repeated skin tests. Those patients who had a positive skin test tended to have greater reactions when tested again at the site of injection.

Donovan showed that the level of IgE was raised in polyp fluid irrespective of the results of skin tests. All immunoglobulins are found in polyp oedema and both IgA and IgE levels tending to be higher in polyp fluids than in sera. The levels of IgG, IgA and IgM are variable and elevated levels probably represent a recent upper respiratory tract infection.

Inflammation

Allergy

Allergy has been implicated because of three factors; the histological picture where 90% or more of nasal polyps have an eosinophilia, the association with asthma and finally the nasal findings which may mimic allergic symptoms and signs. Other chapters of this book have described the relationship of allergy and nasal polyps.

Clinically it is easy to consider such symptoms as attacks of anterior rhinorrhoea, sneezing and blockage as allergic when no obvious cause is found and the patients have one or more positive skin tests.

Inflammatory Mediators

Mast cells and other inflammatory cells give rise to a variety of products. Histamine is the easiest to measure and has been measured in polyp oedema[19]. Levels which are between 100 and 1000 times the serum level are encountered. This would suggest that when mast cells degranulate local homeostatic mechanisms may be overcome. (See Chapter VI.)

Arachidonic acid metabolites are not easy to quantify since they are relatively unstable and may be generated by trauma. The results from the four studies which looked at these compounds are difficult to interpret[20–23] for there is little work on normal levels in nasal tissues and two of the studies induced the generation of metabolites by challenge. It appears that the levels of thromboxanes are elevated and that challenge will produce 5, 12, and 15 hydroxyeicosatetraenoic acid (HETE), the most elevated being 15-HETE. There is some suggestion that levels are higher in patients with aspirin sensitivity but whether this is due to a more severe inflammation is not clear. Leukotrienes C4 and D4 may be demonstrated in polyp oedema fluid (see above). Prostaglandins E2, F2α and 6 keto are also present in the oedema. The elevation of certain cytokines such as granulocyte macrophage colony stimulating factor may account in part for the inflammation and attraction of eosinophils. Epithelial growth factor and an insulin like growth factor have also been demonstrated. These may act indirectly on granulocutes and T cells to attract other inflammatory cells and perpetuate the oedema. (See Chapter VI.)

Mast Cells

Mast cells which are a heterogenous collection of cells and have been divided in animals into two main groups: mucosal and connective tissue types, in addition to circulating basophils, may also enter the tissue. Ultrastructural analysis showed that mast cells were degranulated[24] and this has been confirmed but the features may not be consistent with those described in the allergic nose[25]. The mast cells are also degranulated on the inferior turbinate of over half the patients.

Eosinophils

Eosinophils may produce a variety of intensely irritating mediators when activated. It has been suggested that the release of mediators may produce some of the intense inflammation seen in those patients who suffer from both asthma and aspirin hypersensitivity[26]. Major basic protein is in the core of the granule and it has not been demonstrated in polyp oedema fluid (Drake-Lee, unpublished observation). (See Chapter VII.)

Lymphocytes and Macrophages

Lymphocytes and macrophages can easily be demonstrated in the stroma of nasal polyps using light microscopy. Frozen sections have been used to look at the distribution of T- and B-lymphocytes, HLA-DR expressing cells and macrophages[27]. Monoclonal and immunohistological staining demonstrated that T-helper cells were present in greater numbers than T-suppressor lymphocytes and that clumping occured in the former around the glands and sub-epithelialy. This is different from chronic infection where the pattern is reversed. B cells were present but in lesser numbers and macrophages could also be demonstrated. These are easily seen with the transmission electron microscope. Lymphocyte subpopulations and the levels of antigen-specific IgE in nasal polyps were not different between the allergic and non-allergic subjects which supports a non-allergic hypothesis in the pathogenesis of polyps.[28]

Allergen Challenge to Polyp Tissue

The first report of pollen allergen challenge to nasal polyps tissue was by Kaliner and his colleages in 1973. They used a heterogeneous collection of tissue, including that taken from children with cystic fibrosis, and either challenged allergic tissue or passively sensitised non allergic tissue with pollen extract and demonstrated that it was possible to release histamine. Challenge with mixed grass pollen and house dust mite extracts to non sensitised tissue has released histamine. Polyp tissue is less re-

active than peripheral blood and then only releases histamine rarely on direct challenge suggesting that allergic reactions are not common[29].

Local Nasal Allergy

It is possible that a local allergy occurs in the nasal cavity that is not manifest systemically. Levels of IgE in polyp oedema have been shown to be higher than the corresponding values in serum in several studies[18,19]. Although some authors feel that this may be related to the presence of an allergic response, others feel that the production is purely a function of local plasma cells, because elevated levels of IgE may be found in nasal secretions in non atopics[30]. Polyps are capable of local production and this has been shown by comparing the levels of IgE with those of either albumin or α_2-macroglobulin which are produced elsewhere. Serum values for these compounds are usually below those in polyp oedema.

Allergen Specific IgE

RAST levels in polyp fluid and sera are raised only infrequently[31]. This would suggest that allergic reactions may occur but are infrequently encountered in patients with nasal polyps.

INFECTION

In the last century, there were two main types of maxillary sinusitis here described; "purulent" and "hyperplastic" to differentiate infection from inflammation. This division is broadly applicable today.

Purulent sinusitis results from infection usually by bacteria following a viral upper respiratory infection. The ethmoid mucosa may become polypoidal secondarily.

Hyperplastic sinusitis is associated with mucus hypersecretion in which organisms may be found and cultured. Infection may exacerbate the condition as in chronic bronchitis, but it does not cause it. This could be what occurs in the majority of cases with nasal polyps. An inappropriate inferior antrostomy into maxillary sinus leaves an ostium through which the diseased mucosa subsequently prolapses. Polyps may appear from both the middle and inferior meatus.

The cause of inflammatory reactions is uncertain. Mucus washed out and cultured may grow an organism. The commonest organism is the noncapulsated Haemophilus influenzae[32]. This study was confirmed by Daws et al[33] which also showed that pus cells and bacteria were only found in 16 percent of antral irrigations. Pus cells were found in 25% and bacteria were cultured in 31%.

Unfortunately, it is difficult to implicate any further relationship because antibiotics have little effect on the course or recurrence of the disease but merely modify the infectivity of the mucus. Corticosteroids improve the symptoms in over half of the cases. It may be possible that patients are allergic to bacteria. As mentioned previously, the lymphocyte pattern is also not typical of an infective process in the polyps themselves. (See Chapter XV.)

Culture

Nasal polyp homogenates have been cultured for organisms and 24 out of the 40 grew aerobic bacteria, gram negative cultures were obtained in 6 cases whereas 14 were completely sterile[34]. Streptococci were cultured most frequently and were more common in asthmatics and patients on inhaled steroids. If the polyps showed a polymorph infiltration then bacteria were more likely to be cultured. Cultures were completely negative for mycobacteria, mycoplasmata and viruses.

The presence of bacterial specific IgE in nasal polyp oedema fluid has been investigated by Calenoff and his co-workers[35]. They stated that 59 of the 61 patients had bacterial specific IgE in the polyp oedema and the most commonly raised immunoglobulin was to proteus. They defined a positive result on the basis of count of 150% above background noise. It would appear from their studies that the activity was lost on incubation of sera at 56°C. The results appear to be inconclusive. They have looked at the sera of patients with polyps, chronic sinusitis and allergic rhinitis and using a modified RAST found that bacteria-specific IgE was raised in the two former groups but not the latter and concluded that bacterial sensitization is possible[36].

Nasal polyp tissue has been challenged with bacteria to release histamine[37] and a wide and variable release of histamine was released with anti IgE. The study concluded that although there was some response to challenge with streptococcal and staphylococcal extracts that bacterial allergy was only a possibility.

ALTERATION IN THE CONNECTIVE TISSUE POLYSACCHARIDES

An inherent alteration in the polysaccharides of ground substances was postulated by Jackson and Arihood in 1971[38]: the abnormality was present in the ground substance. Analysis of polyps have shown them to be oedematous[17] with little alteration in the collagen. The collagen appears normal on analysis though tends to be recently formed and therefore less mature.

ALTERATION IN THE MUCOUS GLANDS

Tos considered that an alteration in the mucous glands was the initiating factor in the pathogenesis of nasal polyps[39]. Dilatation and cystic changes occured along with epithelial changes and the subsequent break in the epithelium allowed herniation of the submucosa through and subsequent polyp development. The epithelium regrew over the denuded stroma.

ANATOMICAL VARIATIONS

Considerable attention has been paid in the past few years to the middle meatus of the nose and its impact on the presentation of nasal disease. The collective term for the area is the ostiomeatal complex. Some surgeons considerer that the variations here are the most important factor in the development of nasal polyps and that the correction of these variations is the main stay of therapy.

Variations include aggar nasi cells, choncha bullosa, paradoxical middle turbinate, over pneumatised ethmoid bulla and bent uncinate process. The frequency of these variations would seem similar in patients with and without nasal polyps[40]. Surgical treatment is aimed at correcting the anatomical variations and opening out the ethmoid cells into a large unit, an ethmoidectomy, often aided by the endoscope. Correct radiographic imaging with computerised tomorgraphy is essential before surgery but a limited series of cuts of four or five coronal sections at 5mm intervals and two axial cuts through the orbits may be all that is necessary[41]. Any CT scan increases the dose of radiation to the orbit but is limited by decreasing the number of cuts.

The reductio ad absurdum of the anatomical argument is the idea that there is only one precise place in the nose that polyps develop, viz the junction of the ethmoid sinus and the nasal cavity. This hypothesis is dealt with in the next chapter.

BERNOULLI PHENOMENON

As a result of the Bernoulli phenomenon, the pressure falls next to a deviation or narrowing and this sucks the ethmoid mucosa into the nose. The Bernoulli's equation describes reversible velocity changes when pressure alters:

$$P + \tfrac{1}{2}\rho V^2 = \text{constant.}$$

ρ is the density.

The nose always has some viscous forces in operation and so the Bernoulli equation is not strictly applicable. The nose has a variable cross section and so the pressure and velocity will alter continuously within the system. The inspiratory phase lasts approximately 2 seconds and reaches a pressure of -10mm dPa and expiration lasts about 3 seconds and reaches a pressure of 8mm dPa. The respiratory rate is between 10–18 cycles a minute in adults at rest. If this were the only or a major factor, then the mucosa nearest the nasal valve would be polypoidal in the normal nose. It may account why polypoidal changes are seen occasionally in the middle meatus anteriorly on both sides at post mortem.

NEUROVASCULAR CHANGES

Vascular Development

There has been little work done on the vascular flow through the nose and sinuses, and, that which has, has used relatively insensitive techniques. Direct inspection of the nasal cavity will show the well developed blood supply which can be compared directly by endoscopy with the sinus mucosa both in the ethmoid complex and the maxillary antrum. The sinus mucosa is a pale almost transparent lining and the feeding vessels can be seen through the yellowish mucosa.

This picture is confirmed by histological examination. Sections through the nasal cavity show how well adapted the mucosa is to fulfill its physiological function of warming and humidifying the inspired air. The blood supply has both capacitance and resistance vessels together with venous sinusoids whereas the vascularity of the sinuses is much less well developed. This means that there is less reserve in the blood supply in the sinuses to transport away compounds released by cellular reactions: homeostasis is less easy to maintain. Inflammation results in venous congestion and/or increased blood flow in intranasal disease whereas persistant oedema occurs in the sinuses.

Plain radiographs of the paranasal sinuses demonstrated by the conventional three view will show the extent of the disease in the nose and paranasal sinuses to some extent. A CT scan will give more information, particularly the anatomical detail. Other features seen include, loss of radio translucency in the nose, hypertrophy of the turbinates and deviation of the bony septum and intranasal masses. The ethmoid complex is usually opaque to a variable extent on the side of the polyps and these changes may occur on the other side where there are no visible polyps. The maxillary sinus will have changes in most cases with mucosal thickening of a variable degree until the antrum becomes opaque. Fluid levels are encountered and may be due to retained secretion alone or purulent material since blockage of the maxillary ostium by polyps will prevent the migration of mucus from the sinus.

Expansion of the ethmoids will be encountered in children with polyps since polyps developed before the bones of the mid face and anterior cranial fossa have fused. Bony erosion although highly suggestive of malignancy may be found in patients who have polyps and is usually due to previous surgery. Previous surgery is often implicated when mucoceles develop. They are most commonly frontal or ethmoid; primary sphenoid mucocele are rare.[42]

Loss of Autonomic Control

Vasomotor imbalance is implied because the majority of cases are not atopic and no obvious allergen can be found. Patients frequently have a prodromal period of rhinitis prior to occurrence of polyps. Polyps themselves often have a very poor nerve supply since they may be palpated freely and insensitively. Blood vessels are encountered in polyps but they are infrequent and are usually venules. Larger ones have little smooth muscle within them. Vasomotor problems may cause polyps but this is just conjecture.

CLINICAL SYMPTOMS

Nasal Symptoms

All patients suffer from nasal obstruction or blockage which is constant although it will vary with the size and position of polyps. In its mildest form, there is nasal congestion. Patients complain frequently of cold-like symptoms.

About half the patients suffer from attacks of either clear rhinorrhea and/or sneezing similar to hay fever but symptoms are perennial and have no obvious triggers.

Partial loss of the sense of smell and alterations in taste are common complaints. These do not tend to recover following treatment except in some cases treated by corticosteroids particularly when taken orally when there may be a general improvement in respiratory function.

Although not frequent, pain does occur. It is usually over the bridge of the nose, in the forehead and in the cheeks. It is worse when the nose is congested or when the post nasal drip changes in colour and the sinuses are infected secondarily.

Three quarters of patients complain of a post nasal drip which is usually white or yellow. It may become green following exacerbation of nasal symptoms and sinusitis. The post nasal drip may improve following surgery or improve in colour following antibiotic therapy.

When epistaxis is a major symptom, it indicates a more sinister pathology.

Chest Symptoms

About one third of patients will have symptoms from the lower respiratory tract. These are usually related to intermittent bronchospasm or more severe asthma. Complaints commonly include wheezing and chronic cough which may be productive. Diet may induce exacerbations if the patient has aspirin hypersensitivity. Mucociliary disfunction and immunodificiency also produce similar symptoms.

Signs

Patients have a distinctive hyponasal voice. When the blockage is severe, polyps may be seen externally. Mouth breathing and occasionally flaring of the alar cartilages occur with complete obstruction. This later sign is usually produced by the polyps themselves. If polyps develop before the nasal facial bones fuse, hypertelorism will develop in more florid cases: it is seen in children with cystic fibrosis. The intranasal signs have been mentioned earlier.

RECURRENCE

The natural history suggests that recurrence is common. Two studies have looked at this phenomenon in some detail[10,42]. The severity of recurrence is established in ten years[10]. Larsen and Tos followed their patients up for up to eight years with a median of five years. Even so it is possible to make some comments on the severity of recurrence based on these two studies. Approximately five percent have severe recurrent disease. Over 60% of patients will require only one polypectomy in a five period, many other patients will only require one other polypectomy over this time.

Regression techniques were only able to identify under 50% of the factors associated with resurrence. These included the length of history, the presence of asthma and severity of sinus diseased measured by previous surgery[10]. It is important to bear the natural history of recurrence in mind when studying treatment for nasal polyps.

CONCLUSIONS

Polyps are not a disease and therefore do not have a pathogenesis in the true sense of the word. It is possible to make some comments on their distribution within the population and factors associated with their development. Oedema and inflammation are present in nasal polyps and are probably not caused by allergy. Corticosteroids will work since oedema and inflammation are present. The anatomy of the ethmoids predisposes to their formation and so surgery here will help patients symptoms to improve. Careful clinical trials conducted for ten years are required to evaluate the best approach to therapy.

REFERENCES

1. Schwachman H, Kulczychi I L, Mueller H L, Flake C G (1962). Nasal polyposis in patients with cystic fibrosis. *Paediatrics* **30**, 389–410.

2. Jacobs R, Lux G, Spielvogel R, Eichberg J, Gleiser C. Nasal polyposis in a chimpanzee. Journal of Allergy and Clinical Immunology. 1984. **74**, 61–3.

3. Drake-Lee A. Nasal Polyps. In: Allergic and non-allergic rhinitis. Eds Mygind N, and Naclerio R. Munksgaard. Copenhagen. Chapter 20. 167–173.

4. Berdal P (1954). Serological examination of nasal polyp fluid. *Acta Otolaryngologica*, **115**,

5. Maloney J, Oliver R. (1980). HLA antigens, nasal polyps and asthma. *Clinical Otolaryngology* **5**, 183–189.

6. Drake-Lee A. Nasal polyps in identical twins. Journal of Laryngology and Otology. 1992. **106**, 1084–1085.

7. Burger J, Macek M, Stuhrmann M, Reis A, Krawczak M, Schmidtke J. (1991). Genetic influences in the formation of nasal polyps. *Lancet* 337 974 (letter).

8. Maloney J R and Collins J (1977). Nasal polyps and bronchialasthma. *British Journal of Diseases of the Chest*, **71**, 1–6.

9. Settipane G A and Chafee F G (1977). Nasal polyps in asthma and rhinitis. *Journal of Allergy and Clinical Immunology*, **58**, 17–21.

10. Drake-Lee A B, Lowe D, Swanston A, Grace A. (1984). Clinical profile and recurrence of nasal polyps. *Journal of Laryngology and Otology*, **98**, 783–793.

11. Maloney J R (1977). Nasal polyps, nasal polypectomy, asthma and aspirin sensitivity. *Journal of Laryngology and Otology*, **91**, 837–846.

12. Samter M and Beers R F (1968). Intolerance to aspirin. Clinical studies and consideration of its pathogenesis. *Annals of Internal Medicine*, **68**, 975.

13. Sczeklik A, Gryglewski R J, Czerniawska-Mysik G (1975). Relationship of inhibition of prostaglandin biosynthesis by analgesics to asthma attacks in aspirin-sensitive patients. *British Medical Journal*, January, 67–69.

14. Bodian M. (1952). Pathology in fibrocystic disease of the pancreas. Chapter 5. *London: Heineman Medical Books* 67–146.

15. Lurie H. (1959). Cystic fibrosis of the pancreas and the nasal mucosa. *Annals of Otology, Rhinology and Laryngology.* **68**, 478.

16. Drake-Lee AB, Pitcher Willmott R. (1982). The clinical and laboratory correlates of nasal polyps in cystic fibrosis. *International Journal of Paediatric Otolaryngology.* **4**, 209–214.

17. Taylor M. (1963). Histochemical studies on nasal polyps. *Journal of Laryngology and Otology*, **77**, 326–341.

18. Donovan R, Johansson SGO, Bernich H, Soothill J P (1970). Immunoglobulins in nasal polyp fluid. *International Archives of Allergy and Applied Immunology*, **37**, 154–166.

19. Drake-Lee A B, McLaughlan P. (1982). Clinical symptoms, free histamine and IgE in patients with nasal polyps. *International Archives of Allergy and Applied Immunology*, **69**, 268–271.

20. Salari H, Borgeat P, Steffenrud S, Richard J, Bedard P, Hebert J, Pelletier G. (1986). Immunological and non-immunological release of leukotrienes and histamine from human nasal polyps. *Clinical and Experimental Immunology* **63**, 711–7.

21. Nigam S, Kunkel G, Herold D, Baumer F, Jusuf L. (1986). Nasal polyps and their content of arachidonic acid metabolites. *N Engl Reg Allergy Proc* **7**, 109–12.

22. Smith D, Gerrard J, White J. (1987). Comparison of arachidonic acid metabolites in nasal polyps and eosinophils. *International Archives of Allergy and Applied Immunology* **82**, 83–88.

23. Jung T, Juhn S, Hwang D, Stewart R. (1987). Prostaglandins, leukotrienes and other arachidonic acid metabolites in nasal polyps and nasal mucosa. *Laryngoscope* **97**, 184–189.

24. Cauna N, Hindover K H, Manzethi G W, Swanson E W (1972). Fine structure of nasal polyps. *Annals of Otolaryngology*, **81**, 41–58.

25. Drake-Lee A B, Barker THW, Thurley K (1984). Nasal polyps II. Fine structure of mast cells. *Journal of Laryngology and Otology*, **98**, 285–292

26. Sasaki Y, Nakahara H. (1989). Granule core loss in eosinophils from a patient with aspirin induced asthma: an electron microscope study. *Ann Allergy* **63,** 306–8.

27. Linder A, Karlsson-Parra A, Hirvela C, Jonsson L, Koling A, Sjoberg O. (1993). Immunocompetent cells in human nasal polyps and normal mucosa. *Rhinology* **31** 125–129.

28. Liu C, Shun C, Hsu M. (1994). Lymphocyte subsets and antigen-specific IgE in nasal polyps. *Annals of Allergy* **72** 19–24.

29. Drake-Lee A B, McLaughlan P. (1988). The release of histamine from nasal polyp tissue and peripheral blood when challenged with anithuman IgE, house dust mite extract and mixed grass pollen extract and compared with positive skin tests. *Journal of Laryngology and Otology.* **102,** 886–889.

30. Mygind N, Ullman S, Weeke B (1975). Quantitative determination of immunoglobulins in nasal secretions. *International Archives of Allergy and Applied Immunology* **49,** 99–107.

31. John A C and Merrett T G (1979). The radioallergosorbent test (RAST) in nasal polyposis. *Journal of Laryngology and Otology,* **93,** 889–898.

32. Majumdar B and Bull PD (1982). The incidence of maxillary sinusitis in nasal polyposis. *Journal of Laryngology and Otology,* **96,** 937–941.

33. Dawes P, Bates G, Watson D, Lewis D, Lowe D, Drake-Lee A. (1989). The role of bacterial infection of the maxillary sinus in nasal polyps. *Clinical Otolaryngology* **14** 447–450.

34. Dunnette S, Hall M, Washington J, Kern E, McDonald T, Facer G, Gleich G. (1986). *Journal of Allergy and Clinical Immunology* **78,** 102–8

35. Calenoff E, Guilford T, Green J, Engelhard C. (1983). Bacterial specific IgE in patients with nasal polyps. *Archives of Otolaryngology* **109** 372–375.

36. Calenioff E, McMahan J, Herzon G, Kern R, Ghadge G, Hanson D. (1993). Bacterial allergy in nasal polyps. A new method of quantifying specific IgE. *Archives of Otolaryngology* **119** 830–836.

37. Baenkler H, Schaubschlager W, Behnsen H. (1983). Antigen induced histamine release from the mucosa in nasal polyposis. *Clinical Otolaryngology* **8** 227–230.

38. Jackson R J and Arihood S A (1971). The acid mucopolysaccharides and collagen content of human nasal polyps, and perinasal nasal mucosa. *Annals Of Otolaryngology,* **80,** 586–592.

39. Tos M, Morgensen C. (1977). Pathogenesis of nasal polyps. *Rhinology* **15** 87–95.

40. Lloyd GAS (1990). CT of the paranasal sinuses: study if a control series in relation to endoscopic sinus surgery. *Journal of Laryngology and Otology* **104,** 477–481.

41. White P, Cowan I, Robertson M. (1991). Limited CT scanning techniques of the paranasal sinuses. *Journal of Laryngology and Otology* **105,** 20–23.

42. Larsen K, Tos M. (1994). Clinical course of patients with primary nasal polyps. *Acta Otolaryngologica* **114** 556–559.

42. Lund V J and Lloyd GAS (1983). Radiological changes associated with benign nasal polyps. *Journal of Laryngology and Otology,* **97,** 503–510.

Chapter IX

Early Stages of Polyp Formation

Mirko Tos, M.D., Ph.D.

ABSTRACT

In 1977 we described the epithelial rupture theory on formation of nasal polyps[24,27]. We postulated that polyp formation can start with a rupture of the epithelium caused by pressure from the edematous and infiltrated lamina propria. The lamina propria protrudes through the epithelial defect and the mucosa tends to cover it by migration of the epithelium from the edges of the defect. If the regeneration of the epithelium does not occur soon enough to cover the prolapse, or if the prolapse of the lamina propria continues to grow, the polyp will be formed and the vessel stalk established. During the early growth of the polyp some special long tubulous glands are found. These glands have a completely different structure, shape and size than the nasal seromucous glands and are a definitive proof that the polyp is not a prolapse or protrusion of the nasal or sinus mucosa.

The polyp pathogenesis is divided into the following stages: 1) Epithelial damage, necrosis and rupture due to tissue pressure by inflammatory edema and infiltration of the cells of the nasal mucosa leading to a prolapse of the lamina propria. 2) Epithelialization of the prolapse. 3) Gland formation. 4) Enlargement due to gravity with elongation of the glands. 5) Changes of the epithelium and stroma of the well-developed polyp.

The first two stages are difficult to prove in the human nose, but experimentally we have been able to demonstrate, in three different models, including experimental acute otitis and long term tubal occlusion, that the epithelial necrosis in fact takes place during the infection. These experiments are briefly described.

Pathogenesis of nasal polyps explains how polyps form. It is related to the etiology which is multifactorial. Neither pathogenesis nor etiology are fully clarified, although several etiological factors, such as chronic infection[1], allergy[2], aspirin idiosyncrasy with abnormal response of the vascular bed[3,4], nasal mastocytosis[5] and cystic fibrosis[6,7] as well as air flow blockage are important in the development of nasal polyps.

PATHOGENETIC THEORIES AND NASAL POLYPS

During the last century several pathogenetic theories of nasal polyp formation have been published[8–16], all are based upon the presence of edema of the mucosa, several upon the presence of mucous glands and gland cysts in the polyps. A critical analysis of the pathogenetic theories[16] reveals that all published theories are based on investigation of "grown out" polyps removed at surgery and none on investigation of the nasal mucosa at the time of polyp formation. Furthermore no theory explains why a polyp may occur in one particular place in the nose, and not in another.

Studying the glands in nasal polyps allowed us to apply a completely new view on pathogenesis of nasal polyps. We have found special long tubulous mucous glands (Fig. 1) running along the surface of the nasal polyps[17,18]. These glands have a completely different structure, shape and size from the nasal seromucous glands[19]. They must have formed during formation of the nasal polyp, strongly indicating that the nasal polyps are not just a prolapse of the nasal mucosa or of the nasal epithelium, as indicated in previous theories. Besides the long glands, other shapes of tubulous glands have been found (Fig. 2), such as small simple tubulous glands, branched tubulous glands and long branched tubulous glands also named "cork screw-like" glands. All these glands are formed during the process of polyp formation by division of the epithelial basal cells, producing a solid cylinder subepithellialy followed by duct formation, further division and growth of the gland. The shape and development of long "cork screw-like" gland illustrates their origin from the polyp epithelium being influenced

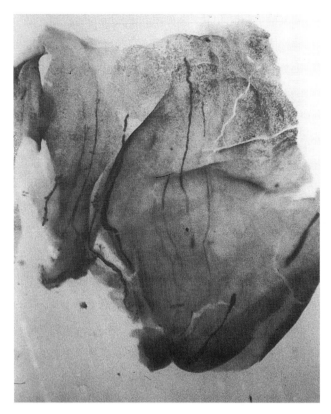

Figure 1. Several long tubulous glands in a nasal polyp. The glands are arranged parallel with top the stalk–top axis of the polyp. Stalk is superior. PAS alcian blue whole mount × 20.

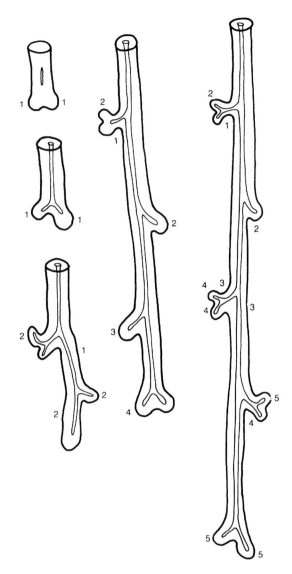

Figure 3. Development and growth pattern of a "cork screw-like" gland influenced by growth and elongation of the polyp during the generation of dichotomous divisions of the gland. A solid cylinder with incipient duct formation and first dichotomous division (1) into two side-ducts. One of the side-ducts elongates and grows faster than the other, resulting in an asymmetrical gland. During the second dichotomous division into two side-ducts (2) and during the third (3) fourth (4) and fifth (5) divisions the same phenomenon is taking place, resulting in the "cork screw-like" shape of the gland.

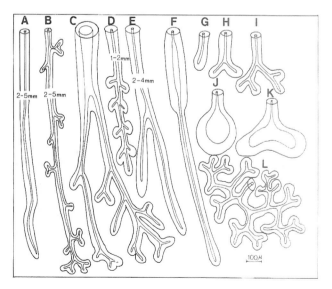

Figure 2. Schematic illustration of various shapes of tubulous glands in nasal polyps. A-F) Long tubulous. G-I) short tubulous glands. B) "cork screw-like" gland.

by the growth of the polyp (Fig. 3). The density, distribution and structure of the nasal glands from the lateral wall of the middle turbinate and the middle meatus[19], which are considered the most common places of origin of nasal polyps[20–22], are completely different from the polyp glands in the following characteristic ways:

INFERIOR TURBINATE

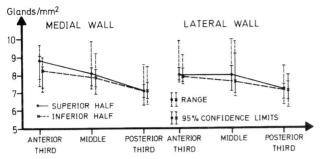

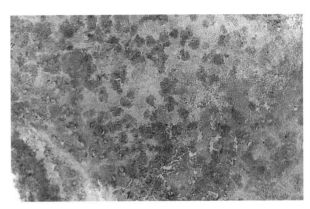

Figure 6. The superficial layer of nasal glands in the whole mount (PAS alcian blue staining).

MIDDLE TURBINATE

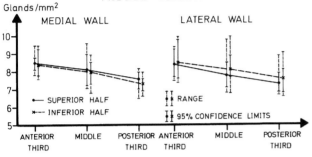

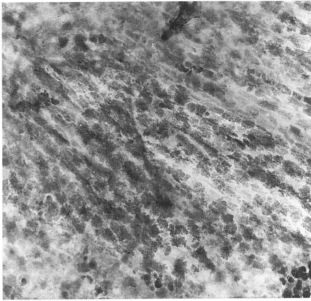

Figure 4. Density of nasal glands in the turbinates from 10 normal human adults.

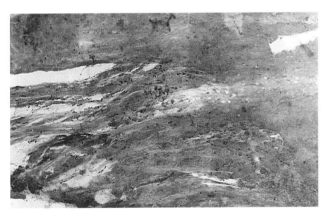

Figure 7. The deep layer of the nasal glands seen in the whole mount (PAS staining).

Figure 5. Distribution of gland ostia in the middle turbinate mucosa in the whole mount. Ostia are visible as small holes or small rings.

1) *Density of glands* in the middle turbinate mucosa is high, 7 glands/mm^2 (Fig. 4). In most nasal polyps it is much lower, less than 0.2 glands/mm^2.

2) *Distribution of the ostia of nasal glands* on the surface of the turbinate mucosa is regular whereas (Fig. 5) on the polyp surface only a few ostia are visible, simply because there are only few glands.

3) *Distribution of the gland mass* in the nasal mucosa is regular in two layers, the superficial and the deep layer (Figs. 6, 7). In the nasal polyps the few glands are irregularly distributed, although the long tubulous glands run along the polyp axis (Fig. 1), but they do not originate in the polyp stalk region.

4) *Shape and structure of the glands.* The nasal glands are tubulo-alveolar consisting of a main duct and two side ducts, connecting several tubules and ending in several seromucous acini (Fig. 8). The nasal polyp glands are tubulous glands with long and small tubules each with one or two divisions, thus differing completely from the nasal glands (Figs. 1–3).

Since most pathogenetic theories are based on a prolapse of edematous nasal mucosa, the nasal tubulo-alveolar glands should be found in the nasal polyps. Thus in the mucosal exudate theory of Hayek[9], further elaborated by Eggston and Wolff[23], edema, associated with

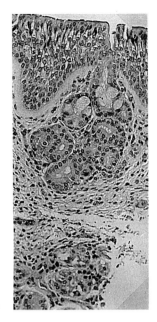

A

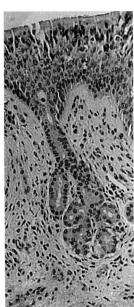

B

Figure 8. Structure of nasal glands in two neighbouring sections. The gland consists of the main duct and two side-ducts with several tubuli and acini. A) This shows mainly the side-duct with tubuli and acini. B) The main duct. (Haematoxylin-eosin).

exudate localized deep in the nasal mucosa (Fig. 9A) should push the mucosa caudally as a polyp. The nasal glands should therefore be visible on the superior surface of the polyp (Fig. 9B), which is definitely not the case. In none of the investigated 105 polyps[17] the glands were found at the superior surface of the polyp. In case of edema occurring centrally in the mucosa, between the two layers of glands (Fig. 9C), causing prolapse of the

superficial layer of the mucosa, such a layer should be found in the top of the polyp, which is not the case. In the case of subepithelial edema of the mucosa (Fig. 9D), leading to protrusion and prolapse of the epithelium, the extended glands tubules should be found within the polyp. The tubules should have connection to the gland mass in the base of the polyp. We have not found any such structures in the nasal polyps[17].

EPITHELIAL RUPTURE THEORY

Since none of the published pathogenetic theories could explain the histopathology of the nasal polyp glands, we presented in 1977[20] the "epithelial rupture theory" or "new gland formation" theory. We postulated that polyp formation can start with a rupture of the epithelium caused by tissue pressure from the edematous and infiltrated lamina propria. The lamina propria protrudes through the epithelial defect (Fig. 10A), and the mucosa tends to cover it by migration of the epithelium from the edges of the defect (Fig. 10B). If the regeneration of the epithelium does not occur soon enough to cover the prolapse, if epithelial covering is not sufficient, or if the prolapse of lamina propria continues to enlarge, a polyp will be formed and the vascular stalk established (Fig. 10C). The author believes that epithelial defects are not uncommon during inflammation or infection of the nasal mucosa, but the vast majority of the defects are soon covered by epithelium during the healing process, with no further consequences.

If a small polyp with a stalk is established, it may remain, even if complete re-epithelialization has taken place (Fig. 10D). The polyp may grow further, mainly due to the gravity (Fig. 10E).

During the epithelialization and growth of the polyp, the previously described and characteristic tubulous glands form (Fig. 10D), strongly indicating that nasal polyps are not just a prolapse of the nasal mucosa or epithelium.

EARLY STAGES OF POLYP FORMATION

To understand this theory of polyp pathogenesis we have divided polyp formation into several stages, the first three being the early stages. They have been further documented in three experimental studies which we have conducted in rat middle ear:

1) Epithelial damage, necrosis and rupture due to tissue pressure by inflammatory edema and infiltration of the cells of the nasal mucosa at the site of the polyp formation, leading to a prolapse of the lamina propria (Figs. 10A and B).
2) Epithelialization of the prolapse (Figs. 10B and C).
3) Gland formation (Fig. 10D).

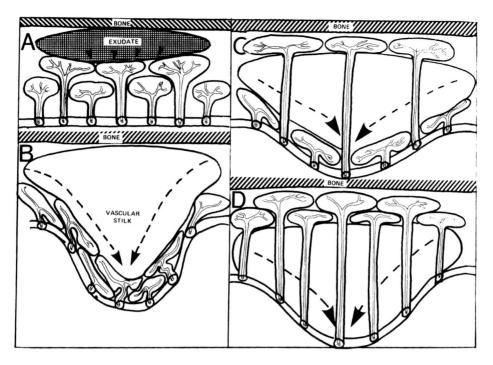

Figure 9. Schematically illustration of the mucosal exudate theory and hypothetical appearance of glands in nasal polyps if they were formed as a prolapse of the nasal mucosa caused by exudate[9,23]. A) Exudate deep in the nasal mucosa, B) displacing the nasal glands outwards (arrows). C) Exudate between the deep and superficial glandular layers, pushing the glands outwards (arrows). D) Edema predominantly subepithelially.

4) Enlargement due to gravity and elongation of the glands (Fig. 10E).
5) Changes of the epithelium and stroma of the well-developed polyp, such as transformation of pseudostratified to stratified epithelium, changes of density of goblet and ciliary cell, changes of cell infiltration, edema and vascularity of the stroma.

The first stage of polyp formation, the epithelial rupture, is difficult to prove histologically, particularly in a human nose. This stage is of short duration, and it is impossible to obtain biopsies from the appropriate locality of the nose at the correct time, which is in the very beginning of polyp formation. Experimental polyp formation is, however, described in rabbits with acute maxillary sinusitis, infected with Streptococcus pneumoniae[1,25] causing localized epithelial defects and epithelial necrosis. Proliferation of the fibroblasts through the defects were already found after the beginning of the infection, and fully developed polyps could be found 3–4 weeks later. The epithelialization of the polyp as we indicated nearly 20 years ago[24] has thus been verified by these studies. Furthermore it has been demonstrated in rabbits with experimental sinusitis that epithelial necrosis and defects are common features and the resultant prolapse of fibrous tissue which occurs as a conse-

quence of this infection will most often be covered by newly formed epithelium.

Epithelial necrosis and polyp formation are common histologic findings in the middle ear mucosa. Experiments of tubal occlusion in rats have shown polyp-like protrusions of the modified respiratory middle ear epithelium[26]. Further studies on the initial stages of polyp formation in rat middle ear after experimental long-term tubal occlusion have demonstrated epithelialization of polyps which originally lacked epithelial covering[27]. In 65 rats the Eustachian tube was occluded on the left side for up to 20 months while the right, unoccluded ear served as a control. Signs of initial polyp formation (Fig. 11) or fully developed polyps (Fig. 12) were seen in 14 middle ears (22%). The polyps were only seen in middle ears with signs of actual or previous infection. It was established in this middle ear experiment that the first stages of polyp formation include epithelial rupture, proliferation of fibrous tissue through the epithelial defect and complete epithelialization of prolapsed fibrous tissue by proliferation and migration of epithelial cells from the surrounding epithelium. The trigger for polyp formation was in this material exudate and the inflammatory cells that accumulated in the middle ear cavity (Fig. 11). A similar trigger may be one of the causes of nasal polyp formation.

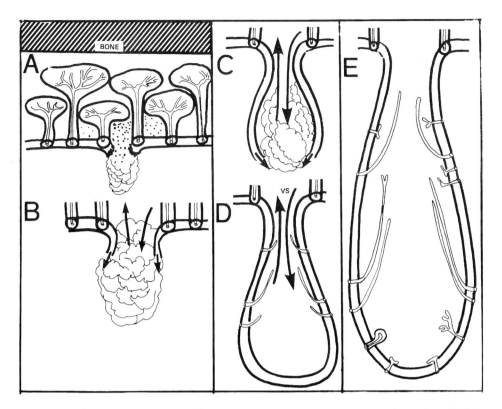

Figure 10. Schematic illustration of the epithelial rupture theory of polyp formation. A) Cellular infiltration and edema of the inflammed nasal mucosa, causing the epithelial defect with protrusion of lamina propria, containing inflammatory cells. B) Initial epithelialization of the protruded tissue from the edges of the epithelial defect (small arrows). C) Establishment of the vascular stalk (large arrows) of a small, nearly fully epithelialized polyp (small arrows). D) Growth of the polyp and formation of new glands - glands being elongated. The glands are becoming stretched and elongated. E) Further growth and elongation of the glands during growth of the polyp.

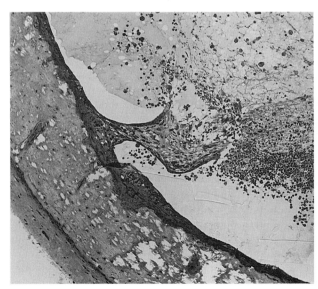

Figure 11. Initial, partly epithelialized polyp protruding into the middle ear cavity after 17 months tubal occlusion, to eliminate the inflammatory exudate from the cavity.

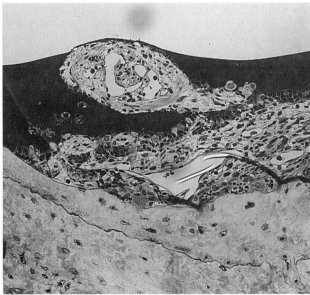

Figure 12. A fully epithelialized polyp in the middle ear after 20 months of tubal occlusion.

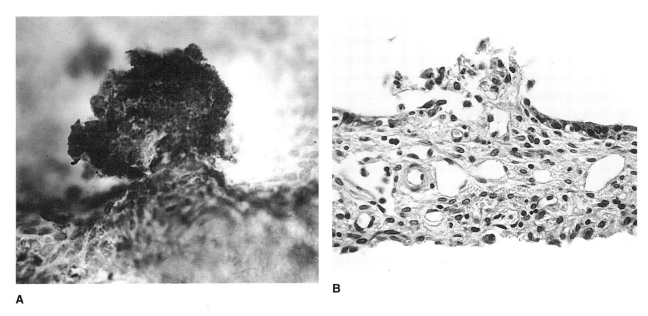

Figure 13. A) Small polypoid prominence seen in a whole mount × 400. B) Section of the same polyp as shown in A, illustrating epithelial rupture, incipient prolapse of the fibrous tissue from the lamina propria and re-epithelialization × 400.

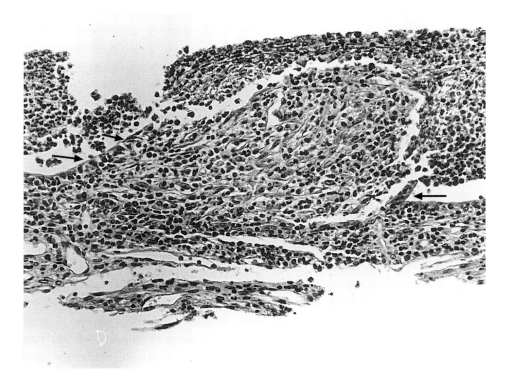

Figure 14. Epithelial defect with prolapse of lamina propria infiltrated by inflammatory cells and incipient re-epithelialization (arrows) × 200.

In a third experiment study 25 rat middle ears were infected with pneumococcus type 3, causing an acute otitis, initial polyp formation was found in 15 ears[28]. We have clearly demonstrated that polyp formation starts with epithelial defect, with protrusion of the lamina propria, containing luminally migrating inflammatory cells, stromal cells and fibrous components (Figs. 13 and 14). Epithelial microruptures were seen in serial sections from days 4 and 18 after inoculation, the microrupture was found adjacent to neutrophils lying just under and between the cells of the epithelial lining. At other localities large epithelial defects with protrusion of lamina propria were seen (Fig. 13). In some instances this polypoid protrusion showed signs of incipient or advanced re-epithelialization (Fig. 14).

Thus our experiments have histologically substantiated the epithelial rupture theory of polyp formation. Even if there may be several other causes of polyp formation with various pathogeneses, the epithelial rupture with prolapse of the lamina propria and re-epithelialization of the prolapse, is the most common pathogenesis of early polyp formation with an inflammatory aetiology.

LITERATURE

1. Nordlander T, Fukami M, Westrin KM, Stierna P, Carlsöö B. Formation of mucosal polyps in the nasal and maxillary sinus cavities by infection. Otolaryngol Head Neck Surg 1993; 109:522–529.
2. Settipane GA, Klein DE, Settipane RJ. Nasal polyps: state of the art. Rhinology 1991;(Suppl)11:33.
3. Pepys J, Duveen G E. Negative skin tests in allergic rhinitis and nasal polyposis. Int Arch Allergy 1951;2/2:147–160.
4. Caplin I, Haynes J T, Spahn J. Are nasal polyps an allergic phenomenon? Ann Allergy 1971;29:631.
5. McKenna EL. Nasal mastocytosis. Laryngoscope 1974;84:112–125
6. Schramm VL Jr, Effron MZ. Nasal polyps in children. Laryngoscope 1980;90/9:1488–1495.
7. Tos M. Cystic fibrosis (Mucoviscidosis). In: English CM (ed) Otolaryngology. Harper and Row (Philadelphia) 1985;Vol.2;Chapt.49.
8. Woakes E. Über nekrotisierende Ethmoiditis und ihre Beziehung zur Entwicklung von Nasenpolyppen. Brit Med J 1885;4:701–705.
9. Hajek M. Über die pathologischen Veränderunen der Siebbein-Knochen im Gefolge der entzündlichen Schleimhauthypertrophie unter der Nasenpolypen. Arch Laryng Rhinol 1986;4:277–300.
10. Yonge ES. Observations on the determing cause of the formation of nasal polypi Brit Med J 1907;12:964–968.
11. Jenkins J. Blockade theory of polyp formation. Laryngoscope 1932;42:703–704.
12. Krajina Z. A contribution to the aetiopathogenesis of nasal polyps. Pact Oto-Rhino-Laryng 1963;25:241–246.
13. Rulon JT, Brown HA, Logan GB. Nasal polyps and cystic fibrosis of the pancreas. Arch Otolaryng 1963;78:192–199.
14. Takasaka T, Kaku Y, Hozawa K. Mast cell degranulation in nasal polyps Acta Otolaryngol (Stockh) 1986;suppl. 430:39–48.
15. Sasaki C. Distribution of the degranulated and non-degranulated mast cells in nasal polyp. Acta Otolaryngol (Stockh) 1986;430:34–38.
16. Tos M. The pathogenetic theories on formation of nasal polyps. Am J Rhinol 1990;4:51–56.
17. Tos M, Mogensen C. Mucous glands in nasal polyps. Arch Otolaryngol 1977;103:407–413.
18. Tos M, Mogensen C, Thomsen J. Nasal polyps in cystic fibrosis. J Otol 1977;91:827–835.
19. Tos M, Mogensen C. Density of mucous glands in normal adult nasal turbinates. Arch Oto-Rhino-Laryng 1977;215:101–111.
20. Larsen P, Tos M. Origination of nasal polyps. Laryngoscope 1991;101:305–312.
21. Tos M, Larsen PL. Origin of nasal polyps. Am J Rhinol 1994;8:297–298
22. Larsen PL, Tos M. Anatomic site of origin of nasal polyps. Endoscopic nasal and paranasal sinus surgery as a screening method for nasal polyps in an autopsy material. Am J Rhinol 1996;10:211–216.
23. Eggston A A, Wolff D. Histopathology of the ear, nose and throat. Williams and Wilkens, Baltimore, 1947.
24. Tos M, Mogensen C. Pathogenesis of nasal polyps Int Rhinology 1977;15:87–95
25. Westrin KM, Stierna P, Kumlien J, Carlsöö B, Nord CE. Induction, course and recovery of maxillary sinusitis: a bacteriological and histological study in rabbits. Am J Rhinol 1990;4:61–64.
26. Larsen PL, Tos M. Polyp formation by experimental tubal occlusion in the rat. Acta Otolaryngol (Stockh) 1991;111:926–933.
27. Larsen PL, Tos M, Kuijpers W, van der Beek JMH. The early stages of polyp formation. Laryngoscope 1992;102:670–677.
28. Cayé-Thomasen P, Hermansson A, Tos M, Prellner K. Polyp Pathogenesis - A histopathological Study in Experimental Otitis Media. Acta Otolaryngol (Stockh) 1995;115:76–82.

Chapter X

Basic Sinus Imaging and Radiological Aspects of Nasal Polyposis

Patrick J. Oliverio, M.D., Mark L. Benson, M.D., and S. James Zinreich, M.D.*

ABSTRACT

Coronal CT scanning is the imaging modality of choice in patients with sinus disease. CT scanning provides an initial screening of these patients and can display both anatomy and pathology both before and after surgery. CT is essential in surgical planning, and it provides an operative "roadmap". Close cooperation between the radiologist and otolaryngologist-head & neck surgeon allows for more accurate diagnosis and brings to light findings predisposing the patient to operative complications. When complications occur, the radiologist can provide assistance in evaluation using CT, MR, and nuclear medicine studies. Interactive image guided-computer assisted surgery now exists and holds great promise in objectively and directly integrating the imaging information with the endoscopic view and thus improve the accuracy and safety of the operative management of patients undergoing sinus surgery.

INTRODUCTION AND HISTORICAL PERSPECTIVE

Inflammatory sinus disease is a serious health problem, affecting an estimated 30-50 million people in the United States alone[1]. Because the physical examination can be nonspecific in these patients, radiologic evaluation has been relied upon for many years in the diagnosis of paranasal sinus pathology. Traditionally, conventional radiography was the modality of choice in the evaluation of the paranasal sinuses. In recent years, however, due to technologic advance in imaging and a change in the therapeutic approach, computed tomography has supplanted conventional radiography as the primary diagnostic modality.

While most patients are initially medically treated, medical therapy alone often does not resolve the problem. With the advent of Functional Endoscopic Sinus Surgery (FESS) the surgical treatments of refractory inflammatory sinus disease have undergone revolutionary changes. These changes are due to the combination of several factors: 1. An improved understanding of the mucociliary clearance pathways in the nasal cavity and paranasal sinuses. 2. Improved endoscopes which afford direct access to nasal cavity and ethmoid sinus drainage portals. 3. The availability of high resolution coronal CT images which provide an accurate display of the regional anatomy.

Our objective in this chapter is to: discuss the available imaging modalities for patients with inflammatory sinus disease and nasal polyposis, describe the pertinent radiographic anatomy and anatomic variants of the paranasal sinuses, review the radiographic appearance of inflammatory sinus disease and its complications (including nasal polyposis), and to discuss the expected radiographic appearance in post-operative patients, as well as the appearance of complications that can occur as a result of surgery.

TECHNIQUES OF EVALUATION

Conventional Radiography

The standard radiographic sinus series consists of four views: lateral view, Caldwell view, Waters view, and submentovertex (SMV or base) view[7]. The lateral view demonstrates the bony perimeter of the frontal, maxillary, and sphenoid sinus. The Caldwell view displays the bony perimeter of the frontal sinus. The Waters view will display the outlines of the maxillary sinuses, some of anterior ethmoid air cells, and orbital outline. The submentovertex view can evaluate the sphenoid sinus as well as the anterior and posterior walls of the frontal sinuses.

*S. James Zinreich, M.D. is a grant recipient and consultant for ISG Technologies.

Standard radiographs may be accurate in showing air/fluid levels in the frontal, maxillary, and sphenoid sinus, but they significantly underestimate the degree of chronic inflammatory disease present. Further, the superimposition of fine bony structures precludes the accurate evaluation of the anatomy of the ostiomeatal channels.[6,8-11]

Computed Tomography (CT)

CT is currently the modality of choice in the evaluation of the paranasal sinuses and adjacent structures[6,8-11]. Its ability to optimally display bone, soft tissue, and air facilitates accurate depiction of anatomy and extent of disease in and around the paranasal sinuses[6,8-11]. In contrast to standard radiographs, CT is able to clearly depict the fine bony anatomy of the ostiomeatal channels.

Many authors stress the importance of performing the initial CT scan after a course of adequate medical therapy to eliminate changes of mucosal inflammation and to better evaluate the underlying anatomic structures. Several authors also suggest routine pretreatment with a sympathomimetic nasal spray 15 minutes prior to scanning to reduce nasal congestion[12]. This will minimize the mucosal edema and will allow an improved display of the fine bony architecture.

Imaging in the coronal plane is recommended. The coronal plane optimally displays the ostiomeatal unit, the relationship of the brain and ethmoid roof, and it depicts the relationship of the orbits to the paranasal sinuses[6,8-11]. Coronal images correlate with the surgical approach and, therefore, should be obtained in all patients with inflammatory sinus disease who are surgical candidates[7].

The patient is placed prone, with the chin hyperextended, on the bed of the CT scanner. The scanner gantry is angled to be as perpendicular as possible to the hard palate (Fig. 1). The angulation of the scan plane is very important. Melhem et al showed that variations in angulation greater than 10° from the plane perpendicular result in significant loss of anatomic detail of the structures of the ostiomeatal unit[13].

Scanning is performed from the anterior wall of the frontal sinus through the posterior wall of the sphenoid sinus. **Contiguous** 3mm thick images are obtained. It is important to scan with contiguous images to avoid loss of information through "skipped" areas[13]. The field of view is adjusted to include only the areas of interest. This helps reduce artifact from the teeth and associated metallic restorations, as well as, magnifying the small structures of the nasal cavity and adjacent paranasal sinuses[9].

In patients who cannot tolerate prone positioning (children, patients of advanced age), the "hanging head" technique can sometimes be utilized. Here, the patient is placed in the supine position and the neck maximally extended. The CT gantry is angled to be as perpendicular as

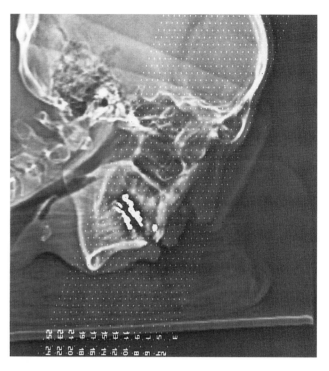

Figure 1. Scout radiograph for coronal CT of the paranasal sinuses. The plane of scanning is perpendicular to the hard palate.

possible to the bony palate. However, it is not always possible to obtain direct coronal images with this technique.

In patients who are intubated or have tracheostomy sites, it is not technically feasible to position them for coronal scans. Also, young children, patients with severe cervical arthropathy, and patients who are otherwise debilitated usually will not tolerate the examination. In such patients, thin section, contiguous axial images with coronal reconstructions are performed.

Originally, the exposure settings for sinus CT were: kVp of 125 and mAs of 450 (5 second scan time). Babbel et al[12] showed that there was no compromise of the images when the mAs was reduced to 200 (2 second scan time), while recent work of Melhem et al[13] showed no significant loss of diagnostic quality with mAs settings of 160 or even 80 (2 second scan time for both). We therefore recommend exposure settings of 125 kVp and 80-160 mAs.

A full discussion of radiation dosimetry and the biologic effects of medical radiation is beyond the scope of this chapter. Suffice it to say that for a given examination, radiation dose equivalent is dependant on the kVp and mAs. For a given kVp, radiation dose equivalent will vary linearly with the mAs. At 125 kVp, the radiation dose equivalent for a CT slice is approximately 1.1-1.2 cSv/100 mAs (1.1-1.2 rem/100 mAs). The actual dose will vary slightly from machine to machine. The radiation dose equivalent for a CT slice can be considerably reduced using low mAs technique and, the effective dose to the patient will be less than the radiation dose equivalent received by the area scanned[14,15].

CT windows are chosen to highlight the air passages, the bony detail, and the soft tissues. Our experience shows that a window width of +2000 Houndsfield Units (HU) with a level of −200 HU is the best starting point. The potentiometers can then be manually manipulated to optimally display the anatomic detail of the uncinate process and ethmoid bulla. This same setting is then used to film the entire study[6,8-11].

Axial reconstructions can be helpful in displaying the position of the internal carotid arteries and optic nerves with respect to the bony margins of the posterior ethmoid and sphenoid sinuses.

Magnetic Resonance Imaging (MR)

While MR imaging provides better visualization of soft tissue than CT,[9,10] its disadvantage is its inability to display cortical bone. Since both cortical bone and air have no mobile protons, they yield no MR signal. This results in an inability to discern the intricate anatomic relationships of the sinuses and their drainage portals. Thus MR imaging cannot be reliably used as a operative "roadmap".

There is a reciprocal cyclic variation in the thickness of the nasal mucosa known as the "nasal cycle". The signal intensity of the mucosal lining of the nasal cavity and ethmoid sinuses varies in concert with the nasal cycle[17,18]. During the edematous phase of the nasal cycle the mucosal signal intensity on T2-weighted images (T2WI) in these two areas is similar to the appearance of mucosal inflammation[11,12] and this limits the usefulness of MR imaging. Interestingly, there is no cyclic variation of the mucosal signal in the frontal, maxillary, or sphenoid sinuses. Increased mucosal thickness and increased signal on T2WI is always abnormal[17,18].

To date, with respect to sinus imaging, MR imaging has proven most helpful in the evaluation of regional and intracranial complications of inflammatory sinus disease and their surgical treatment, detection of neoplastic processes, and an improved display of anatomic relationships between the intra and extraorbital compartments. For example, MR imaging is helpful in diagnosing fungal concretions, as they often demonstrate low signal/signal void on T2WI[19-22]. MR is also useful in the evaluation of mucoceles and cephaloceles[23].

When evaluating the paranasal sinuses with MR imaging, our standard protocol includes sagittal and axial T1-weighted images (T1WI) and axial T2WI. Following the intravenous administration of Gadolinium-diethylenetriaminepentaacetic acid (DTPA), axial and coronal T1WI may be obtained.

SYSTEMATIC READING PATTERN OF CT SCANS

Normal Anatomy

An understanding of the anatomy of the lateral nasal wall and its relationship to adjacent structures is essential[26-28] (Fig. 2) and in interpreting a CT scan of the sinuses, it is helpful to utilize the systematic approach. We favor reading from anterior to posterior and as one reads the study, a mental "check list" of important structures should be made. The reading pattern includes three steps:

I. *Identify and describe the important structures of the nose and paranasal sinuses, and their anatomic variants.* A radiological report should mention the status of the following structures on both the right and left side.

Frontal Sinus	Uncinate process
Frontal recess	Infundibulum
Agger nasi region & anterior ethmoidal sinuses	Maxillary sinus
Ethmoid Roof	Middle meatus
Ethmoid bulla	Nasal septum & turbinates
Ground lamella of middle turbinates	Posterior ethmoidal sinuses
Lateral sinus	Sphenoid sinus

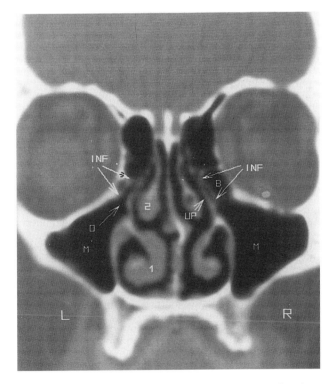

Figure 2. Coronal CT image of the ostiomeatal unit: ethmoid bulla (B), infundibulum (INF), uncinate process (UP), maxillary sinus (M), inferior turbinate (1), and middle turbinate (2). A small spur of the nasal septum with associated deviation of the nasal septum is noted.

Anatomic variant

Even though the nasal anatomy varies significantly from patient to patient, certain anatomic variations are observed commonly in the general population and are often seen more frequently in patients with chronic inflammatory disease in which the anatomic variant may play a role by virtue of obstruction to sinus drainage[6,8–10,24,35–39].

Concha bullosa
Nasal septal deviation
Paradoxic middle turbinate
Variations in the uncinate process, e.g. atelectatic, everted.
Haller cells
Onodi cells
Giant ethmoid bulla
Extensive pneumatization of the sphenoid sinus
Medial deviation and/or dehiscence of the laminar papyracea
Pneumatization of the posterior nasal septum

It should also be remembered that congenital abnormalities such as an encephalocele may be present[40] (Fig 3).

II. *Evaluate the critical relationships.* In addition to describing findings related to the diagnosis of inflammatory sinus disease, it is important for the radiologist to evaluate several critical areas that aid in surgical planning. The symmetry of the ethmoid roof should be noted. Discrepant heights of the ethmoid roof may lead to inadvertent penetration of the cranial vault if not recognized prior to FESS[41].

Careful attention should be paid to the status of the lamina papyracea, and any dehiscence or excessive medial deviation of this bone should be reported. The relationship of the sphenoid sinus and posterior ethmoid air cells with the internal carotid artery and optic nerves should be clearly mentioned. Findings that put either of these structures at increased risk during endoscopic surgery should be conveyed to the referring surgeon. In particular, extensive expansion of the sinuses around the internal carotid artery or the optic nerve as well as bony dehiscences adjacent to either structure should be noted. The incidence of bony dehiscence around the presellar and juxtasellar portions of the internal carotid artery ranges from 12-22%[42-44]. It is quite frequent to find the carotid canal penetrating into the aerated portion of the sphenoid sinus, and in many such cases the sphenoid sinus septations will adhere to the bony covering of the carotid canal. The surgeon needs to be aware of this variation to prevent the fracture of the sphenoid sinus septum-carotid canal junction and avoid puncturing the carotid canal.

The relationship between the posterior paranasal sinuses and the optic nerves is important to note in order to avoid operative complications. DeLano et. al. classified the relationship into four discrete categories[44]. Type 1 in-

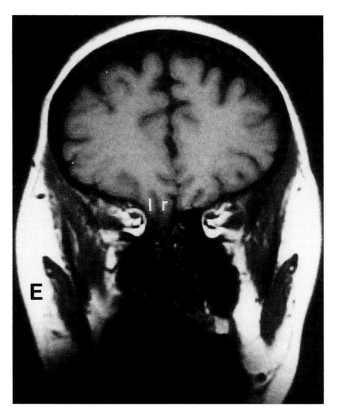

Figure 3. Coronal T1-weighted image of the brain demonstrates an encephaloceole of the right frontal lobe. Both the gyrus rectus (r) and the medial orbital gyrus (l) are seen to herniate into the paranasal sinus cavity.

cludes those optic nerves coursing immediately adjacent to the sphenoid sinus without indentation of the wall or contact with the posterior ethmoid air cell. This is the most common type, occurring in 76% of patients. Type 2 nerves course adjacent to the sphenoid sinus causing indentation of the sinus wall, without contact with the posterior ethmoid air cell. Type 3 nerves course through the sphenoid sinus with at least 50% surrounded by air. Type 4 course immediately adjacent to the sphenoid sinus and posterior ethmoid sinus. The optic nerve was dehiscent in all cases where it travelled through the sphenoid sinus (type 3) and in 82% of cases where the nerve impressed on the sphenoid sinus wall (type 2). Delano et. al. also found that 85% of optic nerves associated with a pneumatized anterior clinoid process were of type 2 or 3 configuration and 77% were dehiscent. Therefore, the presence of anterior clinoid pneumatization is an important indicator of optic nerve vulnerability during FESS due to frequent associations with both bony dehiscence as well as type 2 and 3 configurations[44].

III. *Evaluate the bony outline of the nasal cavity and paranasal sinuses.* Lastly, the "character" of the bony framework of the nasal cavity and paranasal sinuses should be evaluated. Our experience has shown that a prominent thickening of the bone surrounding the paranasal sinuses occurs, especially in patients who have undergone several surgical procedures and those with repeated exacerbations of chronic infection probably related to the underlying inflammatory process and periosteal stimulation.

Bone erosion or absence of bone may have three etiologies. 1) Bone may have been removed during a previous surgical procedure. 2) These changes may be due to the erosion secondary to a mucocele or neoplasm. The associated mass will be a clue as to the etiology and an MR imaging evaluation may afford a distinction between these two processes. 3) Bony dehisences may also be developmental and, in the absence of prior surgery and/or additional pathology, this possibility should be considered.

RADIOGRAPHIC EVALUATION OF PATIENTS FOLLOWING ENDOSCOPIC SINUS SURGERY

This systematic approach using a mental "check list" is particularly important in patients who have already undergone surgery, not only to establish persistent pathology but also to assess the extent of previous surgical interventions which place important adjacent structures at risk. Attention should particularly be paid to the following areas:

1. Frontal recess.
2. Ostiomeatal unit.
3. Lamina papyracea.
4. Ethmoidal roof.
5. Sphenoid sinus.

Chronic Sinusitis and Nasal Polyposis

Chronic sinusitis is diagnosed when the patient has repeated bouts of acute infection or persistent inflammation[35,45]. The responsible pathogens include *staphylococcus, streptococcus, corynebacteria, bacteroides, fusobacteria,* and other anaerobes[38]. Anaerobes are more commonly involved in chronic sinusitis than in acute sinusitis[35,45]. The radiographic findings are quite variable (Fig. 4, 7, 10, and 11). Signs suggestive of chronic sinusitis include mucosal thickening or opacification, bone remodeling and thickening due to osteitis from adjacent chronic mucosal inflammation, and polyposis[23,45,46]. The anterior ethmoid air cells are the most common location involved with chronic sinusitis.

Opacification of the OMU has been found to predispose to the development of sinusitis. Zinreich et al found middle meatus opacification in 72% of patients with chronic sinusitis. In this study, 65% of these patients had mucoperiosteal thickening of the maxillary sinus[6,8,9]. All of the patients with frontal sinus inflammatory disease had opacification of the frontoethmoidal recess[6,8,9].

Frontal sinus opacification involving the OMU without frontal, maxillary, or anterior ethmoid sinus inflammatory disease was rare[6,8,9]. Yousem et al. found that when the middle meatus was opacified, there were associated inflammatory changes in the ethmoid sinuses in 82% and in the maxillary sinuses in 84% of patients[39]. Bolger et al. found that when the ethmoid infundibulum was free of disease, the maxillary and frontal sinuses were clear in 77% of patients[38].

Babbel et al, reviewed 500 patients with screening sinus CT scans and defined five recurring patterns of inflammatory sinonasal disease[47]. The five anatomic patterns included: Infundibular, OMU, sphenoethmoidal recess, sinonasal polyposis, and sporadic or unclassifiable. The infundibular pattern (26% of patients) referred to focal obstruction within the maxillary sinus ostium and ethmoid infundibulum which was associated with maxillary sinus disease. The OMU pattern (25% of patients) referred to ipsilateral maxillary, frontal, and anterior ethmoid sinus disease. This pattern was due to obstruction of the middle meatus. Sparing of the frontal sinus was sometimes seen due to the variable location of the nasofrontal duct insertion in the middle meatus. The sphenoethmoidal recess pattern (6% of patients) resulted in sphenoid or posterior ethmoid sinus inflammation due to sphenoethmoidal recess obstruction. The sinonasal polyposis pattern (10% of patients) was due to diffuse nasal and paranasal sinus polyps. Associated radiographic findings included infundibular enlargement, convex (bulging) ethmoid sinus walls, and attenuation of the bony nasal septum and ethmoid trabeculae[27,47,48].

Polyps in the paranasal sinuses result from a local upheaval of the sinus mucosa with mucous membrane hyperplasia secondary to chronic inflammation (Figs. 10, 11, 12, and 13)[35,47]. If large or numerous, polyps can cause local problems due to obstruction of the important ostiomeatal channels including the sinus ostia. On CT and MR imaging, polyps are often indistinguishable from mucous retention cysts. Patients with extensive polyposis can demonstrate bony resorption and destruction (Figs. 11, 12, and 13).

When sinus secretions are acute and of low viscosity, they are of intermediate attenuation on CT images (10-25 HU). In the more chronic state, sinus secretions become thickened and concentrated, and the CT attenuation increases with density measurements of 30-60 H.U.[20].

On MR imaging, the appearance of chronic sinusitis is quite variable due to the changing concentrations of protein and free water protons[20,21]. Initially, the watery secretions appear on MR imaging as hypointense on T1WI and hyperintense on T2WI[20,21]. According to Som, when sinonasal secretions become obstructed two important physiologic events occur. Namely, the number of glycoprotein-secreting goblet cells in the mucosa increases, and the

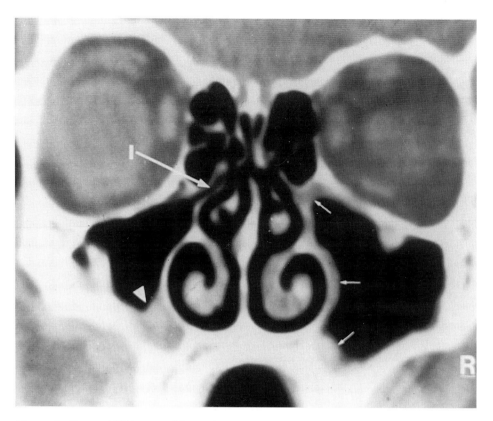

Figure 4. Coronal CT image of the ostiomeatal unit in a patient with mucoperiosteal thickening occluding the ostium of a maxillary sinus (small white arrows). This can occur in chronic inflammatory sinus disease as well as in the acute phase of inflammatory sinus disease. There is a more prominent focus of mucoperiosteal thickening in the base of the contralateral maxillary sinus (arrowhead). The infundibulum (I) of this maxillary sinus is widely patent.

mucosa resorbs free water. This results in a transition from a thin serous fluid, to a thicker mucous, and ultimately to a desiccated stone-like plug[20]. As the protein concentration increases, the signal intensity on T2WI decreases. These charges are presumably due to cross-linking that occurs between glycoprotein molecules. Som describes four patterns of MR signal intensity that can be seen with chronic sinusitis: 1. Hypointense on T1WI and hyperintense on T2WI with protein concentration less then 9%. 2. Hyperintense on T1WI and hyperintense on T2WI with total protein concentration increased to 20-25%. 3. Hyperintense on T1WI and hypointense on T2WI with total protein concentration of 25-30%. 4. Hypointense on T1WI and T2WI with protein concentration >30% and inspissated secretions in an almost solid form[7,20]. A potential pitfall exists on MR imaging of inspissated secretions (i.e. those with protein concentrations over 30%) since the signal voids on T1 and T2 WI may look identical to normally aerated sinuses[20,21].

Fungal Sinusitis

Fungal sinusitis may be suspected clinically when the patient fails to respond to standard antibiotic therapy.

While fungal infection in the paranasal sinuses is uncommon, the fungal pathogens most commonly encountered are *Aspergillus* species, *mucormycosis,* and *Candida* species[29,39]. Although mucormycosis and aspergillus are both part of the normal respiratory flora[35], their involvement in the paranasal sinuses can often be differentiated on clinical grounds. Aspergillus sinusitis usually occurs in an otherwise healthy patient in a noninvasive, saprophytic form. Allergic fungal sinusitis is usually seen in patients with a history of atopy and/or asthma. There is an association between this entity and marked nasal and sinus polyposis. This process may expand the sinuses bordering the orbits, thus causing proptosis or optic nerve compression[51]. The invasive form of aspergillus infection can occur in immunocompromised hosts[35]. The involvement is much more extensive than that seen in the allergic or saprophytic forms and deep extension into the mucosa and bone often occurs.

Mucormycosis is caused by various genera (Rhizopus, Mucor, Absidia) of the family mucoraceae. Spores of these organisms are ubiquitous in our environment and organisms are part of the normal respiratory flora. Infection only occurs in immunocompromised hosts, with poorly controlled diabetics accounting for 50-75% of cases[19,20,52].

On imaging, the presence of an air-fluid level is uncommon. The maxillary and ethmoid sinuses are the most common sites of involvement[20]. The imaging findings are quite variable depending on the aggressiveness of the fungus. Nonspecific mucosal thickening or sinus opacification may occur. The allergic form of aspergillus is associated with recurrent sinonasal polyps. With more invasive fungi, sinus opacification with a central mycetoma and associated bony thickening or erosion may occur[20]. With both mucormycosis and invasive aspergillus, vascular invasion may occur which leads to intra- and extra-cranial thrombosis and infarction.

Several imaging characteristics are suggestive of fungal sinusitis[19,20,22] (Figs. 5 and 6). On CT, a focal hyperdense lesion may be seen with surrounding hypodense mucoid material (Fig. 5). On MR imaging, low signal intensity on T1WI and a signal void on T2WI have been found in a high proportion of patients with fungal sinusitis (Fig. 6). This is thought to be due to the presence of paramagnetic metals (iron and manganese). Even

though a similar MR appearance can be seen in chronic bacterial infection due to desiccated secretions, the decreased signal is not as pronounced as that found with fungal disease.

According to Som, two other circumstances can be seen which can suggest the presence of fungal infections: soft tissue changes in the sinus with thickened, reactive bone and localized areas of osteomyelitis[20,21]. Also suggestive of fungal infection is the association of inflammatory sinus disease with involvement of the adjacent nasal fossa and the soft tissues of the cheek. These signs of aggressive infection are not associated generally with bacterial pathogens.

Mucous retention cyst: This is a cyst that most commonly occurs in the maxillary sinus floor in patients with a history of previous inflammatory disease. It occurs in 10% of the population. It is the result of inflammatory obstruction of a seromucinous gland within the sinus mucosal lining[7,27]. On CT, this will appear as a homogenous, well circumscribed hypo-to isodense mass (Figs. 7 and 10). On MR imaging, it is usually hypointense on T1WI and hyperintense on T2WI. When these lesions are large

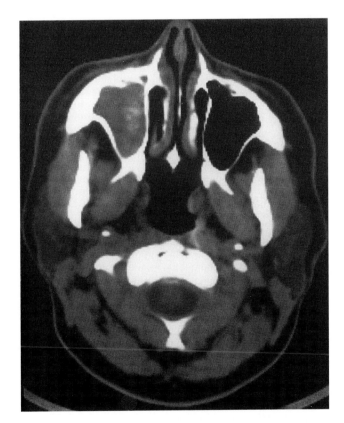

Figure 5. Fungal Sinusitis. Axial CT image at the level of the maxillary sinuses shows complete opacification of the right maxillary sinus. Note that there is hyperattenuation of the material within the mid-portion of the sinus. This is consistent with fungal sinusitis.

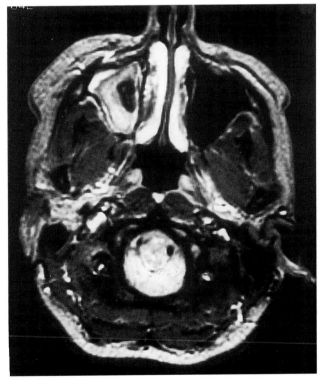

Figure 6. Fungal Sinusitis. Axial T2-weighted image of the same patient seen in Figure 5. The area in the mid-portion of the right maxillary sinus is depicted as an area of signal void on the T2-weighted image. This is thought to be due to the presence of paramagnetic material within the fungal concretion.

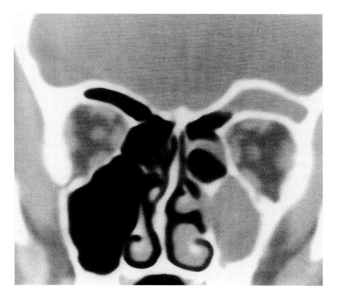

Figure 7. Coronal CT scan shows opacification of the left maxillary sinus (including its ostium). The density is homogeneous. The sinus is not expanded. This lesion could represent a large mucous retention cyst or a polyp. Associated inflammatory change involving the ipsalateral ethmoids is noted. The left frontal sinus is completely opacified to a level near the frontal recess. This nonspecific finding could be related to acute or chronic inflammatory disease.

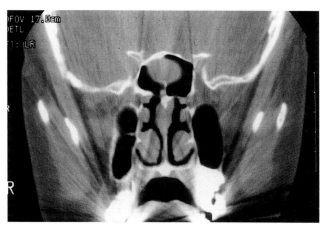

Figure 8. Coronal CT scan demonstrates an opacified and expanded posterior ethmoid air cell. The presence of an expansile lesion is consistent with a mucoceole.

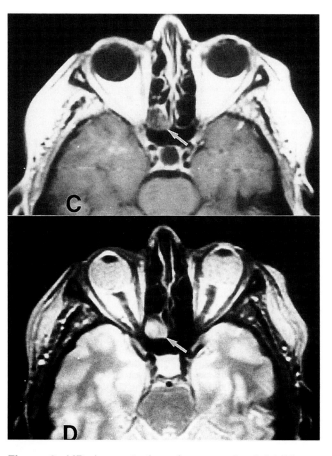

Figure 9. MR demonstration of mucoceole. Axial T1-weighted (top) and axial T2-weighted (bottom) images demonstrate a small lesion which fills and expands a posterior ethmoid air cell. The signal characteristics show the lesion has a relatively high water content. The signal characteristics of mucoceoles are quite variable.

they can be difficult to separate radiologically from mucoceoles and polyps.

Mucocele: This is a dilated mucous-filled sinus that is lined by mucous membrane. It is the result of a chronically obstructed sinus ostium with resulting enlargement of bony walls due to mucous secretions filling the sinus cavity[20,48] (Fig. 7, 8, and 9). It is most commonly caused by inflammatory obstruction of the ostium, but can also be secondary to trauma, tumors, or surgical manipulation[46]; 66% of mucoceles occur in the frontal sinuses with 25% and 10% occurring in the ethmoid and maxillary sinuses, respectively[35]. On CT, this will appear as a hypodense, non-enhancing mass that fills and expands the sinus cavity. On MR imaging, the appearance is variable due to alterations in protein concentration of the obstructed mucoid secretions.

An infected mucocele, a mucopyocele, may demonstrate rim enhancement[47].

OPERATIVE COMPLICATIONS

The radiologist may be called upon to assist in the evaluation of complications arising from surgical intervention for nasal polyposis. Most minor complications such as periorbital emphysema, epistaxis, synechiae and pain do not require specific imaging. Major complications are rarer but can occur with all surgical approaches to nasal

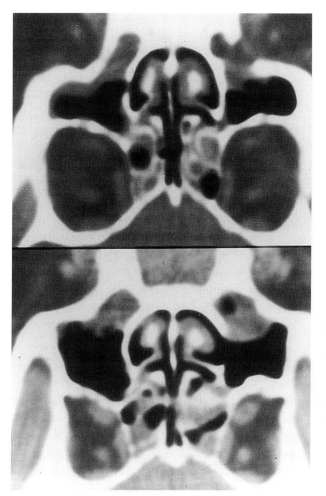

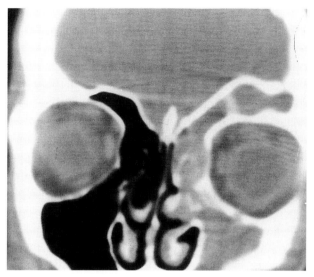

Figure 11. Coronal CT scan demonstrates complete opacification of the left frontal, ethmoid, and maxillary sinuses. Thickening of the left lamina papyracea and left orbital floor indicate that the findings are chronic. Resorption of bone in the ethmoid air cells is also seen. The findings are compatible with polyposis involving the ethmoid and frontal air cells with associated maxillary sinus polyposis or mucoperiosteal thickening. Mucoceole formation in the ethmoid and frontal air cells is also a possibility.

Figure 10. CT demonstration of complex sinus disease. Top image shows a classic appearing mucous retention cyst in the floor of the right maxillary sinus. The patient has had a nasal-antral window on the right. Mucoperiosteal thickening is seen in the floor of the left maxillary sinus. Extensive ethmoid opacification is noted. These changes may be due to mucoperiosteal thickening or a small amount polyposis. Bottom image is taken slightly anterior and it shows opacification of the ethmoid air cells. Again, this may be due to mucoperiosteal thickening or a small amount polyposis. Mucoperiosteal thickening is noted in the inferior portion of both maxillary sinuses. The patient has also undergone a Caldwell-Luc procedure on the right.

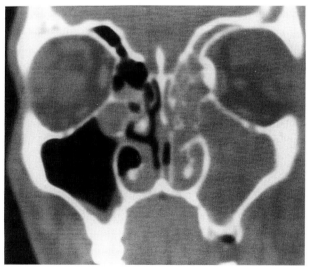

polyps. The radiologist may be called upon to image the orbit in an attempt to establish the exact cause of blindness, diplopia or epiphora following surgery[59]. Similarly transgression of the skull base may lead to a CSF leak, meningitis, intracranial hemorrhage and death[33,34,59,61]. In the presence of a persistent CSF leak, in many institutions a radionuclide CSF study is utilized as the initial radiologic screening examination in such patients[36,62]. When the radionuclide test is positive, a contrast CT cis-

Figure 12. Coronal CT scan demonstrates extensive opacification with aggressive bony resorption and destruction throughout the ethmoid air cells. A small polypoid lesion in the region of the right OMU is compatible with an inflammatory polyp. The soft tissue material filling the left ethmoid air cells is felt to be due to inflammatory polyposis. The opacification of the left frontal sinus is due to obstruction of the left frontal recess. Left maxillary sinus opacification may be due to obstruction of the OMU or to inflammatory polyposis extending into the sinus.

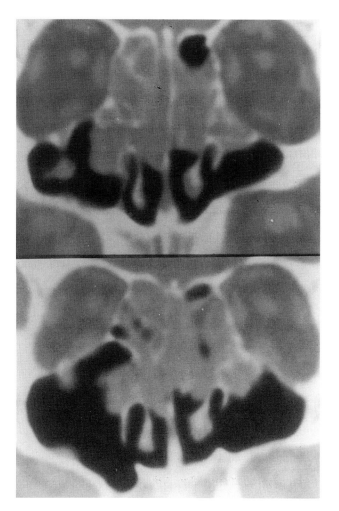

Figure 13. Coronal CT scans: Both images reveal very extensive polypoid appearing ethmoid sinus and OMU opacification. There has been significant bony resorption/destruction. These findings are classic for inflammatory nasal polyposis. Incidental note is made of prior, bilateral nasal antrostomies.

ternogram in the coronal and axial planes is done to define the anatomy and to pin-point the site of leakage, facilitating closure.

COMPUTER ASSISTED SURGERY

A study performed by Kennedy for the American Academy of Otolaryngology and Head and Neck Surgery showed that there is an increasing number of major surgical complications (i.e. death and orbital and intracranial damage) as the number of FESS procedures has increased[63]. Even though CT provides a "road map" for the surgeon, the information that is provided is remote and the surgeon must mentally transfer information from the image to the operative site.

Given the extreme variations in anatomy, extensive inflammatory disease, and at times the copious amount of intraoperative bleeding which can make landmarks difficult to identify, it is not surprising that inadvertent injuries to the orbital and intracranial compartments occur.

Thus, the need for an objective and interactive correlation of the image data with the actual operative site in the patient. Over the past five years, we have successfully achieved this goal utilizing an ISG Allegro multimodality computer (ISG Technologies, Mississauga, Ontario, Canada) attached at first to a mechanical sensor manufactured by Farro Medical Technologies and more recently using the Pixys infrared sensor technology[64]. Prior to CT scanning, 5-10 external markers are placed on the patients face. These are used to register the data in the computer so that they can be applied to the patient in vivo on the surgical table. With the registration complete and the patient immobilized, the mechanical arm holding a probe can be placed into the nasal cavity. The tip of the probe is the location of the sensor. Axial, coronal, and sagittal reformatted images at the tip of the sensor are generated by the computer and the location of the sensor in the patient is thus provided, and shown by cross hairs on these images. The Pixys sensors may be directly placed on the surgeon's instrument. Furthermore, additional sensors may be directly attached via a head band to the patient's head. Thus, two separate sets of sensors are available. One is used to follow the position of the surgeon's instrument and the other is used to update the computer with the patient's head motions. This new sensor technology affords the use of this instrumentation while performing the surgery with either general or local anesthesia.

In this manner, it is intended that the probe be used to confirm the location of specific anatomic structures and thus avoid penetration of the ethmoid roof and lamina papyracea or to identify the relationship of the sphenoid sinus to the optic nerves and carotid canals. The accuracy of this device has been shown to be approximately 2 mm[64].

BIBLIOGRAPHY

1. Moss A and Parsons V. Current estimates from the National Health Interview Survey, United States-1985. Hyattsville, Maryland: National Center for Health Statistics, 1986.
2. Messerklinger W. Endoscopy of the nose. Urban and Schwartzenberg, Baltimore, 1978.
3. Messerklinger W. Zur Endoskopietchnik des mittleren Nassenganges. Arch Otorhinolaryngol 1978, 221: 297-305.
4. Wigand ME, Steiner W, Jaumann MP. Endonasal sinus surgery with endoscopic control: from radical operation to rehabilitation of the mucosa. Endoscopy 1978, 10: 255-260.
5. Kennedy DW, Zinreich SJ, Rosenbaum AE, Johns ME. Functional endoscopic surgery. Theory and diagnostic evaluation. Arch Otolaryngol 1985, 111: 576-582.

6. Zinreich S, Kennedy D, Rosenbaum A, Gayler B, Kumar A, and Stammberger H. Paranasal sinuses: CT imaging requirements for endoscopic surgery. Radiology, 1987. 163(3): 769-775.

7. Som P. Sinonasal cavity. In: Head and Neck Imaging. Som P and Bergeron T, Editors. 1991, Mosby: p. 51-168.

8. Zinreich S. Paranasal sinus imaging. Otolaryngol Head Neck Surg, 1990. 103(5/2): 863-868.

9. Zinreich S. Imaging of chronic sinusitis in adults: X-ray, computed tomography, and magnetic resonance imaging. J Allergy Clin Immunol, 1992. 90 (3/2): 445-451.

10. Zinreich S. Imaging of inflammatory sinus disease. Otolaryngol Clin North Am, 1993. 26(4): 535-547.

11. Zinreich S, Abidin M, and Kennedy D. Cross-sectional imaging of the nasal cavity and paranasal sinuses. Operative Techniques in Otolaryngol Head Neck Surg, 1990. 1(2): 93-99.

12. Babbel R, Harnsberger HR, Nelson B, Sonkens J, Hunt S. Optimatization of techniques in screening CT of the sinuses. AJR 157: 1093-1098, 1991.

13. Melhem ER, Oliverio PJ, Benson ML, Leopold DA, Zinreich SJ. Optimal CT screening for functional endoscopic sinus surgery. (In Press)

14. Beck, D.Sc. Thomas. Radiation Physicist, Dept. of Radiology, The Johns Hopkins Hospital, Baltimore, MD. Personal communication.

15. Curry TS, Dowdey JE, Murry RD. Christensen's Physics of Diagnostic Radiology, 4th Edition. Lea & Febiger, Philadelphia, 1990, p. 372-391.

16. Jones DJ, Wall BF. Organ Doses from Medical X-ray Examinations Calculated Using Monte Carlo Techniques, National Radiological Protection Board, NRPB-R186 (HMSO, London), 1985.

17. Zinreich SJ, Kennedy DW, Kumar A, Rosenbaum A, Arrington J, and Johns M. MR imaging of normal nasal cycle: comparison with sinus pathology. JCAT, 1988. 12(6): 1014-1019.

18. Kennedy D, Zinreich S, Kumar A, Rosenbaum A, and Johns M. Physiologic mucosal changes within the nose and ethmoid sinus: imaging of the nasal cycle by MRI. Laryngoscope, 1988. 98(9): 928-933.

19. Zinreich S, Kennedy D, Malat J, Curtin H, Epstein J, Huff L, Kumar A, Johns M, and Rosenbaum A. Fungal sinusitis: diagnosis with CT and MR imaging. Radiology, 1988. 169(2): 439-444.

20. Som P and Curtin H. Chronic inflammatory sinonasal diseases including fungal infections. The role of imaging. Radiol Clin North Am, 1993. 31(1): 33-44.

21. Som P. Imaging of paranasal sinus fungal disease. Otolaryngol Clin North Am, 1993. 26(6): 983-994.

22. Som P, Dillon W, Curtin H, Fullerton G, and Lidov M. Hypointense paranasal sinus foci: differential diagnosis with MR imaging and relation to CT findings. Radiology, 1990. 176: 777-781.

23. Weber A. Inflammatory diseases of the paranasal sinuses and mucoceles. Otolaryngol Clin North Am, 1988. 21(3): 421-437.

24. Shankar L, Evans K, Hawke M, Stammberger H. An atlas of imaging of the paranasal sinuses. Imago Publishing Ltd. p. 41-72, 1994.

25. Stammberger H. Functional Sinus Surgery. BC Decker, Philadelphia, 1991, p. 273-282.

26. Kennedy DW, Zinreich SJ. The functional endoscopic approach to inflammatory sinus disease: current perspectives and technique modifications. Am J Rhinol 1988. 2(3): 89-93.

27. Harnsberger R. Imaging for the sinus and nose, in Head and Neck Imaging Handbook. 1990, Mosby Yearbook: p. 387-419.

28. Hosemann W. Dissection of the lateral nasal wall in eight steps. In: Endoscopic Surgery of the Paranasal Sinuses and Anterior Skull Base, M.E. Wigand, Editor. 1990, Thieme Medical Publishers, Inc.: New York. p. 36-41.

29. Yousem D. Imaging of sinonasal inflammatory disease. Radiology, 1993. 188(2): 303-314.

30. Buus D, Tse D, and Farris B. Ophthalmic Complications of Sinus Surgery. Ophthalmology, 1990. 97: 612-619.

31. Hudgins P. Complications of endoscopic sinus surgery-the role of the radiologist in prevention. Radiol Clin North Am, 1993. 31(1): 21-31.

32. Hudgins P, Browning D, and Gallups J. Endoscopic paranasal sinus surgery: radiographic evaluation of severe complications. AJNR, 1992. 13: 1161-1167.

33. Maniglia A. Fatal and major complications secondary to nasal and sinus surgery. Laryngoscope, 1989. 99: 276-283.

34. Maniglia A. Fatal and other major complications of endoscopic sinus surgery. Laryngoscope, 1991. 101: 349-354.

35. Laine F and Smoker W. The ostiomeatal unit and endoscopic surgery: anatomy, variations, and imaging findings in inflammatory diseases. AJR, 1992. 159(4): 849-857.

36. Benson ML, Oliverio PJ, Zinreich SJ. Techniques of imaging of the nose and paranasal sinuses. In: Advances in Otolaryngology-Head and Neck Surgery, Volume 10. Mosby Year Book, 1996. (in Press)

37. Mafee M. Preoperative imaging anatomy of the nasalethmoid complex for functional endoscopic sinus surgery. Radiol Clin North Am, 1993. 31(1): 1-20.

38. Bolger W, Butzin C, and Parsons D. Paranasal sinus bony anatomic variations and mucosal abnormalities: CT analysis for endoscopic sinus surgery. Laryngoscope, 1991. 101(1/1): 56-64.

39. Yousem D, Kennedy D, and Rosenberg S. Ostiomeatal complex risk factors for sinusitis: CT evaluation. J Otolaryngol, 1991. 20(6): 419-424.

40. Laine FJ, Kuta AJ. Imaging the sphenoid bone and basiociput: pathologic considerations. Semin Ultra CT MRI, 14(3): 160-177, 1993.

41. Dessi P, Moulin G, Triglia JM, Zanaret M, Cannoni M. Difference in height of the right and left ethmoidal roofs: a possible risk factor for ethmoidal surgery. Prospective study of 150 CT scans. The Journal of Laryngology and Otology 1994, 108: 261-262.

42. Johnson DW, Hopkins RJ, Hanafee WN, Fisk JD. The unprotected parasphenoidal carotid artery studied by high-resolution computed tomography. Radiology 1985, 155: p. 137-141.

43. Kennedy DW, Zinreich SJ, Hassab MH. The internal carotid artery as it related to endonasal sphenoethmoidectomy. AJR 1990; 4(1): 7-12.

44. Delano M, Fun FY, Zinreich SJ. Optic Nerve Relationship to the Posterior Paranasal Sinuses: a CT anatomic study. AJNR (in Press).

45. Evans F, Sydnor J, Moore W, and Moore G. Sinusitis of the maxillary antrum. N Engl J Med, 1975. 293(15): 735-739.

46. Gullane P and Conley J. Carcinoma of the maxillary sinus. A correlation of the clinical course with orbital involvement, pterygoid erosion or pterygopalatine invasion and cervical metastases. J Otolaryngol, 1983. 12: 141-145.

47. Babbel R, Harnsberger H, Sonkens J, and Hunt S. Recurring patterns of inflammatory sinonasal disease demonstrated on screening sinus CT. AJNR, 1992. 13(3): 903-912.

48. Scuderi A, Babbel R, Harnsberger H, and Sonkens J. The sporadic pattern of inflammatory sinonasal disease including postsurgical changes. Semin Ultrasound CT MR, 1991. 12(6): 575-591.

49. Stammberger H and Wolf G. Headaches and sinus disease: the endoscopic approach. Ann Otol Rhinol Laryngol Suppl, 1988. 134: 3-23.

50. Lidov M and Som P. Inflammatory disease involving a concha bullosa (enlarged pneumatized middle nasal turbinate): MR and CT appearance. AJNR, 1990. 11(5): 999-1001.

51. Moloney J, Badham N, and McRae A. The acute orbit, preseptal cellulitis, subperiosteal abscess and orbital cellulitis due to sinusitis. J Laryngol Otol, 1987. 12: 1-18.

52. Centeno R, Bentson J, and Mancuso A. CT scanning in rhinocerebral mucormycosis and aspergillosis. Radiology, 1981. 140(2): 383-389.

53. Osguthorpe J and Hochman M. Inflammatory sinus diseases affecting the orbit. Otolaryngol Clin North Am, 1993. 26(4): 657-671.

54. Walters E, Waller P, Hiles D, and Michaels R. Acute orbital cellulitis. Arch Ophthalmol, 1976. 94: 785-788.

55. Weber A and Mikulis D. Inflammatory disorders of the paraorbital sinuses and their complications. Radiol Clin North Am, 1987. 25(3): 615-631.

56. Patt B and Manning S. Blindness resulting from orbital complications of sinusitis. Otlaryngol Head Neck Surg, 1991. 104(6): 789-795.

57. Vinning EM, Kennedy DW. Surgical Management in Adults-Chronic Sinusitis. Immunology and Allergy Clinics of North America, 1994. 14(1): 97-112.

58. Panje WR, Anand VK. Endoscopic Sinus Surgery Indications, Diagnosis, and Technique. In: Practical Endoscopic Sinus Surgery. Anand VK and Panje WR, editors. McGraw-Hill, New York, 1993, p. 68-86.

59. Neuhaus R. Orbital complications secondary to endoscopic sinus surgery. Ophthalmology, 1990. 97: 1512-1518.

60. Stankiewicz J. Complications in endoscopic intranasal ethmoidectomy. Laryngoscope, 1987. 97: 1270-1273.

61. Stankiewicz J. Complications in endoscopic intranasal ethmoidectomy: an update. Laryngoscope, 1989. 99: p. 668-670.

62. Mettler FA, Guiberteau MJ. Essentials of Nuclear Medicine Imaging. 3rd Edition. WB Saunders, Philadelphia, 1991, p. 73-74.

63. Kennedy D, Shaman P, Hen W, Selman H, Deans D, Lanza D. Complications of ethmoidectomy: a survey of fellows of Otolaryngology-Head & Neck Surgery. Otolaryngology-Head & Neck Surgery (in Press).

64. Zinreich S, Tebo S, Long D, Brem H, Mattox D, Loury M, Vander Kolk C, Koch W, Kennedy D, Bryan R: Frameless stereotaxic integration of CT imaging data: accuracy and initial applications. Radiology 1993, 188(3): 735-742.

Chapter XI

The Immuno Histopathology and Pathophysiology of Nasal Polyps
(The Differential Diagnosis of Nasal Polyposis)

Joel M. Bernstein, M.D., Ph.D.

ABSTRACT

Monoclonal antibodies were used to identify macrophages, lymphocytes and plasma cells. The remainder of the polyps and turbinates were treated with protease to achieve disaggregation of the epithelial cells. Transepithelial potential differences and resistance were measured daily. At the time of maximal transepithelial potential difference, the epithelial cells were mounted and modified in Ussing chambers and exposed to a sodium positive channel blocker (amiloride hydrochloride) and to selected chloride negative channel agonists (isoproterenol bitartrate and adenosine triphosphate).

Middle turbinates and polyps were found to have more macrophages, lymphocytes, plasma cell, HLA-DR positive cells and eosinophils than the inferior turbinates. IgA represents the most common immunocyte and is distributed primarily around glands and in general outnumber IgG producing immunocytes 5-10 to 1.

Epithelial cells obtained from polyps exhibited higher transepithelial potential differences and equivalent short circuit currents than turbinate cell cultures. The responses to amiloride, isoproterenol and adenosine triphosphate were also greater for polyp than for turbinate cultures.

A theory for the pathogenesis of nasal polyps is proposed. Local release of inflammatory mediators could cause sodium absorption and chloride permeability to be higher in polyps than in turbinate epithelia. Increased sodium absorption is consistent with the hypothesis that epithelial fluid absorption contributes to the development of nasal polyps and is secondary to the increased recruitment of inflammatory cells which are present in nasal polyps.

Finally, the differential diagnosis of unilateral and bilateral nasal masses is reviewed.

INTRODUCTION

Despite recent advances in basic science, particularly immunology and molecular biology, the etiology and pathogenesis of nasal and paranasal polyposis have still not been completely clarified. In the last decade, our laboratory has been addressing two aspects of this problem; namely, (1) the distribution of antigen presenting cells, immunocompetent cells, eosinophils and basophiloid cells in nasal polyps and have compared these findings to the inferior turbinate and middle turbinate mucosae which act as intrinsic controls from the same patient and, (2) the ion flux of Na^+ and Cl^- in these same tissues. The results of these studies and the review of the literature suggest that nasal polyps represent a de novo inflammatory growth arising from the lateral wall of the nose or the anterior ethmoidal air cells.

The purpose of this chapter is to summarize our work and review the concept of the microenvironmental differentiation hypothesis of nasal airway inflammation[1]. In addition, this chapter will address the differential diagnosis of both benign and malignant lesions of the nose which may mimic nasal polyposis.

DEFINITION

Nasal polyps represent macroscopically, edematous tissue, very often yellow-white in appearance and soft in consistency in comparison to the more pink, firm middle turbinate. Histologically the polyps are very clearly different than normal nasal mucosa, consisting of respiratory epithelium covering very edematous stroma infiltrated by a number of inflammatory cells with eosinophils predominating in most specimens. One of the critical differences between normal nasal mucosa and the nasal polyp is the number and cytoarchitecture of the glands. The density of the glands in nasal polyps is significantly less than in the normal turbinate mucosa and demonstrates no evidence of true seromucinous gland development as in the inferior and middle turbinates. Finally, the density of eosinophilic and basophiloid cells is markedly greater in the nasal polyp than in the inferior turbinate.[2]

All of these findings taken together suggest that the nasal polyp is an inflammatory growth which is controlled by the local micro-environment. This concept has been championed by the McMaster group over the last decade.[3,4,5,6,7] These investigators in elegant molecular biological studies have demonstrated consistently that various colony stimulating factors and interleukins produced by constitutive cells such as epithelial cells, and fibroblasts of the nasal polyp result in the up-regulation of inflammatory cells. These colony stimulating factors and interleukins recruit, stimulate and prolong the survival of various inflammatory cells such as eosinophils and mast cells. Our laboratory has recently sought evidence that this microenvironmental hypothesis of airway inflammation is under some type of genetic control, either systemically or at the level of the nasal airway.

HISTOLOGY AND IMMUNOHISTOLOGY OF NASAL POLYPS

The conventional histology of the inferior and middle turbinates is well known and has been eluded to in several chapters in this text. The inferior turbinates contain stratified squamous epithelium or pseudo stratified columnar ciliated epithelium under which a thickened basement membrane is noted in 70% of the samples that we have observed (Figure 1,2). Multiple seromucinous glands are present in both superficial and deep layers and are separated by large venous sinusoids. In contrast to this, the histological appearance of nasal polyps varies from extremely edematous tissue with very few glands to tissue that has scattered glands. The unique features of nasal polyps are: (1) an irregularity of the morphology of the cystically dilated glands, (2) a virtual absence of true seromucinous glands as found in the inferior and middle turbinates and, most importantly, (3) a large accumulation of inflammatory cells, particularly eosinophils (Figure 3).

Our laboratory has studied the distribution of antigen presenting cells such as macrophage, B-cells, plasma

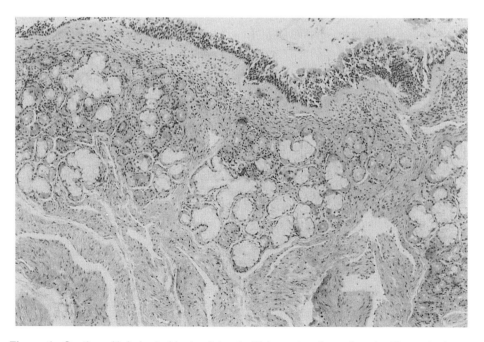

Figure 1. Section of inferior turbinate stained with hematoxylin and eosin. The typical morphology of the inferior turbinate is shown with pseudostratified squamous epithelium, and typical seromucinous glands. Note the large arterioles at the bottom of the photograph (H and E, x100).

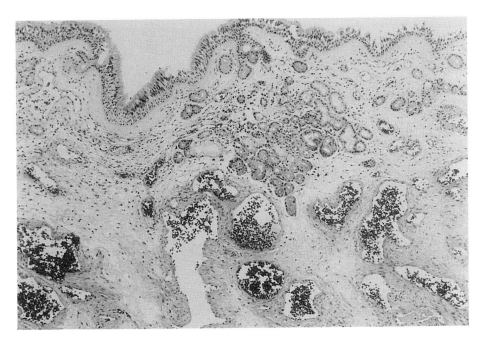

Figure 2. Section of middle turbinate showing respiratory epithelium covering seromucinous glands and dilated sinusoids (H and E, x100).

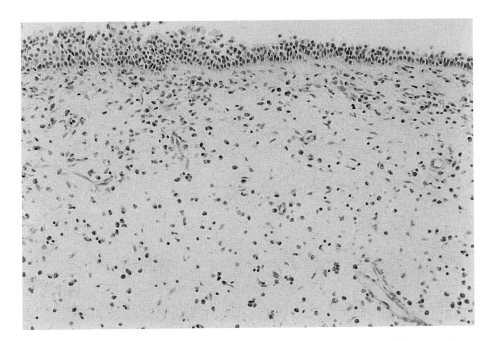

Figure 3. Typical morphology of a nasal polyp with respiratory epithelium covering a very edematous stroma with multiple inflammatory cells which are mainly eosinophils (H and E, x200).

A.

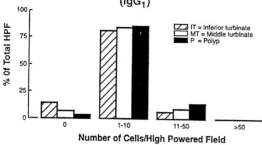

B.

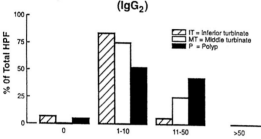

C.

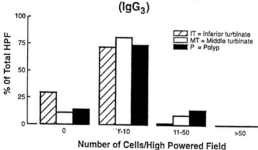

D.

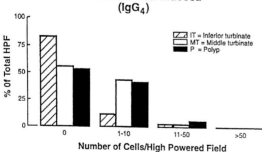

HPF: High Power Fields

cells, HLA-DR cells, and secretory component. In addition, using appropriate stains, we have quantified the distribution of eosinophils and metachromatic staining cells. In general, there is a significant increase in the number of antigen presenting cells such as macrophage and HLA-DR positive cells in the lateral wall of the nose compared to the inferior turbinates of the same patient. This is true for all IgG subtypes except for IgG_4 which is found in extremely small numbers. IgA represents the most common immunocyte present and is distributed primarily around the glands and, in general, outnumber IgG producing immunocytes 5-10 to 1. The distribution of IgG subclasses and IgA subclasses is summarized in Figures 4 and 5.

Antigen presenting cells such as macrophage are found in highest numbers in nasal polyps in comparison to both the middle turbinates and inferior turbinates. Most importantly, there appears to be a significant up-regulation of macrophage not only in pure numbers of cells, but blood vessels in the polyps are literally lined

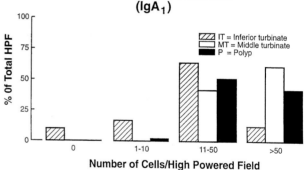

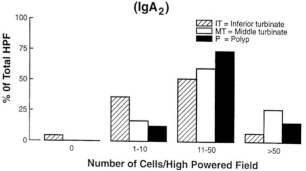

HPF: High Power Fields

Figure 4A–D. Periglandular distribution of cells in different locations of the nasal mucosa involving IgG subclasses. The figure represents a semi-quantitative distribution of the immunocytes in the inferior turbinate, middle turbinate and polyp. The figure demonstrates the number of cells per high powered field related to the percentage of total high powered field. In general, there are more IgG_1 cells and IgG_2 cells in the polyps than in the inferior turbinates.

Figure 5 Top and Bottom. Periglandular distribution of IgA_1 and IgA_2 subtypes in the inferior turbinate, middle turbinate and nasal polyps. Many more IgA positive immunocytes are present in the middle turbinates and polyps compared to the inferior turbinates.

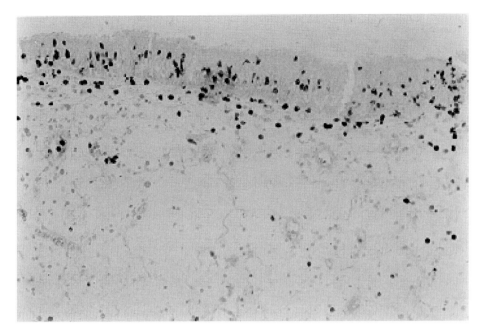

Figure 6A. MAC 387 staining for macrophage in the nasal polyp showing significant staining of inter-epithelial cells as well as in the lamina propria (Immunoperoxidase, x200).

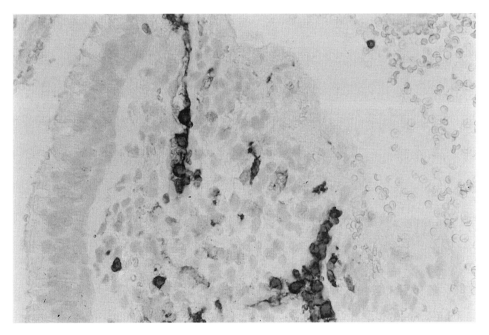

Figure 6B. MAC 387 staining in nasal polyp showing significant margination of macrophage in blood vessels of the nasal polyp (Immunoperoxidase, x400).

with macrophage suggesting that there is an up-regulation of adhesion molecules for these inflammatory cells and that they are being recruited into the nasal polyp interstitial tissue (Figure 6A and 6B). Furthermore, macrophage are known to produce a significant amount of tumor necrosis factor alpha which can cause cytotoxic changes in the nasal polyp.

Recruitment of eosinophils and basophiloid cells into the nasal polyp is also demonstrated in the histological sections of nasal polyps where eosinophils, lymphocytes

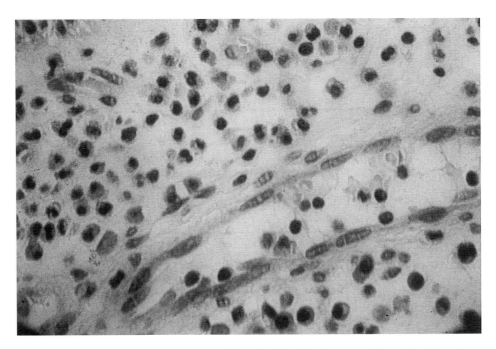

Figure 7. High power photomicrograph of nasal polyp showing a small venule with various cells lining up against the basement membrane of the endothelial wall. One of these cells is an eosinophil and one is a lymphocyte.

and granulocytes are seen to be present in the microvasculature (Figure 7).

Thus, there appears to be a recruitment of immunocompetent cells and inflammatory cells into the nasal polyp in contrast to the inferior turbinate where all of these cells are found in markedly fewer numbers.

These findings extend the elegant studies performed by the McMaster group who have demonstrated with southern blotting and in situ hybridization that macrophage granulocyte colony stimulating factor (MG-CSF) is present in eosinophils as well as in the constitutive cells of the nasal polyp including the epithelium and the fibroblasts of the stroma of the nasal polyps. In this way, they have compared nasal polyps to the mucosa found in the nose in patients with allergic rhinitis and in the tracheal mucosa of patients with bronchial asthma. Therefore in allergic rhinitis mucosa, bronchial mucosa of patients with asthma and nasal polyposis, there are similarities including increased message for colony stimulating factors, various other cytokines and, most importantly, the presence of eosinophils.

Taken together then, the nasal polyps appear to be an inflammatory tissue where there is an up-regulation of antigen presenting cells, immunocompetent cells such as B-cell and immunocytes and, most importantly, a significant increase in the number of eosinophils, mucosal and connective tissue mast cells as compared to the inferior turbinates. Furthermore, the presence of eosinophils and mast cells does not appear to be related to the presence or

absence of allergy in these patients. There is extensive epidemiological evidence to suggest the lack of relationship between IgE-mediated hypersensitivity and the presence of inflammatory cells in nasal polyps.

BIOELECTRIC PROPERTIES OF CULTURED POLYP AND TURBINATE EPITHELIAL CELLS (Pathophysiology of Nasal Polyps)

In collaboration with Dr. James Yankaskas, our laboratory has studied the voltage (V_t) resistance (R_t) and the short circuit current (I_{eq}) of cultured polyp and turbinate epithelial cells.[8,9] Most polyp specimens cultured in collagen matrix support dishes produce measurable and significant bioelectrical properties. The maximal voltage, resistance, and short circuit currents of these cultures are summarized in Table 1. The most striking observation is the increased

Table 1. Maximal Bioelectric Properties of Cultured Human Nasal Polyp and Turbinate Epithelial Cells

	n	V_t (mV)	R_t ($\Omega.cm^2$)	I_{eq} $\mu A/cm^2$
Polyp (12 patients)	37	−11.2 ±1.5	243 ±15	43.6 ±4.2
Turbinate (7 patients)	9	−5.3 ±1.4	187 ±24	28.5 ±5.7

Table 2. Bioelectric Properties of Cultured Human Nasal Polyp and Turbinate Epithelial Cells

	Polyps (n = 21)			Turbinates (n = 3)		
	V_t (mV)	R_t ($\Omega.cm^2$)	I_{eq} ($\mu A/cm^2$)	V_t (mV)	R_t ($\Omega.cm^2$)	I_{eq} ($\mu A/cm^2$)
Basal	−7.8 ±1.2	173 ±16	44.1 ±6.2	−2.4 ±1.0	103 ±17	20.8 ±6.6
Amiloride (10^{-4} M)	−4.0* ±0.5	208* ±20	20.6* ±2.0	−1.1 ±0.3	104 ±15	10.4 ±1.5
Isoproterenol (10^{-5} M)	−4.3* 0.5	194 ±15	22.8* ±2.2	−1.3 ±0.4	100 ±16	12.7 ±2.9
ATP (10^{-5} M)	−6.7 ±1.1	142* ±13	64.0* ±11.4	−1.7 ±1.8	77 ±15	30.6 ±11.1

*Significant change from preceding value, p < 0.01, paired t-test. Mean ± S.E.

voltage and short circuit current in polyp cells as compared to turbinate cells. We have found this to be the case in both polyps from patients with cystic fibrosis and in non-cystic fibrosis polyps. To evaluate the regulatory pathways of ion transport, specimens have been evaluated in Ussing chambers in basal conditions and during exposure to selected chemicals such as amiloride, isoproterenol and ATP. The overall results are summarized in Table 2. The basal current was significantly decreased by amiloride and was increased by both isoproterenol and ATP. Turbinate cultures had similar, but smaller, responses. Similar studies in cystic fibrosis cultures (data not shown), demonstrated the ion transport regulatory properties that characterize CF. In particular, amiloride caused a dramatic decrease in I_{eq} and there was no response to isoproterenol, but the ATP response was retained.

These findings suggest that there is a significant increase in Na+ absorption across the cell in nasal polyps from both CF and non-CF patients. Furthermore, the chloride channel in patients who do not have CF is normal because it responds to Isoproterenol. It is possible that the increased Na+ absorption could be one of the fundamental defects in nasal polyps. The increased Na+ absorption would then allow water to be absorbed through the epithelium into the interstitial space and might account for the edema which is the classic hallmark of the nasal polyp.

Based on our immunohistopathological findings and the bioelectrical properties of nasal polyps, we propose a hypothesis for the development of nasal polyps which is summarized in Figure 8. Turbulent flow of air in the lateral wall of the nose, or viral-bacteria host interactions produce an inflammatory change in the mucosa of the lateral wall of the nose. According to the theory of Tos[9a], there may be ulceration and prolapse of the submucosa with re-epithelialization and new gland formation. This may be the beginning of the nasal polyp. However, the structural cells of the nasal polyp, including epithelial cells and fibroblasts in the stroma, all have the ability to synthesize mRNA for granulocyte-monocyte colony stimulating factor (GM-CSF). Furthermore, there is early evidence from our laboratory that the macrophage can produce message for TNF α in the nasal polyp. Stimulation of such an effector capability by both structural cell-derived cytokines and inflammatory cells would undoubtedly represent a major amplification pathway for the inflammatory response in nasal polyps. This microenvironmental structural inflammatory response in the nasal polyp, in turn, can affect the bioelectrical integrity of the Na+ and Cl− channels at the luminal surface of the respiratory epithelial cell. The change in the Na+ absorption which has been demonstrated in our studies may result in an increased movement of water into the cell and into the interstitial fluid. The resultant edema can lead to growth and enlargement of the nasal polyp. The rapid recurrence of nasal polyps despite adequate surgery may reflect some intrinsic phenotypic characteristic of nasal epithelial cells in the lateral wall of the nose which is likely to be under genetic control.

DIFFERENTIAL DIAGNOSIS OF NASAL POLYPOSIS

Although nasal polyps represent by far the most common inflammatory growth found in the nose of adults and some children, the presence of a unilateral nasal mass should alert the clinician to the many benign sinonasal lesions that can occur in this area. The nose and sinuses represent one of the regions of greatest histological diversity in the body with any tissue capable of producing benign and malignant tumours which can mimic nasal polyposis. In

A Multivariate Hypothesis for the Pathogenesis of Nasal Polyposis

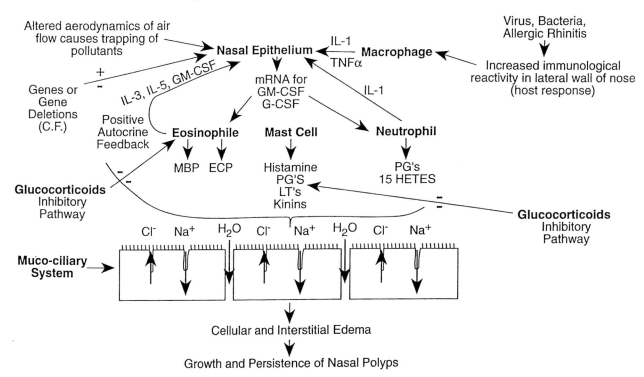

Figure 8. Schematic diagram of a multi-variant hypothesis for the pathogenesis of nasal polyps. The nasal epithelium in the lateral wall of the nose is altered by the change in the aerodynamics of airflow allowing trapping of pollutants. In addition, virus bacteria or allergic disease may cause an increased immunological reactivity in the lateral wall of the nose. Macrophages are abundant in the epithelium and the lamina propria of the nasal polyp. These can alter the nasal epithelium and upregulate messenger RNA for the synthesis of granulocyte, monocyte colony stimulating factor or granulocyte colony stimulating factor (GM-CSF and G-CSF). These colony stimulating factors increase the recruitment of eosinophils, mast cells and neutrophils. In addition, there may be a genetic background for the upregulation of the production of these cytokines as well. The inflammatory cells release various inflammatory mediators such as ECP (eosinophilic cationic protein), MBP (major basic protein), PGs (prostaglandins), LTs (leukotrienes) and kinins. These may feedback on the nasal epithelium in a positive autocrine feedback mechanism and cause more synthesis of cytokines. Glucocorticoids may inhibit all of these inflammatory cells from releasing these cytokines. Finally, these inflammatory mediators may play a role in alteration of sodium and chloride, ion transport (increase sodium absorption and/or increase chloride secretion). This increased ion transport may cause water tension in the cell or in the lamina propria of the polyp leading to cellular interstitial edema and eventual growth and persistence of the nasal polyps.

addition certain congenital and anatomical conditions may simulate a polyp, emphasizing the need for pre-operative imaging even when only a biopsy is being considered.

Conversely, benign nasal polyposis may be associated with significant bone skull base erosion[10] and in exceptional cases, with intracranial invasion.

Benign Lesions in an Adult

Anatomic

Pneumatisation of the middle turbinate (concha bullosa)[12] can produce a large mass in the nose which might on first examination simulate a fleshy polyp or tumour.

This pneumatisation may be present on one or both sides but its true nature is readily resolved by palpation and if any confirmation is required, by CT scanning (Table 3).

Tumours

1. Inverted Papilloma[13]

These are the commonest true tumours occurring in the nose, arising within the middle meatus from where extension may occur into the nasal cavity and any of the sinuses. The tumour has been a source of concern due to its reportedly high recurrence rate and association with malignant transformation. The recurrence rate is entirely related to inadequate removal and

Table 3. Benign Lesions Simulating Nasal Polyps

Anatomic
Concha bullosa

Tumours
Epithelial
    Papilloma—inverted, everted, cylindric
    Minor salivary—pleomorphic adenoma
Mesenchymal
    Neurogenic— meningioma, schwannoma,
      neurofibroma
    Vascular— haemangioma, angiofibroma
    Fibro-osseous— ossifying fibroma
    Muscular— leiomyoma, angioleiomyoma

Granulomatous/Inflammatory
Wegener's granulomatosis
Sarcoidosis
Crohn's disease

---

whilst the malignant transformation rate ranges from 0-55% in the literature, this is almost due to a failure to recognize the presence of squamous cell carcinoma *ab initio*. The true potential for malignant transformation in carefully examined large series is less than 5%. However, inverted papilloma may occur in association with nasal polyposis, may be bilateral and may infiltrate adjacent bone which has led to diagnostic and management problems in the past and reinforces the need for submission of all tissue removed at surgery to histopathological examination.

2. *Angiofibroma*[14]

Juvenile angiofibroma occurs almost exclusively in male children or adolescents who present with nasal obstruction and epistaxis. This may be combined with dacrocystitis, serous otitis media, swelling of the cheek and occasionally visual loss. The tumour arises within the sphenopalatine foramen presenting in the nasal cavity and nasopharynx from whence it may extend into the sphenoid. The lesion will spread laterally through the pterygopalatine region compressing the back wall of the maxillary sinus to dumb-bell into the infratemporal fossa and from thence may affect the orbit via the infraorbital fissure. Biopsy of the lesion may result in life threatening hemorrhage but fortunately a combination of CT and MRI allows both the diagnosis and extent of the lesion to be determined accurately.

A number of other benign tumors may occur in the nose all of which are extremely rare and in which a combination of biopsy and imaging will determine the histology, extent and the most appropriate surgical approach for excision.

Benign Epithelial Tumours
a. Other papillomas—everted (fungiform)
              —cylindric (transitional)
b. Minor salivary gland tumours eg. pleomorphic adenomas[15]

Benign Mesenchymal Tumours
a. Fibro-osseous-ossifying fibroma
b. Vascular-haemangioma
c. Neurogenic eg. schwannomas[16], neurofibromas, meningioma[17]
d. Leiomyoma, angioleiomyoma[18]

Inflammatory/Granulomatous Condition

Diseases such as Wegener's granulomatosis[19], sarcoidosis and very rarely Crohn's disease[20] may present with granulomatosis changes within the nose and sinuses. It is exceptional, however, for these to simulate nasal polyps and are more usually manifest by a friable granular mucosa associated with crusting and bleeding, pansinusitis and ultimately loss of nasal stucture and support.

Malignant Lesions In Adults

Any malignant tumour may mimic nasal polyposis as lesions such as mucinous adenocarcinoma which may affect both ethmoid labyrinths, producing bilateral lesions. **Squamous cell carcinoma** remains the commonest tumour of the sinonasal region but once again the whole spectrum of histological types may occur of which the commonest simulating localized nasal polyps are adenocarcinoma, olfactory neuroblastoma and malignant melanoma (Table 4).

Differential diagnoses of a nasal mass in children

The differential diagnosis of a unilateral mass in the nose of a child would include congenital lesions such as an

---

Table 4. Malignant Lesions Simulating Polyps

Epithelial
Squamous cell carcinoma
Adenocarcinoma [27]
Adenoid cystic carcinoma
Acinic cell carcinoma [28]
Mucoepidermoid carcinoma
Olfactory neuroblastoma [26]
Malignant melanoma [23]
Metastatic tumours eg. kidney [33], breast [34], pancreas
Undifferentiated carcinoma [32]

Mesenchymal Tumours
Lymphoreticular —lymphoma [25]
               —plasmacytoma [29]
Rhabdomyosarcoma [24]
Chondrosarcoma [31]
Ewing's Sarcoma [30]

Table 5. Differential Diagnosis of a Nasal Mass in a Child

Congenital
Encephalocoele
Glioma
Dermoid cyst
Nasolacrimal duct cyst

Neoplasia
Benign   —craniopharyngioma
           —haemangioma
           —neurofibroma
Malignant—rhabdomyosarcoma

encephalocele, glioma, dermoid cyst and nasolacrimal duct cyst[21] and lesions such as craniopharyngioma[22], haemangioma, neurofibroma and rhabdomyosarcoma. Imaging prior to any intervention is mandatory, optimally a combination of CT and MRI. In particular this will define the skull base defect and determine the most appropriate surgical approach. True nasal polyposis can of course occur in children in whom cystic fibrosis must be suspected until proven otherwise (Table 5).

REFERENCES

1. Denburg J, Dolovich J, Ohtoshi T, Cox G, Gauldie J, Jordana M. The microenvironmental differentiation hypothesis of airway inflammation. Am J Rhinol 1990; 4:29-32.

2. Ohnishi M, Ruhno J, Bienenstock J, Milner R, Dolovich J, Denburg J. Human nasal polyp epithelial basophil/mast cell and eosinophil colony-stimulating activity: The effect is T-cell dependent. Am Rev Respir Dis 1988; 138:560–564.

3. Ohno I, Lea R, Finotto S, Marshall J, Denburg J, et. al. Granulocyte/macrophage colony-stimulating factor (GM-CSF) gene expression by eosinophils and nasal polyposis. American Journal of Respiratory Cell Molecular Biology 1991; 5:505–510.

4. Denburg J, Gauldie J, Dolovich J, Ohtoshi T, et. al. Structural cell-derived cytokines and allergic inflammation. Arch Allergy Appl Immunol 1991; 94:127–132.

5. Ohnishi M, Ruhno J, Bienenstock J, Dolovich J, Denburg J. Hematopoietic growth factor production by cultured cells of human nasal polyp epithelial scrapings: Kinetics, cell source, and relationship to clinical status. J Allerg Clin Immunol 1989; 83:1091–1100.

6. Gauldie J, Jordana M, Cox G, Ohtoshi T, Dolovich J, Denburg J. Fibroblasts and other structural cells in airway inflammation. Am Rev Respir Dis 1992; 145:14–17.

7. Otsuka H, Dolovich J, Richardson M, Bienenstock J, Denburg J. Metachromatic cell progenitors and specific growth and differentiation factors in human nasal mucosa and polyps. Am Rev Respir Dis 1987; 138:710–717.

8. Bernstein JM, Cropp GA, Nathanson I, Yankaskas JR: Bioelectric properties of cultured nasal polyp and turbinate epithelial cells. Am J Rhinol 1990; 4:45–48.

9. Bernstein JM, Yankaskas JR. Increased ion transport in cultured nasal polyp epithelial cells. Arch Otolaryngol Head Neck Surg 1994; 120:993–996.

9a. Tos M, Mogensen C. Pathogenesis of nasal polyps. Rhinol 1977; 15:87-95.

10. Som PM, Lawson W, Lidov MW. Simulated aggressive skull base erosion in response to benign sinonasal disease. Head and Neck Radiology 1991;180:755–759.

11. Reddy PK, Rao GP, Prakasham A, Purnanand A, et al. Intracerebral polyposis. J Neurosurg 1993;78:294–296.

12. Yellin SA, Weiss MH, O'Malley B, Weingarten K. Massive concha bullosa masquerading as an intranasal tumor. Ann Oto Rhinol Laryngol 1994;103(8Pt 1):658–659.

13. Tsunoda R, Takooda S, Nishijima W, Ogawa M, Terada S. Inverted papillomas in the nose and paranasal sinuses. Nippon Jibiinkoka Gakkai Kaiho (Journal of the Otorhinolaryngological Society of Japan) 1994;97(5):912–918.

14. Jamal MN. Imaging and management of angiofibroma. Eur Arch Otorhinolaryngol 1994;251(4):241–245.

15. Nonomura N, Niijima H, Kimura O, et al. Immunohistochemical study of pelomorphic adenoma of the nasal septum. Auris Nasas Larynx 1992;19(2);125–131.

16. Klossek JM, Ferrie JC, Goujon JM, et al. Nasosinusal schwannoma. Apropos of 2 cases. Value of nasal endoscopy for diagnosis and treatment: Review (French). Ann Otolaryngol Chir Chervicofac 1993;110(6):341–345.

17. Perez Villa J, Maristany M, Sabater F, Olmo A, Biurrun O, Traserra J. Primary Meningioma of the nasal cavity (Spanish). Anales Otorrinolaringologicos Iberoamericanos 1994;21(4):369–380.

18. Trott MS, Gewirtz A, Lavertu P, Wood BG, Sebek BA. Sinonasal leiomyomas (Review). Otolaryngol Head Neck Surg 1994;111(5):660–664.

19. Verschuur HP, Struyvenberg PA, et al. Nasal discharge and obstruction as presenting symptoms of Wegener's granulomatosis in childhood. Pediatr Otorhinolaryngol 1993; 27(1):91–95.

20. Ernst, A, Preyer S, Plauth M, Jenss H. Polypöse pansinusitis als eine ungewöhnliche, extraintestinale manifestation des morbus Crohn. HNO 1993;41–:33–36.

21. Reilly JR, Koopman CF, Cotton R. Nasal mass in a pediatric patient (clinical conference). Head Neck 1992;14(5): 415–418.

22. Bret P, Beziat JL. Sphenoido-nasopharyngeal craniopharyngioma. A case with radical excision by LeFort I-type maxillotomy: Review. Neurochirurgie 1993;39(4): 235–240.

23. Grijalba Uche M, Mozota Ortiz JR, Puente Lopez G, Dot Saldana J. Amelanotic mucous melanoma of the nasal cavity. Report of a case: Review (Spanish). Acta Otorrinolaringol Esp 1994;45(5):365–367.

24. Maier W, Laubert A, Weinel P. Acute bilateral blindness in childhood caused by rhabdomyosarcoma and malignant lymphoma. J Laryngol Otol 1994;108(10):873–877.

25. Zrunek M, Kürsten, Erlacher L, Wagner A, Knoflach B, et al. Manifestation der malignen lymphomatösen polyposis im nasopharynx. Laryngorhinootologie 1993;72:178–180.

26. Som PM, Lidov M, Brandwein M, Catalano P, Biller HF. Sinonasal esthenioneuroblastoma with intracranial exten-

sion: marginal tumore cysts as a diagnostic MR finding. American Journal of Neuroradiology 1994;15(7): 1259–1262.

27. Morais D, Benito JI, Bachiller J. Alonso-Vielba J, Alvarez T. Adenocarcinoma of the nasal cavities and paranasal sinuses. On low-grade adenocarcinoma (Spanish). Anales Otorrinolaringologicos Iberoamericanos 1994;21(2): 185–192.

28. Valerdiz-Casasola S, Sola J, Pardo-Mindan FJ. Acinic cell carcinoma of the sinonasal cavity with intracytoplasmic crystalloids. Histopathology 1993;23(4):382–384.

29. Kautzky M, Susani M, Steurer M, Youssefzadeh S. Plasmacytoma of the nose and paranasal sinuses with intracranial and orbital extension (German). Laryngorhinootologie 1993;72(7):352–355.

30. Howard DJ, Daniels HA. Ewing's sarcoma of the nose. Ear Nose Throat J 1993;72(4):277–279.

31. Steurer M, Kautzky M, Zrunek M. Chondrosarcoma of the nose and paranasal sinuses. Status of diagnostic imaging and therapeutic concept (German). HNO 1993;41(1):30–32.

32. Zoppi J. Avagnina A, Elsner B, Terzian A, Kaimen M. Undifferentiated carcinoma of the nose and paranasal sinuses. A clinicopathologic and immunohistochemical study (Spanish). Medicina 1991;51(3):222–226.

33. Szlenk Z, Osuch-Wojcikiewica E, Janczewski G. The head and neck metastases from clear cell carcinoma of the kidney (Polish). Otolaryngol Pol 1994;48(2):203–208.

34. Wanamaker JR, Kraus DH, Eliacher I, Lavertu P. Manifestations of metastatic breast carcinoma to the head and neck. Head Neck 1993;15(3):257–262.

Chapter XII

The Clinical Relationship of Nasal Polyps to Asthma

Knud Larsen, M.D.

ABSTRACT

From a meta-analysis on the clinical related literature on asthma and nasal polyps, it was found that patients with asthma had polyps in 7–15% with the highest frequency in the age group above 50 years. Between 36–96% of acetylsalicylic acid (ASA) intolerant patients had polyps.

Patients with nasal polyps had asthma at an average of 29.9% in those referred to ENT-departments, and more than 70% in those referred to allergy departments. An average of 12.8% had ASA intolerance. Male to female ratio showed a tendency towards lower values in the series with the highest frequency of asthma and ASA intolerance. Not all polyp patients had an associated lower airway disease, neither as manifest asthma, nor as hyperreactive airways on challenge test. Females with polyps were more likely to have asthma than males. Patients with polyps, asthma and ASA intolerance showed a later onset of both asthma and polyps compared to those from unselected series. Asthma developed before polyps in an average of 69% of the series.

Most patients showed improvement or at the least were unchanged in the control of their asthma after surgery. Bronchospasm during endonasal surgery was observed in less than 2%. Active asthma before treatment and surgery under local anaesthesia have been factors considered to be of importance. Control of polyps and sinus disease showed a poorer outcome in patients with asthma, and this was even more pronounced in patients having ASA intolerance.

This survey give support to the believe that the eosinophilic nasal polyp patients include patients with different aetio-pathogenetic factors and with different clinical outcome both regarding the upper and lower airways. Identification of such entities is still needed through basal and clinical research to improve treatment.

THE FREQUENCY OF POLYPS IN ASTHMATICS

The true incidence of nasal polyps is not known. It has been estimated that 0.2–1% of the adult population in UK have nasal polyps at some time in their lives[1]. In a Danish county we found an estimated incidence of patients with nasal polyps who sought treatment at ENT-practices to be between 0.3 and 0.49 per thousand per year during 1986–88. A crude annual incidence in a Swedish population was estimated to be 0.43 per thousand per year[2]. However, in a study on cadavers, 42% were found to have nasal polyps[3].

In DK the incidence of asthma was 0.5 per hundred in 1978–79, and 5.2 per hundred had had or still had asthma. In a comprehensive study by Settipane[4] on the relationship between asthma, rhinitis, atopy and nasal polyps, the overall frequency of nasal polyps in asthmatics was 6.7% and in rhinitis 2.2%, in both groups with an overrepresentation of patients with negative allergy skin test. When related to age the frequency of polyps in asthmatics were 7% in the ages 10–50 years, and in a subgroup of asthmatics, over 40 years old, or those with negative skin tests the frequency ranged from 10–15%[5]. In patients with acetysalicylic acid (ASA) intolerance the frequency of nasal polyps ranged from 36–96%[6–12].

These data suggest that nasal polyposis is a relatively common disease and may be even more common if asymptomatic patients were included. In asthmatics the frequency of polyps increases with age and make up 15%

at the age over 50 years old, and it is more frequent in non-atopic than in atopic patients and reaches a peak frequency in patients with ASA intolerance, mainly of the bronchospastic type[4–6,13–15].

THE FREQUENCY OF ASTHMA IN NASAL POLYPOSIS

From a number of studies selected on the basis of the presence of nasal polyps as a main criteria for inclusion in the individual study, the frequency of asthma, ASA intolerance and sex ratio can be depicted. Table 1 shows the results from this meta-analysis. The referral pattern and type of intended treatment is shown as these factors might influence the judgment of the observed frequencies. There are two large series with selected triad cases[16,17]. Two series from allergy clinics showed a very high frequency of asthma, 71–72%[4,18], and in one series the asthmatics were included among those with chronic obstructive pulmonary disease[19]. Those referred to ethmoidectomy might be thought to be the more severe cases, but generally those included were fairly comparable with the remaining series, and from these an average fre-

quency of asthma was 29.9% and the corresponding average frequency of ASA intolerance was 12.8%. A tendency towards a higher male to female ratio is observed in the series with the lowest frequencies of asthma, a finding also present for the ASA intolerant patients, where the male to female ratio approximates to 1. Interpretation of such observations is dependent on the definition of asthma and ASA intolerance and variations between the series might be explained by this. It has been stated that asthma will evolve at one time or another in all polyp patients[18], that aspirin intolerance will inevitably evolve in some with only asthma or nasal polyps, in others will first begin in those with sensitivity to aspirin[20], and finally that those with polyps without asthma are an incomplete group[21]. Those statements, although theoretically possible, do not seem to be quite in accordance with the clinical findings as presented, where an average of more than two thirds of the patients from several series did not have asthma and an average of more than eighty percent did not show evidence of ASA intolerance. Other sources of investigation do not give support to the opinion that all polyp patients are prone to asthma or ASA intolerance. Metacholine challenge in

Table 1

	Year	Note	N total	M/F ratio	With Asthma			ASA	
					N	%	M/F ratio	N	%
Blumstein & Tuft[18]	1957	allerg.	160	1.6	115	72%	—	—	—
Schenck[20]	1974	p	174	2.2	31	18%	—	24	14%
Delaney[22]	1976	p	100	3.6	25	25%	1.8	3	3%
Moloney[23]	1977	p	445	2.0	95	21%	1.0	25	6%
Holopainen et al[24]	1979	p	109	1.4	23	21%	—	25	23%
Brown et al.[16]	1979	total	1660	—	513	31%	—	182	11%
		p+e,ASA	101	1.2	101	100%	—	101	100%
Drake-Lee et al.[21]	1984	p	200	3.0	58	29%	1.9	11	6%
English[17]	1986	p+e,ASA	205	1.0	205	100%	—	205	100%
Settipane[15]	1987	allerg.	211	1.0	149	71%	—	30	14%
Stevens & Blair[25]	1988	e	87	1.3	35	40%	—	17	20%
Jantti-Alanko et al[26]	1989	p+e	85	—	34	40%	—	22	26%
Vleming et al[19]	1991	e	105	1.7	44	42%	—	—	—
Granstrom et al[27]	1992	p	224	2.9	59	26%	—	10	4%
Wong et al[28]	1992	p	337	2.9	—	36%	—	—	—
Davidsson/Hellquist[2]	1993	p	95	2.2	—	38%	—	22	23%
Larsen & Tos[29]	1994	p	180	2.9	38	21%	2.5	7	4%
Larsen & Tos[30]	1994	p,recur	103	2.8	32	31%	1.7	13	13%

ASA: Acetylsalisylic acid intolerance. Allerg.: Patients referred to allergy clinics. Patients referred for ethmoidectomy (e), and polypectomy (p). Recur: Denotes a subgroup of recurrent polyp patients from that series.

Table 2. Methacholine Challenge in Non-Asthmatics

	N	Test Positive	Test Negative	Comments
Kordash et al, 1978[31]	9	2	7	7 intermediate reaction
Downing et al., 1982[32]	13	0	13	1 transient positive
Miles-Lawrence[33] et al, 1982	15	7	8	2/7 atopics positive 1 asthma excluded from 16
Jacobs et al., 1983[34]	19	11	8	10 prick and RAST positive

Table 3

Series	Year	Males			Females		
		Total	Asthma	%	Total	Asthma	%
Delaney[22]	1976	78	16	20.5%	22	9	40.9%
Moloney[23]	1977	297	47	15.8%	148	48	32.4%
Drake-Lee et al[21]	1984	151	38	25.2%	49	20	40.8%
Larsen & Tos[29]	1994	134	27	20.1%	46	11	23.9%
Larsen & Tos, (recur)[30]	1994	76	20	26.3%	27	12	44.4%

non-asthmatics with nasal polyps in different series did not show a clear-cut evidence of lower airway hyper-reactivity in all patients as presented in Table 2. These findings are in accordance with the statements of Settipane[5] and Connell[35], that not all polyp patients have an associated lower respiratory disease.

Although nasal polyps are 2–3 times more common in men, there are nearly twice as many asthmatics among females in different series (Table 3). In primary polyp patients followed for nearly five years, there were only slightly more females with asthma[29]. while those with recurrent polyps and a longer total polyp history[30] had a male to female ratio close to the findings in the other studies[21–23]. It is therefore possible that the development of asthma after the onset of polyps occurs more often in females compared to males.

AGE AND ONSET OF ASTHMA AND POLYPS

In rather unselected series the mean age of asthma onset varied between 32–38 years with an average of 35 years[21,23,29]. From the same series, the mean age of polyp onset varied between 39–47.5 years with an average of 42 years. There was no difference in the mean age of polyp onset with or without asthma.

In selected groups of patients with ASA intolerance, asthma and nasal polyps, the mean age of asthma onset varied between 39.6–41 years, with an average of 40.5 years[16,20,27], while the mean age of polyp onset varied between 44–45.1 years with an average of 45 years.

From these findings the age of onset of asthma in rather unselected series was about 5 years prior to that found in the selected series with ASA intolerance. The mean age of polyp onset was closer to the mean age of asthma onset in the ASA intolerant patients than in the unselected series.

The relationship between the onset of asthma and polyps has been analyzed in more detail in the studies presented in Table 4. Asthma developed first at a mean of 53% to 88% of the patients with an average of 69%, and the mean interval from onset of asthma to the development of polyps varied between 9 and 13 years[4,17,20,29]. Polyps developed first in 22% to 33% with an average of 28%[4,20,27,29] of the patients. The mean interval from onset of polyps to the development of asthma varied between 2 and 12 years[4,20,29]. In a group of patients followed for 5–26 years, 16% of the patients subsequently developed asthma[31]. A simultaneous development of nasal polyps was observed in 9.2 and 10%[15,27]. The onset of asthma and ASA intolerance usually occurred within one year[13,15].

LOWER AIRWAY RESPONSE TO POLYP TREATMENT

A number of statements in the literature have appeared, where polypectomy was regarded as a causation for the development of asthma[36–38]. The difference between coincidence and causation on that subject has since been highlighted by several authors.

Table 4

	Year	Total N	Asthma N	Asthma First N	%
Blumstein & Tuft[18]	1957	160	115	61	53%
Schenck (ASA)[20]	1974	18	18	10	56%
Moloney[23]	1977	445	95	64	67%
Settipane & Chafee[4]	1977	119	119	73	61%
English (ASA)[17]	1986	205	205	—	86%
Jantti-Alanko et al[26]	1989	85	34	30	88%
Granstrom et al[27]	1992	224	59	40	68%
Larsen & Tos[29]	1994	180	38	27	73%

Most asthmatics as shown before, develop asthma before the polyps. Many patients can have several polypectomies before the asthma develops. A mean of 5 polypectomies before asthma developed within weeks to 8 years after the last polypectomy has been observed, and only in 1.4% of the first polypectomies did it occur within a few months[23]. Development of asthma within 24 hours after polypectomy is rarely reported, but has been observed in 2 cases[20]. The time interval between polyp onset, and the onset of asthma as reported above, does not confirm any causative relationship between polypectomy and the development of asthma. Furthermore the bronchial reactivity on metacholine challenge measured before and after polypectomy did not show any significant deterioration. In one study[32] no change was observed in 6 non-asthmatics, and in 4 asthmatics there was no change in 2, it was increased in one and decreased in another, at a mean of 5 months after polypectomy. In a similar study[33], both the patients negative before were negative after, and among 4 positive patients before there were 2 positive and 2 negative patients one month after polypectomy. Reduction of bronchial reactivity on metacholine challenge has been found in one patient[39] and in 30% of patients having radical sphenoethmoidectomy[40].

These results are also supported by clinical studies on the pulmonary function after surgery[19,40,41], from evaluation of the medical needs to control asthma.[17,20,39–42], and from subjective or more global setting of the control of asthma[16,20,21,26,39,43,44,45]. These results are shown in Table 5. Four groups are included, although not solely polyp patients, but 72–91% of the patients in these series had nasal polyps[39,42,43,45]. It is obvious that most patients had benefit or at least were unchanged in the control of their asthma after surgery. It is not possible to evaluate whether one type of surgery is superior to the other from these figures.

From the literature during more than twenty years there is no reason to believe that either polypectomy or ethmoidectomy should aggravate asthma, or be the cause of the development of asthma. On the contrary most patients seem to benefit from surgery. Deterioration of asthma in the small numbers observed might be explained by variations of an underlying disease process shared by those with polyps and asthma. There is a remarkable lack of studies on this subject after medical treatment for polyps.

A naso-bronchial reflex is still debated. Several nasal reflexes are known[46]. A nasobronchial reflex is thought to cause bronchoconstriction on nasal stimulation with irritants[47,48]. It is unclear whether such a reflex mechanism is involved when acute attacks of asthma develop during nasal surgery. A number of other factors related to the anaesthetic or other medical conditions, as well as exposure of the lower airways to secretions might be involved. Some studies have found nasal obstruction and nasal packing to cause increased bronchomotor tone and decreased oxygen tension[49,50], while others could not demonstrate such a relationship in otherwise healthy young adults, either after packing or after surgery for relieving nasal obstruction[51–54]. A review on these relationships has been done by others[55,56], without finding positive evidence of a reflex mechanism. On the other hand this has not been fully investigated in susceptible individuals including asthmatics. Apart from that, a few studies have shown improvement of the lower airways after topical nasal steroid treatment, especially in respect to exercise-induced asthma in atopic asthmatic children[57]. The importance of the shift from oral to nasal breathing after relieving nasal obstruction, and thereby normalizing the humidification and rewarming of air, seems important for improvement of the lower airway function[56]. A sino-bronchial reflex mechanism is even more difficult to handle. Bronchospasm elicited from stimulation of H1

Table 5

	Year	Note	Asthma N	Method	Control of Asthma		
					Improved	Unchanged	Worse
Schenck[20]	1974	p	18	medi	6%	83%	11%
				subj	28%	39%	33%
Brown et al[16]	1979	p+e,ASA	101	glob	32%	53%	15%
Friedman et al[42]	1982	e	28	medi	93%	7%	0%
Eichel[43]	1982	e	22	subj	41%	32%	27%
Slavin[39]	1982	e	33	medi	83%	—	—
				subj	85%	—	—
Drake-Lee et al[21]	1984	p	58	subj	37%	61%	2%
Settipane et al[41]	1985	p	8	pft	0%	100%	0%
			6	medi	0%	100%	0%
English[17]	1986	p+e,ASA	205	medi	84%	16%	0%
Jantti-A. et al[26]	1989	p+e	85	subj	59%	29%	12%
McFadden et al[44]	1990	e	25	glob	100%	—	—
Vleming et al[19]	1991	e	30	pft	64%	23%	13%
Jankowski et al[40]	1992	e	30	medi	91%	9%	0%
Lawson[45]	1994	e	47	subj	34%	60%	6%

medi: medical need to control asthma. subj: subjective judgement. glob: global judgement. pft; pulmonary function test. p: polypectomy. e: ethmoidectomy.

receptors, irritant receptors or cholinergic receptors via trigminal afferent and vagal efferent pathways has been proposed[41]. Bacterial seeding of the lower airway from infected sinuses and an increased beta-adrenergic blockade caused by lower airway infection are suggested mechanisms[39].

Bronchospasm during simple polypectomy does not seem to have been reported as a specific problem. In series undergoing ethmoidectomy, bronchospasm in the perioperative period in one study was observed in 20 of 101 patients, but 17 of these also had active asthma before surgery[16]. In another study 40% of the patients had bronchospasm in the immediate post-operative period, but most of the patients also had severe asthma before surgery[17]. Both of these studies included selected triad cases. In two other studies 17 of 1163 patients and 2 of 100 patients undergoing endonasal sinus surgery had asthmatic attacks during surgery[58,59]. In a meta-analysis bronchospasm was observed in 1% during traditional endonasal surgery and in 0.12% during endoscopic sinus surgery, while their own results showed a frequency of 1.8% during endoscopic sinus surgery[60]. It has been shown that patients operated under local anaesthesia showed a higher incidence of bronchospasm versus patients operated under general anaesthesia. Exposure of the airways to secretions was thought to trigger laryngo-bronchospasm in patients with reactive airways during local anaesthesia[60]. The number of asthmatic attacks during surgery was minimised when general anaesthesia was used for patients with reactive airways[60,61].

Judging from the literature, the development of asthmatic attacks during the nasal and sinus surgery does not seem to be a quantitatively large problem, but proper medical and anaesthetic care of patients with asthma before and during any surgery for nasal polyps or sinuses is obviously important.

UPPER AIRWAY RESPONSE TO POLYP TREATMENT

The influence of the presence of asthma and ASA intolerance on the outcome of polyp treatment, has been highlighted in several studies. The number of polypectomies observed in the series has been used as a parameter for comparison between groups of patients. A mean number of 4 polypectomies was observed in ASA triad cases versus 2.1 polypectomies in asthmatics[20]. The mean number of polypectomies was 4.5 in asthmatics and 2.9 in nonasthmatics in another study[28]. In two studies on triad cases the mean number of polypectomies was 3.0[16] versus 1.8 with an increase to 2.0 in the most severe asthmatics[17]. Overall control of polyps was found to be 60%

in one study of triad cases and was more likely if post-operative asthma was under control[16], while no recurrences were found in 87% of asthmatics and in 100% of non-asthmatics in another study on ethmoidectomy for nasal polyps[42]. It has been stated that recurrences are more often found in older age groups[20,31], in later onset of polyps[18], or when asthma develops after the polyps[18,23,26,31]. In one study ASA intolerance appeared not to be a factor in response to surgical treatment[42], while others have found a close relationship between a higher number of polypectomies and the presence of asthma and ASA intolerance[21,26]. Re-polypectomy was needed in 59% of patients with ASA intolerance, among whom 91% had asthma and 23% of these needed 3 or more polypectomies[26].

From the author's own studies the number of polypectomies in asthmatics were significantly higher when compared to non-asthmatics (Table 6), and the likelihood of being recurrence free after the first polypectomy within a specified observation time also showed a significant difference. Asthmatics had the poorest outcome (Fig. 1). These findings are in accordance with the observations done after ethmoidectomy for sinus disease, with or without nasal polyps. In seven of ten revision ethmoidectomies the patients had asthma, three with ASA intolerance[62]. A success rate of 91% was found in patients with focal disease, and dropped to 50% in asthmatics with panpolyposis. Recurrences were found in 41% in patients with triad cases[45]. From another series[59] the recurrence rate of hyperplastic disease after intranasal sphenoethmoidectomy in asthmatics was 18.2%, and in non-asthmatic 14.2%. From the same series a similar difference was observed in patients with an antral approach, and two thirds of ASA intolerant patients had the same results as asthmatics without ASA intolerance. From another study the improvement was nearly the same in patients with and without asthma, 78.9% versus 85.1%, but showed lower figures in triad cases, 69.3%[63]. When using a detailed grading system those with the ASA triad had the poorest outcome with 35% success, polyposis and asthma 39%, no polyposis but with asthma 55%, and otherwise normal patients with or without polyposis showed 65% and 68% suc-

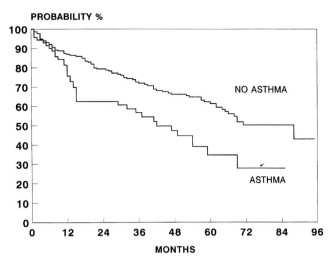

RECURRENCE PROFILE AFTER FIRST POLYPECTOMY

Figure 1. The probability to be recurrence free by time after the first polypectomy. Life-table method. Log rank test: p < 0.001.

cess[64]. Poorer results in asthmatics have been found by others[65,66], and corresponding results was observed in another study, where 39.2% of the cavities in asthmatics were normal versus 62.7% in non-asthmatics, but it was found that the difference primarily was due to a greater extent of disease present in patients with asthma[67]. In a study on revision cases 32.6% were asthmatics and half of these were considered revision failures[68]. The effect of topical and systemic steroid treatment for nasal polyposis in patients with or without asthma or ASA intolerance does not seem to have been studied in a similar way. These pieces of information, although not uniform and not directly comparable in many cases, indicate that the effect of nasal and sinus surgery in patients with polyps generally has the poorest outcome in patients with asthma, and that is even more pronounced in patients also having ASA intolerance. From studies on the effect of ethmoidectomy in chronic sinusitis, with or without polyposis, corresponding observations showed a similar trend.

Table 6

	N	Obs. Time* months	Polypectomies 1	2	≥3	Mean no.	Range	P
Asthma	70	58.3	32	17	21	2.4±SD2.1	1–12	P<0.01
No Asthma	213	57.7	132	44	37	1.7±SD1.4	1–13	

Mann-Whitney test on the mean numbers. *obs = observation time

SUMMARY

A strong relationship between polyps and asthma seen from a clinical and an epidemiological point of view as presented in the literature is well documented. A common underlying disease process for patients who both develop asthma and polyps seems likely. Whether the ASA intolerant patients with asthma and polyps constitute a subgroup within the asthmatics with polyps, make up a separate entity, or are an expression of a higher activity of an underlying disease process cannot be defined from the presented materials. The statement that patients with nasal polyps without asthma and ASA intolerance constitutes an incomplete group must be regarded with reservation. No life-long longitudinal study on such patients exists, and the results from the literature indicate that not all polyp-patients develop lower airway disease. Patients with polyps and no lower airway disease differ from the normal population in having a higher male to female ratio, and when compared to the asthmatics and ASA intolerant patients with polyps, their polyp recurrence seems to be less severe despite the presence of polyp tissue eosinophilia.

Identification of such proposed different subgroups of polyp patients with different clinical characteristics and outcome both regarding the upper and lower airway still needs to be investigated through basal and clinical research.

REFERENCES

1. Drake-Lee AB. Nasal polyps. In: Allergic and Non-Allergic Rhinitis, Mygin N, Naclerio RM(eds). Munksgaard, Copenhagen, 1993.
2. Davidsson Å, Hellquist HB: The so-called "allergic" nasal polyp. ORL 55:30–35, 1993.
3. Larsen PL, Tos M. Anatomic side of origin of nasal polyps: Endoscopic nasal and paranasal sinus surgery as a screening method for nasal polyps in an autopsy material. Am J Rhinol. 10:211–216, 1996.
4. Settipane GA, Chafee, FH. Nasal polyps in asthma and rhinitis, A review of 6037 patients. J Allergy Clin Immunol 59:17–21, 1977.
5. Settipane GA. Nasal polyps. In: Rhinitis (Chap XX). Settipane GA (ed). OceanSide Publications, Inc. Providence, Rhode Island, 1991.
6. Settipane GA, Chafee FH, Klein DE. Aspirin intolerance. J Allergy Clin Immunol 53:200–20, 1974.
7. Chafee FH, Settipane GA. Aspirin intolerance. I. Frequency in an allergic population. J Allergy Clin Immunol 53:193–199, 1974.
8. Weber R, Hoffman M, Nelson HS et al. Incidence of bronchoconstriction due to aspirin, azo dyes, non-azo dyes, and preservatives in a population of perennial asthmatics. J Allergy Clin Immunol 64:32–37, 1979.
9. Caplin, I, Haynes JT. Are nasal polyps an allergic phenomenon? Ann Allergy 29:631–634, 1971.
10. Szczeklik A, Gryglewski RJ, Czerniawska-Mysik G. Clinical patterns of hypersensitivity to nonsteroidal anti-inflammatory drugs and their pathogenesis. J Allergy Clin Immunol 60:276–284, 1977.
11. Spector SL, Wangaard CH, Farr R. Aspirin and concomitant idiosyncrasies in adult asthmatic patients. J Allergy Clin Immunol 64,500–506, 1979.
12. Ogino S, Harada T, Okawachi I, Irifune M, Matsunaga T, Nagano T. Aspirin-induced asthma and nasal polyps. Acta Otollaryngol(Stockh) Suppl 430:21–27, 1986.
13. Settipane GA, Pudupakkam RK. Aspirin intolerance III. Subtypes, familial occurrence, and cross-reactivity with tartrazine. J Allergy Clin Immunol 56:215–221, 1975.
14. Settipane GA. Nasal polyposis. NES Allergy Proc 3:497–504, 1982.
15. Settipane GA. Nasal polyps: epidemiology, pathology, immunology and treatment. Am J. Rhinol 1:119–126, 1987.
16. Brown BL, Harner SG, Van Dellen RG. Nasal polypectomy in patients with asthma sensitivity to aspirin. Arch Otolaryngol 105:413–416, 1979.
17. English GM: Nasal polypectomy and sinus surgery in patients with asthma and aspirin idiosyncrasy. Laryngoscope 96:374–380, 1986.
18. Blumstein Gl, Tuft L: Allergy treatment in recurrent nasal polyposis. Amer J Med Sci 234:269–280, 1957.
19. Vleming M, Stoop AE, Middelweerd RJ, de Vries N. Results of endoscopic sinus surgery for nasal polyps. Am J Rhinol 5:173–176, 1991.
20. Schenck NL. Nasal polypectomy in the aspirin-sensitive asthmatic. Trans Am Acad Ophthalmol-Otolaryngol 78:108–119, 1974.
21. Drake-Lee AB, Lowe D, Swanston, A, Grace A: Clinical profile and recurrence of nasal polyps. J Laryngol Otol 98:783–793, 1984.
22. Delaney JC. Aspirin idiosyncrasy in patients admitted for nasal polypectomy. Clin Otolaryngol 1:27–30, 1976.
23. Moloney JR. Nasal polyps, nasal polypectomy, asthma, and aspirin sensitivity. J Laryngol Otol 91:837–846, 1977.
24. Holopainen E, Makinen J, Paavolainen M, Palva T, Salo OP. Nasal polyposis. Acta Otollaryngol 87:330–334, 1979.
25. Stevens HE, Blair NJ: Intranasal sphenoethmoidectomy: 10-year experience and literature review. J Otolaryngol 17:254–258, 1988.
26. Jantti-Alanko S, Holopainen E, Malmberg H: Recurrence of nasal polyps after surgical treatment. Rhinology Suppl 8:59–64, 1989.
27. Granstrom G, Jacobsson E, Jeppsson P-H. Influence of allergy, asthma and hypertension on nasal polyposis. Acta Otolaryngol(Stockh) suppl. 492:22–27, 1992.
28. Wong D, Jordana G, Denbuurg J, Dolovich J. Blood eosinophilia and nasal polyps. Am J Rhinol 6:195–198, 1992.
29. Larsen K, Tos M. Clinical course of patients with primary nasal polyps. Acta Otolaryngol(Stockh) 114:556–559, 1994.
30. Larsen K, Tos M. Recurrence frequency of nasal polyps. In: Passali D (ed): Rhinology up-to-date. Industria Grafica Romana (Rome) 1994:225–228.
31. Kordash TR, Gleich GJ, Kern EB, O'Fallon WM. Evidence for increased risk of development of asthma in

patients with nasal polyps. J Allergy Clin Immunol 61: 138, 1978.

32. Downing ET, Braman S, Settipane GA. Bronchial reactivity in patients with nasal polyposis before and after polypectomy. J Allergy Clin Immunol 69 (Part 2):102, 1982.

33. Miles-Lawrence R, Kaplan M, Chang K. Methacholine sensitivity in nasal polyposis and the effects of polypectomy. J Allergy Clin Immunol 69 (Part 2):102, 1982.

34. Jacobs RL, Freda AJ, Culver WG. Primary nasal polyposis. Ann Allergy 51:500–505, 1983.

35. Connell T. Nasal disease. N Engl Soc Allergy Proc 3:389–396, 1982.

36. Francis C. The prognosis of operations for removal of nasal polypi in cases of asthma. Practitioner 123:272–278, 1929.

37. Samter M, Lederer FL. Nasal polyps: Their relationship to allergy, particularly to bronchial asthma. Med Clin North Am 42:175–179, 1958.

38. Samter M, Beers RF. Intolerance to aspirin: Clinical studies and consideration of its pathogenesis. Ann Intern Med 68:975–983, 1968.

39. Slavin RG. Relationship of nasal disease and sinusitis to bronchial asthma. Ann Allergy 49:76–80, 1982.

40. Jankowski R, Moneret-Vautrin DA, Goetz R, Wayoff M. Incidence of medico-surgical treatment for nasal polyps on the development of associated asthma. Rhinology 30: 249–258, 1992.

41. Settipane GA, Klein DE, Lekas MD. Asthma and nasal polyps. In Myers E, ed. New Dimensions in Otorhinlaryngology, Head and Neck Surgery. Amsterdam: Excerpta Medica, 1985, pp 499–500.

42. Friedman WH, Katsantonis GP, Slavin RG, Kannel P, Linford P. Sphenoethmoidectomy: Its role in the asthmatic patient. Otolaryngol Head Neck Surg 90:171–177, 1982.

43. Eichel BS. The intranasal ethmoidectomy: a 12-year perspective. Otolaryngol Head Neck Surg 90: 540–543, 1982.

44. McFadden EA, Kany RJ, Fink JN, Toohill RJ. Surgery for sinusitis and aspirin triad. Laryngoscope 100: 1043–1046, 1990.

45. Lawson W. The intranasal ethmoidectomy: Evolution and an assessment of the procedure. Laryngoscope suppl. 64:1–49, 1994.

46. Raphael GD, Meredith SD, Baraniuk JN, Kaliner MA. Nasal reflexes. In: Rhinitis. Settipane GA (ed) OceanSide Publications, Inc. Providence, Rhode Island, 1991.

47. Yan K, Salome C. The response of the airways to nasal stimulation in asthmatics with rhinitis. Eur J Resp Dis 64 (suppl 128):105–108, 1983.

48. Kautman J, Wright GW. The effect of nasal and nasopharyngeal irritation on airway resistance in man. Am Rev Respir Dis 100:626–630, 1969.

49. Cassisi NJ, Biller HF, Ogura JH. Changes in arterial oxygen tension and pulmonary mechanics with the use of posterior packing in epistaxis: a preliminary report. Laryngoscope 81:1261–1266, 1971.

50. Ogura I, Unno T, Nelson JR. Nasal surgery, physiological considerations of nasal obstruction. Arch Otolaryngol 88:288–295, 1968.

51. Jacobs JR, Levine LA, Davis H, Lefrak SS, Druck NS, Ogura JH. Posterior packs and the nasopulmonary reflex. Laryngoscope 91:279–284, 1981.

52. Larsen K, Juul A. Arterial blood gases and pneummatic nasal packing in epistaxis. Laryngoscope 92:586–588, 1982.

53. Larsen K. Oxhøj H. Spirometric forced volume measurements in the assessment of nasal patency after septoplasty. A prospective clinical study. Rhinology 26:203–208, 1988.

54. Larsen K, Kristensen S. Peak flow nasal patency indices and self-assessment in septoplasty. Clin Otolaryngol 15: 327–334, 1990.

55. McFadden ER, Jr. Nasal-sinus-pulmonary reflexes and bronchial asthma. J Allergy Clin Immunol 78:1–3, 1986.

56. McFadden ER, Jr. Physiological and pathological interactions between the upper and lower airways and bronchial asthma. In: Rhinitis and asthma. Mygind N, Pipkorn U, Dahl R (eds). Munksgaard, Copenhagen, 1990.

57. Henriksen JM, Exercise-induced asthma in children. Thesis, University Hospital of Aarhus, 1990.

58. Schaefer SD, Manning A, Close LG, Endoscopic paranasal sinus surgery: Indications and considerations. Laryngoscope 99:1–5, 1989.

59. Friedman WH, Katsantonis G: Intranasal and transantral ethmoidectomy: a 20-year experience. Laryngoscope 100: 343–348, 1994.

60. May M, Levine HL, Schaitkin B, Mester M. Complications of endoscopic sinus surgery. In: Endoscopic Sinus Surgery. Levine HL and May M (eds). Thieme Medical Publishers, New York, 1993.

61. May M, Levine HL, Mester SJ, Schaitkin B. Complications of endoscopic sinus surgery: Analysis of 2108 patients—Incidence and prevention. Laryngoscope 104: 1080–1083, 1994.

62. Eichel BS, Revision sphenoethmoidectomy. Laryngoscope 95:300–304, 1985.

63. Wigand ME, Hosemann WG. Results of endoscopic surgery of the paranasal sinuses and anterior skull base. J Otolaryngol 20:385–390, 1991.

64. May M, Levine HL, Schaitkin B, Mester SJ: Results of surgery. In: Endoscopic Sinus Surgery. Levine HL and May M (eds). Thieme Medical Publishers, New York, 1993.

65. Ragheb S, Duncavage JA. Maxillary sinusitis: Value of endoscopic middle meatus anstrostomy versus Caldwell-Luc procedure. Operative Techniques in Otolaryngology-Head and Neck Surgery, 3:2:129–133, 1992.

66. Schaitkin B, May M, Shapiro A, Fucci M, Mester SJ: Endoscopic sinus surgery: 4 year follow-up on the first 100 patients. Laryngoscope 103:1117–1120, 1993.

67. Kennedy DW: Prognostic factors, outcomes and staging in ethmoid sinus surgery. Laryngoscope Suppl 57:1–18, 1992.

68. King JM, Caldarelli DD, Pigato JB. A review of revision functional endoscopic sinus surgery. Laryngoscope 104: 404–408, 1994.

Chapter XIII

Nasal Polyps and Immunoglobulin E (IgE)

Guy A. Settipane, M.D.

ABSTRACT

Nasal polyps are usually found in non allergic individuals. However, when nasal polyps and atopy occur together a special interaction exists. Total and specific immunoglobulin E (IgE) are found in significantly greater concentration in nasal polyp tissue than in serum and tonsil tissue. Immunoglobulin A (IgA) is also more concentrated in nasal polyps than serum. Patients with nasal polyps and allergies seem to have a greater recurrence rate after surgical polypectomy. Frequently, polyp recurrence occurs during specific pollen seasons in sensitive individuals. Upper respiratory infections are also a precipitating factor for recurrence. Nasal ciliary beat frequency is inhibited in patients with chronic sinusitis, allergic nasal reactions, and non specific nasal eosinophilia syndromes (NARES, BENARS). Nasal polyps are frequently associated with these conditions, which may predispose the nasal mucosa to infections and increased risk for developing nasal polyps.

When nasal polyps and allergies occur together, it is important to treat the allergic condition. This takes the form of identifying the allergens, eliminating them from the environment (if possible) using antihistamines/decongestants, and nasal antiinflammatory drugs such as topical steroids. Hyposensitization may be considered in resistant cases.

In 1952 Berdal[1] reported that skin sensitivity antibody in nasal polyp fluid was many times more concentrated than that found in sera. In 1974, Chandra and Abrol[2] stated that polyp fluid contains albumin and immunoglobulins (IgA, IgE, IgG, and IgM). The concentration of the secretory immunoglobulin IgA and IgE and in some cases IgG and IgM were greater in the polyp fluid than in the serum. Whiteside et al[3] reported that in five of six cases of nasal polyps in non allergic patients, no IgE bearing lymphocytes were detected in polyp tissue. In 1993, Sheen-Yie Fang [4] stated that about 73% of chronic sinusitis associated with nasal polyps had one or more positive skin tests to 10 common allergens. The type of allergens were not specified. His statistics may be high because they were affected by his equation where bilateral chronic maxillary sinusitis was counted twice (two sinus units) compared to patients who had unilateral maxillary sinusitis (one unit). His data were based on 71 patients, comprising 121 maxillary (chronic) sinusitis units. Counting some patients twice may have had undue influence on his results.

In 1991, Yaremchuk, McCullough, and Ownby[5] studied forty-seven patients undergoing nasal polypectomy and 27 adults undergoing tonsillectomy. At surgery, samples of serum, tissues, and nasal washings were obtained for evaluation of total and allergen-specific IgE. He found that total serum IgE levels were not higher in polypectomy patients compared to tonsillectomy patients. However the total IgE/mg of protein was significantly greater in polyp than tonsil tissue. Also, allergen-specific serum IgE (RAST) levels did not differ in polyp and tonsil patients nor was bacterial specific IgE detected in polyp patients. By skin test 46% of polypectomy patients had positive reactions compared to 13% of tonsillectomy patients. The majority of polypectomy patients had negative allergy skin tests. In addition, they stated that the allergen specific IgG4 levels and the ratios of specific Ig4 to specific IgE did not differ between the two patient groups.

Our own data show that in 211 cases of nasal polyps, 56% had one or more positive allergy skin tests to a standard battery of allergens.[6] However, it is important to note that our patients came from a large hospital allergy clinic and two allergy private practices. In this regard, the basic population was biased in favor of allergies, and may explain the high rate of positive skin tests.

There are two main theories as to why polyps contain higher concentration of total and specific IgE than tonsils and serum. The first is that IgE is a secretory immunoglobulin and is locally produced and accumulated inside the closed polyp sac. Normally, these secretory immunoglobulins would be washed away by nasal secretions. The other secretory immunoglobulin, IgA, is similarly found in higher concentration in nasal polyps tissue than in serum. Another explanation for concentrated immunoglobulins in nasal polyps is that the polyp may act as a dialyzing membrane. Removing the water component of the fluid in the polyp sac concentrates higher molecular structure components such as immunoglobulins inside the polyp. The clinical significance of this increased concentration of IgE may be that only small concentration of aeroallergens are needed to activate the allergic reactions which results in the release and cascade of histamine, prostaglandin and other chemical mediators (Chapter VI). One hypothesis is that these mediators in turn may stimulate the secretory glands, causing the polyp to increase in size and cause recurrences during the pollen season if pollen sensitivity exists.

The overwhelming evidence is that nasal polyps are not caused by the allergic or IgE antibody response. However, when nasal polyps and atopy occur together, allergies aggravate nasal polyps and cause recurrence. Our data in reviewing the frequency of polyp recurrence after surgical polypectomy is shown in Table 1.[7-9] In 167 patients, the number of total surgical polypectomies per patient is directly proportional to the number of positive allergy skin tests to common allergens. It is probable the number of polypectomy may be affected by positive allergy skin tests.[7]

Other data also demonstrate that allergies increase the recurrence rate of nasal polyp, table II.[10,11] In 14 allergic patients there were 15 incidences of recurrence of nasal polyp during the pollen season to which the patient was sensitive. The pathogenic mechanism is thought to be re-

Table 1. Frequency of Polypectomies in Patients with Positive Allergy Skin Tests

No. of Polypectomies	Total Patients*	No. with Positive Allergy Skin Tests	%
None	24	12	50
One or more	143	81	57
Two or more	57	33	53
Three or more	34	20	59
Four or more	22	15	68
Five or more	17	12	71
Six or more	11	8	73

*Total Patients = 167
One patient did not have a skin test
Reprinted from Ref. 9.

lated to increase secretion of goblet cells (rhinorrhea) within the polyp, as a result of hayfever.

Table 2 also shows that in 25 patients with nasal polyps seven recurrences were associated with upper respiratory infections.[10] Again, a plausible pathogenic mechanism may be the increased secretion of mucous cells in the polyps occurring with the common cold.

An infectious and inflammatory relationship to nasal polyps will be discussed in Chapter XVI. Infections of the nose and sinuses as well as inflammation and allergies can cause an inhibition of the nasal ciliary beat frequency. This inhibition of mucous flow may increase the risk of developing nasal infection and perhaps nasal polyp formation. Saito and Tsubokawa[12] reported that ciliary activity in chronic sinusitis showed impairment in both decreased ciliary rate of beating and reduced ciliated area. Chronic sinusitis is frequently found in patients with nasal polyps and this association may be on an infectious and as well as on an obstructive basis.

Holmstrom, Lund, and Scadding[13] reported that nasal ciliary beat frequency was decreased when an allergic reaction was provoked. They concluded that in a nasal allergic reaction it is possible that decreased mucociliary function contributes to nasal obstruction and decreased ventilation of the sinuses. This type of allergic

Table 2. Nasal Polyps & IgE[10-11]
Polyp Recurrence: Precipitating Factors

Condition	Total Patients	Precipitating Factor	Number
Positive Skin Tests to Pollens	14	Pollen Season	15
Upper Respiratory Infections	25	URI	7

reaction may increase the risk of infection and recurrence of polyps.

In 1985, we evaluated 78 consecutive patients with perennial, non allergic rhinitis of at least 3 months duration (mean duration 8 years)[14]. An attempt was made to diagnosis and to characterize these patients, Table 3 and Table 4. Patients with a history of nasal polyps, aspirin intolerance, physical nasal obstruction, rhinitis medicamentosa, and asthma/bronchitis were excluded from this study. We found a significant number of these non allergic patients had nasal eosinophilia.

Table 3. Diagnosis of 78 Patients with Non Allergic Rhinitis

Diagnosis	No.	Totals Considered	%
Vasomotor rhinitis VMR	44	72	61%
Non Allergic Rhinitis with Eosinophils (NARE)	25	75	33%
Sinusitis (X-rays)*	11	68	16%
Possible allergy**	9	76	12%
Blood Eosinophilic Non Allergic Rhinitis (BENAR)*	3	76	4%
Hypothyroidism	1	68	2%

*Overlapping of diagnosis present.
**Elevated serum IgE levels.
Reprinted from Ref. 14.

Table 4. Non Allergic Rhinitis with Eosinophils Syndrome (NARES)

Characteristics	No.	Total Considered	%
Total patients	25	75	33%
Mean age (40 years)	25		
Females	16	25	64%
Males	9	25	36%
Allergy skin test	25	All negative	
IgE*		All normal	
Sinusitus (X-ray)	6	25	24%
Eosinophil nasal smear (≥5%)	25	All positive	
Eosinophil nasal smear (≥25%)	9	25	36%
Elevated blood eosinophils**	3	25	12%

*Three patients with elevated IgE were removed from this group.
**Sub classified as BENAR Syndrome (Table V).
Reprinted from Ref. 14.

Table 5. Statistically Significant Correlation between Nasal Eosinophilia (Eos) and Nasal Circulation Time (NCT) Greater than 25 Minutes ($P = 0.156$)

	Total	NCT > 25 Min	%	P
Eos −	44	8	18.2	
				.0156
Eos +	12	7	58.3	
Total	56	15		

Reprinted from Ref. 26.

In non allergic rhinitis with eosinophilia syndrome (NARES)[14–17] and in blood eosinophilic non allergic rhinitis syndrome (BENARS),[14–18] non specific and non allergic nasal eosinophilia may cause inflammation. This may occur as a result of toxic substances associated with eosinophils such as the major basic protein and other eosinophil granule-derived proteins.[19] These toxic proteins may damage nasal ciliated epithelium and cause a delay in mucociliary clearance.[20–25] In 1992 we reported on fifty-six non allergic patients with rhinitis and found a statistically significant correlation of nasal eosinophilia with prolonged nasal circulation time (saccharine challenge, Table 5.[26]

In summary, nasal allergic reactions/upper respiratory infections and non specific inflammation (eosinophils) can cause a delay in nasal cilary activity. This delay in activity will inhibit mucus flow rate and can increase infections. Recurrent infections are thought to be one cause of nasal polyps. Nasal polyps are frequently associated with nasal eosinophilia. There is some concern that nasal eosinophilia may be a precursor for nasal polyps.[15,16,18]

TREATMENT OF ALLERGIES

Treatment of allergies is important in preventing recurrences in individuals with both nasal polyps and allergies. It is appropriate that all patients with nasal polyps have an allergy evaluation. This consists of having total and specific IgE determination. The latter can be done by allergy skin tests, serum RAST or an enzyme-linked test equivalent to RAST. Once the allergies have been identified, an attempt must be made to remove the offending allergen, if possible. For example, if a patient is found to be allergic to a cat or dog, these animals are best removed from the immediate living conditions. The allergenic proteins from animals are found in the saliva and urine.

House dust mites are another frequent offender. These mites are difficult to eradicate. They live on skin and secretory debris of humans. Mite excreta contain the allergenic substance which becomes embedded in rugs, pillows, mattresses, and stuffed chairs. It is possible to place a barrier such as a plastic cover on the mattress and pillow to prevent the antigenic substance from stimulating the nose. The rugs are a different matter. It is practically impossible to remove all the antigenic material from rugs, despite vacuuming and washing. It is best to remove rugs especially from the bedroom. Besides animals and dust mites, other perennial allergens are molds, especially the indoor molds, Aspergillosis and penicillium, and possibly cockroach antigen. A dehumidifier and eliminating mold source in damp cellars are helpful. Control of these perennial allergens are needed to prevent recurrence of nasal polyps.

Pollens are difficult to avoid. Home and office air filtering systems are effective in reducing these aeroallergens. Other helpful environmental factors are not exercising outdoors especially in the morning during the pollen season. It is best for sensitive individuals not to cut the grass but if one is to work outdoors a pollen mask may render some relief.

Medications such as antihistamines, decongestants, and anti inflammatory drugs may be needed for control in patients with nasal polyps and allergies. It seems logical that the classical antihistamines should be preferred since they have an anti cholinergic factor which will inhibit mucus production.[27] Care should be taken to caution patients about sedatory properties of these older classical antihistamines. Anti inflammatory drugs such as topical corticosteroids and cromolyn/nedocromil are very helpful in controlling allergies. It seems likely that patients with nasal polyps should be on daily treatment with nasal corticosteroid sprays and possibly decongestants. This type of treatment is especially important when nasal polyps are associated with allergies.

Immunotherapy with allergen (hyposensitization treatment) may be used to prevent polyp recurrence in some of these patients who have both nasal polyps and allergies. In patients with allergic rhinitis only (without nasal polyps), immunotherapy is reserved for those individuals who do not respond to allergen elimination procedures, antihistamines, decongestants, and anti inflammatory medications. However, in patients with allergies and recurrent nasal polyps, immunotherapy may be considered more readily than usual. The rationale is that whatever allergies a patient may have is enhanced by the increased concentration of IgE found in polyps as compared to serum.[28]

REFERENCES

1. Berdal P. Serologic investigations on the edema fluid from nasal polyps. J Allergy 23: 11–14, 1952.
2. Chandra RK, Abrol BM. Immunopathology of nasal polypi. J Laryngol Otol 88:1019–1024, 1974.
3. Whiteside TL, Rabin BS, Zetterberg J, Criep L. The presence of IgE on the surface of lymphocytes in nasal polyps. J Allergy Clin Immunol 55:186–194, 1975.
4. Fang, Sheen-Yie. Normalization of maxillary sinus mucosa after FESS. A prospective study of chronic sinusitis with nasal polyps. Rhinology 32, 173–140, 1994.
5. Yaremchuk K, McCullough J, Ownby DR. Immunologic evaluation of nasal polyps. Am. J Rhinol 5:19–23, 1991.
6. Settipane GA, Chafee FH. Nasal polyps in asthma and rhinitis: A review of 6,037 patients. J Allergy Clin Immunol 59:17–21, 1977.
7. Settipane GA, Klein DE, Lekas MD. Asthma and nasal polyps. In: Myers E, Ed. New Dimensions in Otorhinolaryngology, Head and Neck Surgery, Amsterdam: Excerpta Medica, 1987, pp 499–500.
8. Settipane GA. Nasal polyps: Epidemiology, pathology, immunology and treatment. Am J Rhinol I:119–126, 1987.
9. Settipane GA. Nasal polyps in Rhinitis, 2nd Ed. Settipane (Ed), OceanSide Pub, 1991, pp 173–183.
10. Settipane GA. Presented at the ERS 90 Congress, London, 1990.
11. Settipane GA. Aspirin intolerance and other systemic diseases presenting as nasal polyps. Am J Rhinol 8:298–299, 1994, supplement.
12. Saito H, Tsukokawa T. Ciliary activity of nasal polyp and mucous in a chronic sinusitis.
13. Holmstrom M, Lund VJ, Scadding G. Nasal ciliary beat frequency after nasal allergen challenge. Am J Rhinol. 6:101, 1992.
14. Settipane GA, Klein DE. Non allergic rhinitis: demography of eosinophils in nasal smear, blood total eosinophil counts and IgE levels. Allergy Proceedings: 6:363–366, 1985.
15. Mullarkey MF, Hill JS, Webb DR. Allergic and nonallergic rhinitis: their characterization with attention to the meaning of nasal eosinophilia. J Allergy Clin Immunol 65:122–126. 1980.
16. Mullarkey MF. Eosinophilic nonallergic rhinitis. J Allergy Clin Immunol 82:941–949, 1988.
17. Jacobs RL, Freedman PM, Boswell RN. Nonallergic rhinitis with eosinophilia (NARES syndrome). J Allergy Clin Immunol 61:253–262, 1981.
18. Moneret-Vautrin DA, Hsieh V, Wayoff M, Guyot JL, Mouton C, Maria Y. Nonallergic rhinitis with eosinophilia syndrome a precursor of the triad: nasal polyposis, intrinsic asthma, and intolerance to aspirin. Ann Allergy 64: 513–518, 1990.
19. Takasaka T, Kurihara A, Suzuki H, et al. The differentiation of polyps and their musosal ultrastructure. Am J Rhinol 4:159–162, 1990.
20. Bousquet J, Chanez P, Lacoste JY, et al. Eosinophilic inflammation in asthma. N Engl J Med 323:1033–1039, 1990.
21. Hastie AT, Loegering DA, Gleich GJ, Kueppers F. The effect of purified human eosinophil major basic protein on mammalian ciliary activity. Am Rev Respir Dis 135:848–853, 1987.
22. Flavahan NA, Slifman NR, Gleich GJ, Vanhoutte PM. Human eosinophil major basic protein causes hyperreactivity of respiratory smooth muscle. Am Rev Respir Dis 138:685–688, 1988.
23. Venge P, Dahl R, Fredens K, Peterson CGB. Epithelial injury by human eosinophil. Am Rev Respir Dis 138:S54–S57, 1988.

24. Spector SL, English G, Jones L. Clinical and nasal biopsy response to treatment of perennial rhinitis. Am J Allergy Clin Immunol 66:129–137, 1980.
25. Ayars GH, Altman LC, McManus MM, et al. Injurious effect of eosinophil peroxide-hydrogen peroxide-halide system and major basic protein on human nasal epithelium in vitro. Am Rev Respir Dis 140:125–131, 1989.
26. Davidson AE, Miller SD, Settipane RJ, Ricci AR, Klein DE, Settipane GA. Delayed nasal mucociliary clearance in patients with non allergic rhinitis and nasal eosinophils. Allergy Proceedings 13:81–84, 1992.
27. Cooper JW. Classical antihistamines and decongestants in the treatment of chronic rhinitis, in Rhinitis, 2nd Ed. Settipane GA (ed). OceanSide Publications, Providence, RI, 1991, p. 219–223.
28. Shatkin SS, Delsupehe KG, Thisted RA, Corey JP. Mucosal allergy in the absence of systemic allergy in nasal polyposis and rhinitis. A meta-analysis. Otolaryngol-HNS 111:552–556, 1994.

Chapter XIV

Nasal Polyps and Aspirin Intolerance

Guy A. Settipane, M.D., and Russell A. Settipane, M.D.

ABSTRACT

The tetrad of aspirin intolerance (bronchospastic type), nasal polyps, asthma and chronic sinusitis is well established. However, nasal polyps and aspirin intolerance frequently occur alone. There are many similar characteristics between nasal polyps and aspirin intolerance. Both have an increased frequency with increased age, both are not mediated by IgE antibody, both are usually associated with eosinophilia, and both have a familial occurrence. They are most frequently found in association with non allergic asthma. The pathological mechanism of aspirin intolerance is through the inhibition of the cyclo-oxygenase pathway of arachidonic metabolism resulting in increased production of leukotriene, which can cause acute bronchospasm. Nasal polyps do not appear to be associated with this mechanism. However, the effect of the new anti-leukotriene drugs on nasal polyps has not been determined. Surgical removal of nasal polyps does not appear to cause or aggravate asthma. Surgical polypectomy in patients with aspirin intolerance is associated with a shorter interval of polyp recurrence when compared to those patients that are aspirin tolerant.

The medicinal properties of salicylates were well known to ancient physicians who used them mostly for their antipyretic and analgesic effects. Hippocrates used salicylates in the form of willow bark (salix alia). Salican can be extracted from willow bark, and on hydrolysis, liberates glucose and salicylic alcohol. Aspirin or acetysalicylic acid was introduced into medicine in 1899 by Dresel[1]; its name was derived from Spirsaure, German for salicylic acid.

Three years after aspirin's introduction, it was implicated as the cause of an anaphylactic reaction in a report by Hirschberg[2–3] of Pozan, a city presently part of Poland, but which in 1902 was under Prussian control. Hirschberg presented a case report of acute angioedema/urticaria occurring shortly after the ingestion of aspirin. This reaction subsided in 3 days, and the patient survived. Other reports of anaphylactoid reactions to aspirin soon followed. Gilbert[4] in 1911 and Reed[5] in 1914 reported cases of angioedema/urticaria following aspirin ingestion. These first reports were all examples of the urticarial or cutaneous subtype of aspirin intolerance.

There is a second major subtype of anaphylactoid reaction to aspirin manifested as acute bronchospasm which was first reported by Cooke[6] in 1919. In this report, Cooke stated that "symptoms begin as a rule from fifteen to twenty minutes after ingestion of 10 grains of the commercial drug (aspirin). In nine of fifteen cases, violent bronchial asthma was induced and one case was almost fatal from asphyxia." Cooke also demonstrated marked eosinophilia in these patients who had negative skin tests to aspirin. Thus Cooke was one of the first to determine that reactions to aspirin were not mediated by antibody-antigen reaction, although associated with eosinophilia. Other authors have since confirmed this non immunologic reactivity by sophisticated laboratory procedures.[7,8] It is now postulated that anaphylactic reactions due to aspirin are mediated through the arachidonic acid metabolic pathway, specifically inhibition of cyclooxygenase.

Following Cooke's case report of a near fatal reaction to aspirin, Vander Veer[9] in 1920 reported the first death due to aspirin. Other reports of deaths due to aspirin followed: Lamson and Thomas[10] in 1932 and Francis et al.[11] in 1935. In these instances death was attributed to acute bronchospasm following aspirin ingestion.

In modern day science, aspirin intolerance is described as acute bronchial spasm, rhinorrhea, ocular injection or acute urticaria/angioedema occurring within 3 hours after ingesting aspirin. The old term for "aspirin intolerance" was "aspirin allergy." However, this term is no longer used because specific IgE to ASA has not been found[8]. We prefer to use the term "aspirin intolerance" which can be used interchangeably with the term "ASA sensitivity" as used by other authors. The bronchospastic subtype of aspirin intolerance is an important part of the classic syndrome of 1) nasal polyps, 2) aspirin intolerance, 3) asthma and 4) rhino-sinusitis. Widal, et al[12] first described this syndrome and the subsequent desensitization with aspirin in 1922. Parts of this syndrome were first reported by other authors such as Cooke[6] in 1919 (as mentioned above) and Samter and Beers in 1967[13]. These latter authors called the syndrome a triad, leaving out rhino-sinusitis, from their description. It is probably best described as a tetrad.

Since these early publications, a great deal of information has emerged on aspirin sensitivity, including data on epidemiology, further characterization of the two major subtypes of sensitivity (bronchospastic and urticarial types), hereditary aspects, cross-reactions to other nonsteroidal anti-inflammatory drugs, methods of desensitization, and mechanism of action[14-19].

Characteristics of the bronchospastic type of aspirin intolerance are listed in Table 1. The type of aspirin intolerance associated with nasal polyps is the bronchospastic type not the urticaria/angioedema type. Most individuals with aspirin intolerance are not atopic.

Aspirin intolerance is most commonly associated with non allergic (or negative skin test) asthma and a normal serum IgE level. Elevated blood eosinophils and a marked eosinophilia in the nasal secretions are also characteristic of this syndrome. There is a hereditary predis-

Table 1. Characteristics of the Bronchospastic Type of Aspirin Intolerance

Found in asthmatic patients
Correlates with nasal polyposis
Similar age onset as asthma
Severe rhinorrhea with aspirin reactions
Increased frequency in older age groups
Familial occurrence
Eosinophils in nasal smear
Elevated total (blood) eosinophil count
Nonsteroidal anti-inflammatory drug cross-reaction
No specific IgE (anti-aspiryl)
Normal total IgE
Desensitization possible to aspirin
Pathogenic mechanism: Inhibition of cyclo-oxygenase (Arachidonic Metabolism)

position of aspirin intolerance in that clusters of this syndrome are found in certain families[17].

The frequency of aspirin intolerance increases with age, especially over 40. However, it is the bronchospastic type of aspirin intolerance not the urticaria/angioedema type in which this occurs, Table 2[14-15].

It is apparent that there are many similarities between aspirin intolerance and nasal polyps, Table 3[18]. Besides being associated together in the triad of asthma, aspirin intolerance (bronchospastic type) and nasal polyps, both are associated with chronic sinusitis and nasal peripheral eosinophilia. Both conditions increase in frequency with age, both are commonly associated with negative skin test (or non allergic) asthma, and both conditions are associated with a high frequency of steroid-dependent asthma.

Table 2. Frequency of Major Types of Aspirin Intolerance as Determined by History in Various Age Groups of Asthmatic Patients

Asthmatic Patients		Major Type of Aspirin Intolerance			
Age when first seen (Years)	No. With Asthma	No. with bronchospasm	%*	No. With Urticaria/ Angioedema	%†
10–19	358	3	0.8	2	0.6
20–29	351	6	1.7	6	1.7
30–39	342	11	3.2	3	0.9
40–49	357	18	5.0	7	2.0
50 and over	367	17	4.6	2	0.5
Total	1,775	55	3.1	20	1.1

*The trend of progressive differences by decades is statistically significant (P < 0.01)
†The trend of differences is not statistically significant. Included are 3 patients who manifested both bronchospasm and urticaria. Four patients with aspirin intolerance manifested solely by rhinorrhea are not included in this table.
Source: From Ref. No. 14.

Table 3. Similarities Between Routine Nasal Polyps and Aspirin Intolerance

	ASA Intol	Nasal Polyps
Associated with tetrad of ASA Intol., Asthma, Nasal Polyps and Sinsuitis	Yes	Yes
Increased freq in older age group	Yes	Yes
Mediated by IgE	No	No
Familial occurrences	Yes	Yes
Eos. in nasal smear	Yes	Yes
Elevated total eosinophil count	Yes	Yes
Pathogenic mechanisms related to leukotrienes	Yes	?
Associated with other diseases besides asthma and sinusitis	No	Yes

It is important to remember that nonsteroidal anti-inflammatory drugs (NSAID) cross-react with aspirin and cause a similar acute bronchospasm in the aspirin-intolerant asthmatics, Table 4. These drugs also are cyclooxygenase inhibitors. Most of these NSAIDS, such as indomethacin and ibuprofen, cross-react with aspirin in intolerant individuals almost 100% of the time. Some NSAID cross-react with aspirin in intolerant individuals at a somewhat decreased rate, depending on the dose used, and degree of inhibition of cyclooxygenase. There is an inverse relationship between the degree of inhibition of cyclooxygenase and the cross-reactivity rate of the NSAIDs[19].

The surgical removal of nasal polyps does not cause or aggravate asthma. In our laboratory, 10 patients with nasal polyps and no history of asthma were studied, Table 5[20]. Results of methacholine challenge tests done before and about five months after polypectomy were essentially the same. In a report by Miles-Lawrence et al[21], similar data were obtained. They performed methacholine challenge tests 1 month prior to polypectomy and up to 1 year following polypectomy. They found essentially no change in methacholine sensitivity, confirming our conclusion that polypectomy does not cause or worsen asthma.

Table 4. Nonsteroidal Anti-inflammatory Drugs That can React with Aspirin

Cyclo-Oxygenase Inhibitors

Aspirin	Meclofenamate sodium
Etodolac	Mefenamic acid
Fenoprofen	Nabumetone
Ibuprofen	Naproxen
Indomethacin	Piroxicam
Ketorolac Tromethamine	Sulindac

We also evaluated seven steroid-dependent asthmatic patients for steroid requirements before and approximately six months following polypectomy (Table 6)[22–25]. The steroid requirements were essentially unchanged in five patients and decreased in two. Thus, our initial data with methacholine sensitivity essentially has been confirmed with subsequent clinical information. Polypectomy does not make asthma worse but may even cause some improvement, possibly because of less stimulation through the rhinosinobronchial reflex.

Patients with aspirin intolerance and nasal polyps may have similar recurrence rate after surgical polypectomy, as patients who are aspirin tolerant, Table 7[26]. However, the mean interval between recurrence was shorter in aspirin intolerant patients than in aspirin tolerant patients (3.7 years, vs 11.6 years). The recurrence occurred within 1–5 years after polypectomy for aspirin intolerant patients compared with a range 1–24 years in aspirin tolerant patients. Patient education should take into consideration this information when dealing with aspirin intolerant patient polypectomy.

The pathological mechanism of the bronchospastic type of aspirin intolerance has been substantially clarified. The pathogenic mechanism for aspirin intolerance clearly involves its effect on leukotrienes, Fig. 1[24]. In aspirin intolerant individuals, inhibition of the cyclooxygenase pathway by aspirin causes a shunting toward the lipoxygenase pathway resulting in increased production of leukotrienes LTC4, LTD4, and LTE4 which produce bronchospasm, increased airway responsiveness, mucus hypersecretion, airway mucosa edema, and increased neutrophils and eosinophils in the exudate. Both aspirin intolerance and nasal polyps may be associated with increased esoinophils by this mechanism. Lending support to the importance of lipoxygenase pathway shunting is the fact that antagonists of the 5-Lipoxygenase pathway (such as Zileuton® and Accolate®) cause an improvement in asthma and inhibition of bronchospasm induced by

Table 5. Effect of Polypectomy on Methacholine Sensitivity

| Investigators | Total Patients | Diagnosis | Methacholine Sensitivity | | | Time Interval after Polypectomy |
			Same	Increased	Decreased	
Downing, Braman, Settipane	6	No asthma	6	0	0	Mean 20 wk
(1982)[25]	4	Asthma	2	1	1	Mean 20 wk
Miles-Lawrence, Kaplan,	5	No asthma	2	1	2	1 mo*
Chang (1982)[26]	1	Asthma	0	1	0	

*Two patients followed for 6 and 12 months, respectively, had no change in methacholine sensitivity.
Source: From Ref. 20–21.

aspirin intolerant individuals[27–29]. There is also a decrease of urinary LTE4 level. A similar abnormal mechanism involving arachidonic acid and prostaglandins for the formation of nasal polyps has not been developed at this time, but further research is needed in this area.

Acute reactions after the accidental ingestion of aspirin or nonsteroidal antiinflammatory drugs in aspirin intolerant asthmatic patients usually constitute a medical emergency. These reactions may begin with severe rhinorrhea followed rapidly by acute bronchospasm and even shock; an occasional patient may have acute urticarial and/or angioedema with or without respiratory distress. Some reactions may present as acute rhinitis only[30]. Severe reactions involving shock should be treated promptly with epinephrine (adrenalin) 1/1,000, .1–.5 ml. which could be repeated in 20 minutes. Bronchospastic reactions may be treated with aerosolized beta agonists such as albuterol or metaproterenol in repeated dosages. If symptoms persist, aminophylline in intravenous dosages sufficient to achieve or maintain a therapeutic blood levels may be used. Cyanosis should be treated immediately with oxygen (2–5 liters/min via nasal catheter or 34% by Venturi mask). Hypotension should be treated with intravenous fluid administration, volume expanders, dopamine hydrochloride, or norepinephrine

bitartrate. In prolonged reactions, the intravenous administration of methylprednisolone, 125 mg, or hydrocortisone sodium succinate (Solu-Cortef) 100–200 mg, may be needed.

The chronic treatment of asthma in aspirin-intolerant patients frequently requires the use of systemic and inhaled glucocorticoids for the control of respiratory symptoms in addition to the initiation of oral doses of theophylline and aerosolized beta-agonist medication.

Since these patients frequently have associated chronic rhinosinusitis or nasal polyps, treatment should also be directed to the upper airway. Through the rhinobronchial reflex, acute or chronic sinusitis and nasal polyps can aggravate asthma; and successful treatment of the upper airway disease may decrease the asthma. Sinusitis should be treated vigorously with antibiotics, nasal glucocorticoids, and oral or nasal administration of decongestants. Many times the addition of oral glucocorticoids are required to successfully treat the sinusitis especially when polyps are present.

Desensitization with aspirin followed by long-term daily aspirin treatment has recently been demonstrated to result in improvement of both upper and lower airway symptoms in aspirin-sensitive patients[31–33]. Aspirin desensitization may be considered as an alternate treatment

Table 6. Effect of Polypectomy on Steroid-Dependent Asthma (6-Month Interval)

| Patient | Age (yr) | Prednisone | | Change in Asthma |
		Preoperative	Postoperative (6 mo)	
M.S.	48	10 mg alt days	10 mg alt days	Same
P.B.	25	10 mg alt days	10 mg alt days*	Same
L.C.	66	10 mg alt days	2.5 mg daily	Better
P.M.	66	5 mg daily	10 mg alt days	Better
F.S.	42	10 mg alt days	10 mg alt days	Same
V.L.	58	10 mg daily	10 mg daily	Same
J.C.	76	10 mg alt days	10 mg alt days	Same

*Data collected at 9 months.
Source: From Ref. No. 22–25.

Table 7. Polyp Recurrence in Aspirin Intolerance

Condition	Total Patients	Total Polypectomies (surgical)	Mean Interval (yrs)	Range (yrs)
ASA intolerant	5	8	3.7	1–5
ASA tolerant	24	41	11.6	1–24
Total	29	49	6.3	

for aspirin intolerant patients who are not responding well to conventional therapy. This would pertain to patients having increasing problems with sinusitis, nasal polyp recurrence, or exacerbations of asthma requiring doses of systemic glycocorticoids likely to produce significant side effects. Selected patients with aspirin intolerance and resistant arthritis may also be candidates for desensitization. The arthritic symptoms should be severe enough to warrant the inherent risk associated with desensitization procedures, as outlined by Stevenson and his colleagues[34].

Desensitization is initiated immediately following aspirin challenge studies. The 1 day challenge procedure is useful when aspirin sensitivity is not suspected and the

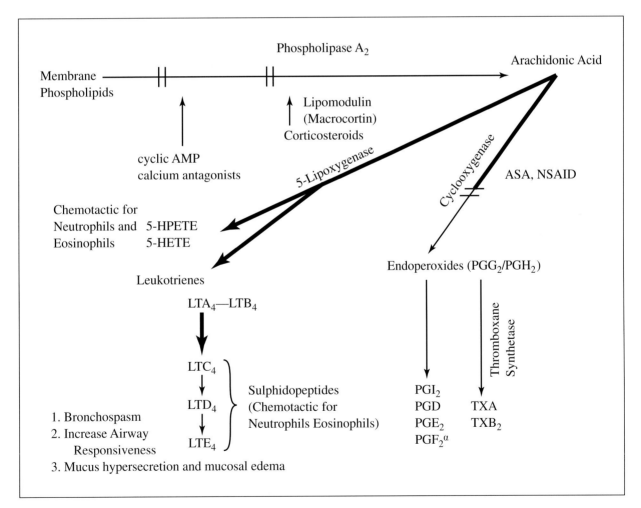

Figure 1. Arachidonic metabolism: pathogenic mechanism for aspirin intolerance. In addition to bronchospasm, LTC$_4$, LTD$_4$, and LTE$_4$ increase cutaneous vasopermeability and elicit a wheal and flare reaction when administered intracutaneously to patients. They also produce increased airway responsiveness, mucus, hypersecretion edema, and mucosal and cellular infiltration of the airways. Elevated cyclic AMP levels, calcium antagonists and glucocorticoids are important inhibitors of arachidonic liberation. (Source: Modified from Reference 24.)

Table 8. One Day Acetylsalicylic (ASA) Acid Challenge

Time	ASA dosage (mg)	Cumulative dosage (mg)
8 AM	30	30
10 AM	60	90
12 PM	100	190
2 PM	325	515
4 PM	650	1,165
6 PM	End*	

*If a reaction does not occur, patient is not ASA sensitive. If forced expiratory volume in 1 sec is reduced 25%, 7 or more days later carry out placebo challenge to confirm specificity. One-day challenge is useful when ASA sensitivity is not suspected and patient has a limited amount of time.
Source: From Ref. 34.

patient has limited time (Table 8). Otherwise, the usual procedure in the patient with a history of aspirin intolerance is the 3-day oral aspirin challenge, (Table 9). It is important to remember that because of the risk involved, challenges should be performed in a hospital setting and that one must start with a 3 mg aspirin dose in patients with a history of severe reactions. If aspirin is continued over ensuing days, the patient will continue to be desensitized to aspirin. However, in rare cases the aspirin reaction may again break through even though the desensitized patient is taking aspirin daily.[35] The refractory period after a positive aspirin challenge usually lasts 2–4 days if aspirin administration is not maintained daily.

Desensitization to aspirin also desensitizes the patient to all other nonsteroidal anti-inflammatory drugs[36–38]. This is also true for weak inhibitors of cyclo-oxygenase such as salsalate and acetaminophen. However because they are weak inhibitors of cyclo-oxygenase these drugs are 1) less likely to cross-react with aspirin, 2) usually require higher challenge doses to induce asthma, and 3) usually result in mild reactions easily treated with beta agonists. Szczezeklik, et al[37] reported that none of their as-

pirin sensitive asthmatics had an adverse reaction except for a possible nasal reaction in one patient when this group was challenged with up to 150 mg of magnesium trisalicylate. Stevenson et al[38] reported that 2 out of 10 aspirin sensitive asthmatics reacted to 2 gm of salsalate. Settipane et al[39] reported that 17/50 (34%) of aspirin sensitive asthmatics reacted when challenged with up to 1500 mg of acetaminophen. This data suggests that low to moderate doses of these analgesics may be cautiously administered in aspirin sensitive patients providing their asthma is in good control and that the first dose is taken under physician observation in a medical setting.

An alternative form of aspirin challenge is by inhalation which is equally sensitive, but is easier to perform and appears safer than oral challenge[40]. Unfortunately lysine-aspirin is not approved for inhalation in the United States. The new antileukotriene drugs may obviate the need for aspirin desensitization or at the very least markedly reduce or abolish the adverse reaction to aspirin. Their effect on the recurrence rate of nasal polyps has not been established as yet.[27]

REFERENCES

1. Gilman Goodman A. The Pharmaceutical Basis of Therapeutics, MacMillan Pergamon Publishing Corp, 8th Edition, 1990.
2. Hirschberg: Mitteillung uber einen Fall von Nebenwirkung des Aspirin. Dtsch Med Wochenschr 28:416, 1902.
3. Settipane GA. Landmark commentary: history of aspirin intolerance. Allergy Proc. 11:251–252, 1990.
4. Gilbert GB. Unusual idiosyncrasy to aspirin. JAMA 56:1262, 1911.
5. Reed EN. Idiosyncrasy to aspirin. JAMA 82:773, 1914.
6. Cooke RA. Allergy in drug idiosyncrasy. JAMA 73:759, 1919.
7. Giraldo B, Blumenthal MW, Spink WW. Aspirin intolerance and asthma. Ann Intern Med 71:479, 1969.
8. Weltman JK, Szaro RP, Settipane GA. An analysis of the role of IgE in intolerance to aspirin and tartrazine. Allergy 33:273, 1978.

Table 9. 3 Day Acetysalicytic Acid (ASA) Challenge

Time	Days 1	2	3
8 AM	Placebo	ASA 30(3) mg	ASA 150 mg
11 AM	Placebo	ASA 60 mg	ASA 325 mg
2 PM	Placebo	ASA 100 mg	ASA 650 mg

Protocol: 1. Discontinue antihistamines, cromolyn and sympathomimetics; 2. Increase gluco-corticoids for 3 days before challenge to produce forced expiratory volume in 1 sec > 70% or a value of 1.5 liters per minute; 3. History of severe reactions; start challenge at 3 mg of ASA (20% of time).
Source: Reprinted with permission of Ref. 34.

9. Vander Veer A Jr. The asthma problem. NY J Med 112:392, 1920.

10. Lamson RW, Thomas R. Some untoward effects of acetyl-salicylic acid. JAMA 99:107, 1932.

11. Francis N, Ghent O, Bullen SS. Death from ten grains of aspirin. J Allergy 8:504, 1935.

12. Widal MF, Abrami P, Lermoyez J. Anaphylaxie et idiosyn-draise, Press Med 30:189, 1922.

13. Samter M, Beers RF. Concerning the nature of intolerance to aspirin. J Allergy 40:281, 1967.

14. Chafee FH, Settipane GA. Aspirin intolerance I. Frequency in an allergic population. J Allergy Clin Immunol 53:193, 1974.

15. Settipane GA, Chafee FH, Klein DE. Aspirin intolerance. II. A prospective study in an atopic and normal population. J Allergy Clin Immunol 53:200, 1974.

16. Settipane RA, Constantine HP, Settipane GA. Aspirin in-tolerance and recurrent urticaria in normal adults and chil-dren. Allergy 35:149, 1980.

17. Settipane GA, Pudupakkam RK. Aspirin intolerance. III. Subtypes, familial occurrence and cross-reactivity with tar-trazine. J Allergy Clin Immunol 56:215, 1975.

18. Settipane GA, Chafee FH. Nasal polyps in asthma and rhinitis: a review of 6,037 patients. J Allergy Clin Immunol 59:17/21, 1977.

19. Szczeklik A, Gryglewski RJ, Czerniawsk-Mysik G. Clini-cal patterns of hypersensitivity to nonsteroidal anti-inflammatory drugs and their pathogenesis. J Allergy Clin Immunol. 60:276, 1977.

20. Downing ET, Braman S. Settipane GA. Bronchial reactiv-ity in patients with nasal polyps before and after polypec-tomy. J Allergy Clin Immunol 69 (part 2):102, 1982.

21. Miles-Lawrence R, Kaplan M, Chang K. Methacholine sensitivity in nasal polyposis and the effects of polypec-tomy. J Allergy Clin Immunol 69 (part 2):102, 1982.

22. Settipane GA, Klein DE, Lekas MD. Asthma and nasal polyps. In: Myers E, ed. New Dimensions in Otorhino-laryngology, Head and Neck Surgery, Amsterdam Excerpta Medica, 449–500, 1987.

23. Settipane GA. Nasal polyps: epidemiology, pathology, im-munology and treatment. Am J Rhinol 1:119–126, 1987.

24. Settipane GA, ed. Nasal polyps. In: Rhinitis, 2nd ed. Prov-idence: Oceanside Publications, 178, 1991.

25. Settipane GA. Nasal polyposis. N Engl Soc Allergy Proc 3:497–504, 1982.

26. Settipane GA, Klein DE, Settipane RJ. Nasal polyps, state of the art. Rhinology 11:33–36, 1991.

27. Israel, E, Rubin P, Kemp JP, Grossman J, Pierson W, Siegel S, Tinkelman D, Murray JJ, Busse W, et al. The effect of inhibition of 5-Lipoxygenase by Zileuton in mild-to-moderate asthma. Annals on Int Med 119:11, 1059–1066, 1993.

28. Laitinen LA, Laitinen A, Haahtela T, Vilkka V, Spur BW, Lee TH. Leukotriene E^4 and granulocytic infiltration into asthmatic airways. Lancet 341:989–990, 1993.

29. Fischer AR, Israel E. Identifying and treating aspirin-induced asthma. Journal Resp. Dis, 16:3, 304–317, 1995.

30. Settipane GA. Aspirin intolerance presenting as chronic rhinitis. RJ Med J 63:63–65, 1980.

31. Zeiss CR, Lockey RF. Refractory period to aspirin in a pa-tient with aspirin-induced asthma. J Allergy Clin Immunol 57:440, 1976.

32. Stevenson DD, Pleskow WW, Simon RA, et al. Aspirin sensitive rhino-sinusitis asthma: a double-blind crossover study of treatment with aspirin. J Allergy Clin Immunol 73:500, 1984.

33. Sweet JM, Stevenson DD, Simon RA, Mathison DA. Long-term effects of aspirin desensitization-treatment of aspirin-sensitive rhinosinusitis-asthma. J Allergy Clin Im-munol 85:59–65, 1990.

34. Stevenson DD. Commentary: The American Experience with aspirin desensitization for aspirin-sensitive rhinosi-nusitis and asthma. Allergy Proc 13,4:185–192, 1992.

35. Danker RE, Wedner HJ. Aspirin desensitization in aspirin sensitive asthma: failure to maintain a desensitized state during prolonged therapy (case report). Am Rev Resp Dis 128:953, 1983.

36. Settipane RA, Stevenson DD. Cross sensitivity with aceta-minophen in aspirin-sensitive subjects with asthma. J Al-lergy Clin Immunol 84:26–33, 1989.

37. Szczeklik A, Nizankowska E, Dworski R. Choline magne-sium trisalicylate in patients with aspirin-induced asthma. Eur Respir J 3:535–539, 1990.

38. Stevenson DD, Houghton AJ, Schrank PJ et al. Salsalate cross-sensitivity in aspirin-sensitive asthmatic patients. J Allergy Clin Immunol 86:749, 1990.

39. Settipane RA, Shrank PJ, Simon RA, Mathison DA, Chris-tiansen SL, Stevenson DD. Prevalence of cross-sensitivity with acetaminophen in aspirin sensitive asthmatics. J Al-lergy Clin Immunol 1995 (In press)

40. Dahlen B, Zetterstrom O. Comparison of bronchial and per oral provocation with aspirin in aspirin-sensitive asthmat-ics. Eur Respir J 3:527–534, 1990.

Chapter XV

Nasal Polyps: Relationship to Infection and Inflammation

Pontus L. E. Stierna, M.D., Ph.D.

ABSTRACT

Since no single predisposing disease can account for the formation of nasal polyps in all patients, medical and surgical therapy has to be directed towards the inflammatory process and/or the underlying infection together with the development of local tissue pathology. Light and electron microscopical studies in experimental models have revealed that the initial polyp formation sequence involves multiple epithelial disruptions with proliferating granulation tissue where immature branching epithelium migrates to cover the mucosal defect. Other branches spread into the underlying connective tissue where intraepithelial microcavities with a differentiated epithelial lining separate the developing polyp body from the adjacent mucosa. Polyp formation and growth is thus activated and perpetuated by an integrated process of mucosal epithelium, matrix and inflammatory cells, which in turn may be initiated by both infectious and non-infectious inflammation. Glucocorticosteroids display a favourable therapeutic profile directly preventing both polyp formation and polyp growth but also by reducing local pathology and inflammatory exudate together with bacterial colonization. Steroids often combined with antibiotics or surgery aimed at specific events in polyp development have to be used in relation to disease progress, and severity as well as differences in clinical behaviour due to the multifactorial pathophysiological events of nasal polyposis.

LOCAL INFLAMMATORY MICROENVIRONMENT

Histologically, the surface mucosal epithelium of the nasal polyp is of the respiratory type with an increase in mucous goblet cells and areas of squamous metaplasia. Epithelial damage, either as an ulceration or area of desquamation is a frequent finding. A thickening and hyalinization of the epithelial basement membrane is also commonly encountered, except in polyps from patients with cystic fibrosis. The stroma of most oedematous polyps varies concerning the amount and degree of amorphous substance and is myxomatous with scattered fibroblasts. The inflammatory cell infiltrate is variable, with a mixture of eosinophils, lymphocytes, plasma cells and activated mast cells that are allergy-independent. Eosinophils are more common as compared to other inflammatory cells, but their role in polyp development is under debate. The neutrophils may be prominent during infection such as in cystic fibrosis where the eosinophil infiltrate is less obvious. Glands are often atypical, few and together with the immature leaky blood vessels lacking normal innervation and thus the vessels are devoid of normal vasomotor regulation[1,2].

In this inflammatory microenvironment many mediators of inflammation such as histamine, prostaglandins, leukotrienes and eosinophil-derived products have been shown to be increased[1]. In ASA-intolerance, a predominance of leukotrienes as compared to prostaglandins may contribute to the development of mucosal oedema. The finding of an increased expression of insulinlike growth factor immunoreactivity in nasal polyps indicates that a continuing growth stimulation of endothelial and epithelial cells may be macrophage dependent[3]. In addition, granulocyte-macrophage colony-stimulating factor (GM-CSF), tumor necrosis factor (TNF α and β) and platelet-derived growth factor (PDGF) appear to initiate eosinophil and neutrophil accumulation, induce further cytokine release and stimulate structural cells, epithelium and endothelial cells directly or indirectly as indicated from in vitro experiments. Both autocrine and paracrine mechanisms are involved[4].

In the already formed polyp, this inflammatory tissue driven response by the activation of structural as well as inflammatory cells has all the characteristics of a chronic inflammation. In this locus minoris both the connective tissue cells, inflammatory cells (eosinophils, neutrophils, macrophages) together with the endothelium and epithelial cells interact to perpetuate the localized tissue inflammation.

CLINICAL BACKGROUND

Predisposing Disease—Inflammation–Infection

As mentioned in previous chapters, the cause of nasal polyps is multifactorial and they are associated with either systemic disease (asthma ASA-intolerance, cystic fibrosis, Kartagener's syndrome) or more localized disease such as chronic sinusitis with a dental or fungal focus of infection/inflammation. The incidence of nasal polyposis in predisposing diseases is given in Table 1.

The frequency of nasal polyps in adults with intrinsic asthma is 13% as compared to 1% in the normal population. In the subgroup of patients with ASA-intolerance it rises sharply to 36%. In this patient group the individual tendency to develop polyps appears to be correlated to activity of basal disease within the upper and lower airways[1]. These patients also deteriorate during an upper respiratory tract infection which adds to the local inflammation, and polyps often grow during purulent rhinosinusitis. Aspirin desensitization may be an effective treatment for aspirin-sensitive rhinosinusitis with asthma and nasal polyps. The need for nasal polypectomies and sinus operations is thereby significantly reduced[5]. The atopy in IgE mediated allergy is not the cause of nasal polyposis and the mast cell activation and local eosinophilia found histologically are not usually allergy dependent[1].

Table 1. Frequency of nasal polyps in predisposing disease indicating the multifactorial basic background to inflammation/infection in sino-nasal polyposis. The incidence of nasal polyps in the normal population is about 1%.

Adult asthma	7%
intrinsic	13%
with ASA-intolerance	36%
atopy	5%
Dental sinusitis	16%
Fungal sinusitis	80%
Cystic fibrosis	18%
Kartagener's syndrome	27%

Treatment Studies

A follow-up study, on patients treated for the first time for nasal polyps, showed a sharp decline in the long-term need for medical or surgical intervention where only 3.9% of patients had 5–10 polypectomies during the follow-up period[6]. These patients, mostly without predisposing disease, needed more medical and surgical intervention, possibly on the individual basis of other local inflammation/infection factors. This patient group thus seems to represent a different clinical entity in which a more aggressive clinical workup as well as therapy may be beneficial. In that study an overrepresentation of polypectomies performed during the winter months was possibly related to upper airway infections as a triggering factor for nasal polyps[6]. In another study on budesonide nasal spray as a prophylactic treatment after polypectomy, only patients with recurrent polyps benefited from treatment by a reduced recurrence rate of polyps following *avulsion*. This could also imply a different etiology or different steroid sensitivity in nasal polyps from the latter group[7]. Interindividual and tissue specific variations on glucocorticoidreceptor regulation in nasal mucosa have been shown by Knutsson[8]. Thus, markers for individual and tissue-specific variations in glucocorticoid responses could possibly be developed.

Importance of Infection–Inflammation

The role of bacterial infection as a cause of nasal polyps has not been thoroughly investigated. However, studies of sinus washouts and antroscopy studies indicate that purulent secretion together with colonizing airway pathogens could activate the disease or make it persistent[9,10]. Treatment studies also indicate that local deposition of an antibiotic together with glucocorticosteroids is more effective than antibiotics alone in reducing local tissue pathology including sinus polyps[11]. Since glucocorticosteroids decrease local inflammatory mucosal pathology, they may also secondarily reduce bacterial colonization and growth. This is indicated in subsequent experimental studies outlined below. Furthermore, bacterial-specific serum IgE has been detected and quantified in most patients with nasal polyposis and/or chronic sinusitis while subjects with only allergic rhinitis are devoid of this. This indicates that multiple bacterial species isolated from chronically infected sinuses are capable of inducing IgE mediated sensitization that may aggravate the disease[12]. The analysis of virus RNA in nasal polyps has proved to be negative, excluding their primary role in polyp growth. Long-term treatment with erythromycin has helped to prevent polyp recurrences after functional endoscopic sinus surgery but as erythromycin also has antiinflammatory effects, the results are hard to interpret.

Patients with cystic fibrosis and Kartagener's syndrome are often colonized with Pseudomonas aeruginosa and the occurrence of nasal polyps appears to some degree to be correlated to this colonization. Intensified and specific pharmacotherapy against Pseudomonas strains, Staphylococcus aureus and mucolytic therapy has been shown to effectively reduce polyp frequency in cystic fibrosis patients to 2–5%. Although theories have been presented to the effect that the basic epithelial defect in cystic fibrosis is responsible per se, there is no clinical evidence for this. In a patient study of chronic sinusitis with dental infectious foci by Melen, the incidence of polyposis was 16% and the dental treatment alone or in combination with minor sinus surgery (polyp removal) gave the best results with healing or improvement in 92% of the patients[13]. An apical and marginal periodontitis may progress slowly over years without any symptoms and eventually induce sinus mucosal inflammation leading to ostial obstruction and bacterial colonization. A marked improvement in oral health has been observed in Sweden and as a result the incidence of nasal polyposis associated with dental infection has decreased.

No single etiologic factor appears to be responsible for the formation of nasal polyps and the final common pathway of inflammation is caused by a variety of mechanisms such as local bacterial colonization or infection secondarily to local induction of mucosal pathology interfering with normal nasal and sinus function[13]. The disturbance in ostial patency alone, as found in acute rhinitis or recurrent sinusitis, is not the sole factor initiating and supporting bacterial growth. An initial low-grade inflammatory response, local lactate production and disturbed gas exchange may together create the appropriate redox potential for growth of pathogenic bacteria in nasal and sinus secretions. The low grade inflammatory response preceding bacterial growth may be the result of a disturbed antral gas exchange and the subsequent bacterial growth may be a phenomenon partly parallel to the increased purulence i.e. recruitment of inflammatory cells[14]. In fact, bacterial colonization or infection by these mechanisms may be the most common cause of nasal polyps in the patient subgroup without predisposing disease and requiring multiple polypectomies as described by Larsen[6].

EXPERIMENTAL STUDIES

Histological examination of nasal polyps has led to several pathogenetic theories[15]. They are all based on the findings of epithelial disruption, atypical gland formation, fibroblast proliferation, inflammatory cell infiltrate and decreased innervation and vascularization leading to loss of homeostasis and control of cell proliferation.

In studies of experimental maxillary sinusitis in rabbits, polyp formation was documented in the sinuses as well as the nasal cavities, irrespective of inducing agent[16,17]. However, in a recent study Pseudomonas aeruginosa was found to be extremely potent in inducing experimental polyps in the rabbit. In mucosal areas with superficial inflammatory mucosal lesions numerous small polyps with an oedematous connective tissue stroma were found. They were covered by an intact epithelial lining and an invasive growth of epithelial cell branches and formation of intraepithelial microcavities were characteristic findings in the underlying connective tissue[16,17]. Polyp formation was also documented in another experimental series where experimental naso-antral windows were surgically created during experimental sinusitis. The tendency for polyp formation in the region of the enlarged ostium was pronounced in sinusitis induced with Bacteroides fragilis and Staphylococcus aureus.

To further verify the role of inflammation/infection in the formation of sinus mucosal polyps, New Zealand White rabbits were subjected to different modes of manipulation intended to induce inflammation of the maxillary sinus. These were a combination of bacterial infection and mechanical surface trauma, or alternatively deposition into the sinus cavity of either agarose (supporting oedema and nasal bacterial colonization) or FMLP, a chemotactic peptide for leukocytes. The majority of these animals developed mucosal polyps which were documented macroscopically and by light electron microscopy[18]. The fully developed polyps were of various sizes, measuring up to 5 mm (Fig. 1). The experimental polyp formation appeared to involve epithelial disruption, connective tissue cell proliferation and migration of immature branching epithelium (Fig. 2). While part of the migrating epithelium eventually covers the

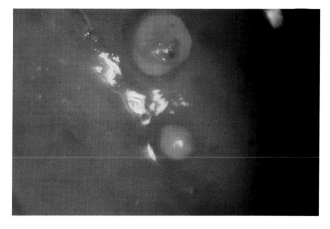

Figure 1. Macroscopical photograph of the rabbit sinus mucosa where a polyp has developed after surface mechanical trauma and pneumococcal infection. 30 × original magnification.

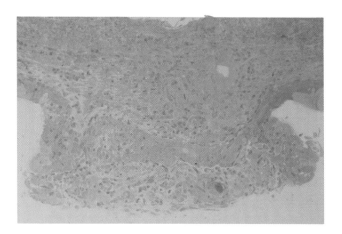

Figure 2. Initial stage of polyp, with granulomatous tissue protruding through an epithelial defect. Regenerating epithelium is migrating from surrounding areas.

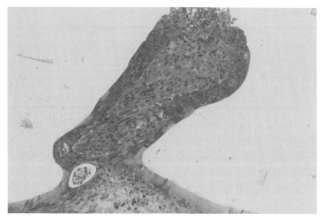

Figure 4. A stalked polyp is formed as a microcavity fuses with the surrounding cavity and the polyp body becomes separated from the sinus wall.

mucosal defect, other branches spread into the underlying connective tissue. Interepithelial microcavities appeared to be formed by the rupture and fusion of intracytoplasmic vacuoles with a cytoplasmic membrane causing communication with the intercellular space. Furthermore, these fusing cavities separated a developing polyp from the adjacent mucosa (Fig. 3 and Fig. 4). On the basis of these findings the polyp forming sequence is schematically illustrated in Fig. 5[18].

The effect of systemic pretreatment with glucocorticosteroids on mucosal polyp formation and local bacterial colonization has been analyzed in our model. This was performed in an experimental study in rabbits combining experimental pneumococcal sinusitis with surface epithelial trauma. Pretreatment with a glucocorticosteroid may reduce polyp formation by specifically inhibiting the migration of epithelium together with microcavity

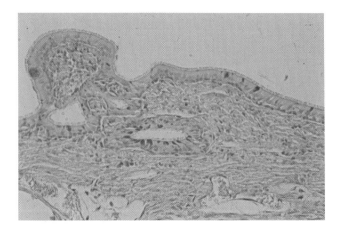

Figure 3. Developing polyp. Microcavities located close to the sinus lumen surface are about to rupture, thereby establishing communication with the surrounding sinus cavity. A cleavage plane is thus created.

formation (epithelial differentiation) and with the concomitant inhibition of colonization by local nasal pathogens[19]. Since the sinus ostium was closed with tissue glue in this study, the inhibition of bacterial colonization was probably secondary to the inhibition of the local inflammatory response (making the local milieu suitable for bacterial growth), rather than promoting sinus drainage. The effect of glucocorticosteroids on an increased bacterial colonization is different from that on an established full blown infection and also dependent upon corticoid dosage and type of bacterium[19].

There are many similarities between the sequence of polyp formation and the normal healing process after surface epithelial trauma. During certain conditions such as a prolonged inflammatory trauma, epithelial regeneration accompanied by interaction with an altered extracellular matrix composition and proliferating connective tissue cells will lead to polyp formation. The behaviour of the regenerating epithelium in our investigations shows morphologic similarities to in vitro studies where cultured human tracheobronchial epithelial cells and epithelial cells from human nasal polyps were cultured on specific collagen matrices, showing that the local expression of extracellular matrix glycoproteins is important for normal and pathological epithelial cell repair, as in the development of polyps[16,20,21]. One such glycoprotein is fibronectin that together with collagen and laminine mediates the cell adhesion and differentiation of epithelial cells. The formation of polyps thus involves a specific cellular sequence with cellular proliferation and differentiation mainly involving epithelial cells, fibroblasts interacting with components of the extracellular matrix. Once formed, polyp growth is dependent on local inflammation as well as oedema formation, stromal cell proliferation perpetuating this localized tissue process. The nature of polyp formation

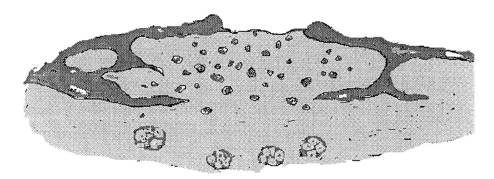

Figure 5A. Schematic illustration of the polyp forming sequence (from 13, reproduced by kind permission of the author, Norlander, T.). At the site of a microscopical epithelial disruption, regenerating epithelium is branching and invading the lamina propria. Microcavities are formed.

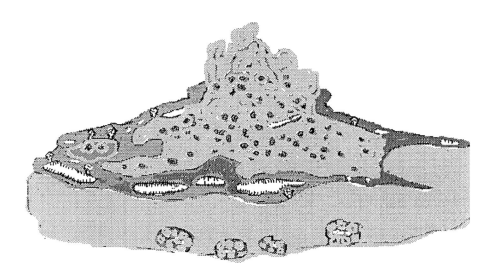

Figure 5B. Granulomatous tissue protruding through the epithelial defect. The microcavities increase in size and develop a ciliary or secretory cell lining.

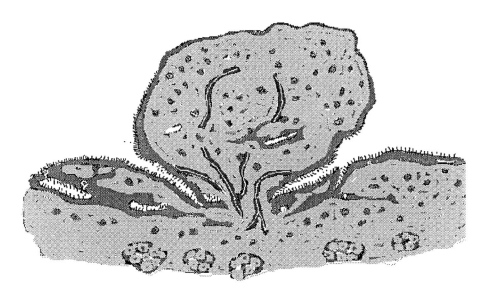

Figure 5C. Fusion of microcavities creating communication with the sinus lumen. A cleavage plane is gained, allowing separation of the developing polyp body from the surrounding mucosa.

Table 2. The basic nature of polyp formation and polyp growth is illustrated as concluded from experimental and clinical studies. This local tissue pathology develops within days to weeks and resolves during months.

Polyp Formation	Polyp Growth
Specific sequence	Local inflammation
Cellular proliferation	Oedema
Cellular differentiation	Stromal proliferation

and polyp growth, respectively, as concluded from experimental and clinical studies is illustrated in Table 2. It is likely that future pharmacological intervention at these two levels may require different strategies, depending on whether therapies are aimed at inhibiting polyp formation or reducing the polyp size of the full-grown polyp.

CLINICAL IMPLICATIONS

Questions, Clinical–Scientific

Both clinical and experimental studies strongly suggest that instead of basic disease, subsequent inflammation together with intermittent bacterial colonization or infection will lead to polyp development and/or polyp growth. To further analyze the connection between basic disease, inflammation, infection and local tissue pathology both basic and epidemiological studies are needed. Experimental studies of rhino-sinusitis could provide further knowledge. These questions have also to be addressed when evaluating treatment modalities and studies designed according to basic scientific data allowing an appropriate design. Basic experimental research on the mechanisms of polyp formation may open avenues to better inhibit the initial stages of formation and also address the role of glucocorticosteroids and antibiotics dur-

ing different stages of disease. The analysis of the polyp microenvironment is an ideal model of chronic inflammation and the nature of these inflammatory and tissue driven responses by the activation of structural cells as well as inflammatory cells may give further clues to the character of polyp growth.

In cadaver studies from Tos and Larsson, polyps were found in 26% of the patients without anamnestic nasal or sinus disease. Most of these polyps originated in the ostia or recesses[22]. This clearly indicates that polyp formation is quite common in the normal population which may signify that smaller sized polyps induced during a viral rhinitis or as a result of normal aging, could involute unless a persisting inflammation continues to challenge the early stage of the polyp. Spontaneous variations in polyp size from day to day has not been analyzed and may vary according to individual differences in the hypothalamic adrenal axis regulatory pattern that shows considerable interindividual variations normally as well as during stress. Our findings from experimental studies also show that certain mechanisms of epithelial differentiation—i.e. branching of epithelial strains and the formation and fusion of intraepithelial cavities are required for the development of an epithelial granulation into a polyp. Since these mechanisms of epithelial proliferation and differentiation display local variations, this may explain the regional tendency towards polyp development in the nasal cavity. In chronic sinusitis, the inflamed sinus mucosa of the sinus ethmoidal cells displays all the stages of polyp formation on histological examination, but possibly due to spatial restrictions polyps can not develop into the sinus cavity. It is also less likely that mucosa should protrude through the ethmoidal cell ostia and thus present itself as a polyp. The most important clinical questions requiring further clinical or scientific investigation in order to understand the influence of infection/inflammation on sino-nasal polyposis are presented in Table 3.

Table 3. Important clinical questions that needs further clinical or scientific investigation in order to understand the influence of infection/inflammation on sino-nasal polyposis.

Clinical Questions

Epidemiological studies
  basic disease, inflammation/infection and tissue pathology

Relation between inflammation, local pathology and bacterial colonization
  specific effects treatment

Mechanisms polyp formation.
  pharmacological intervention, cellular sequence

Basic experimental research on polyp microenvironment.

Site-specific polyp development. Why?

Table 4. Clinical and/or scientific rationale for different modes of intervention in the treatment of inflammation/infection in nasal polyposis.

Clinical Intervention	Rationales
Surgery	Increase patency and reduce inflammatory exudate and possibly bacterial colonization.
Dental measures	Remove local infectious foci.
Glucocorticosteroids	Reduce polyp size and new formation, local pathology and inflammatory exudate together with bacterial colonization.
Antibiotics	Reduce bacterial colonization and thereby polyp formation.
Aspirin desensitization	Reduce inflammation, oedema.

Clinical Intervention–Rationales

In a disease such as nasal polyposis no single etiologic factor can account for the formation of the nasal polyps in all patients and firstline medical therapy has to be directed towards the events of inflammation/infection and often combined with surgery[1,23,24] (Table 4). The development of local tissue pathology in the sinuses or ostia may require surgical intervention to increase patency and thereby reduce inflammatory exudate and possibly bacterial colonization. Surgery may also be aimed at removing a local infectious focus as in chronic dental or fungal sinusitis. Experimental studies supporting the close connection between polyp development and local surgical tissue trauma, especially during infection, suggests the use of corticoids and antibiotics in connection with sinus surgery to prevent polyp formation. Treatment of predisposing disease such as aspirin desensitization may also reduce inflammation and thereby the development of local tissue pathology together with bacterial colonization.

An acute sinusitis in polyp patients should be treated vigorously with antibiotics and glucocorticoids as well as sinus lavage[1]. However, the role of an intermittent bacterial colonization and a low grade infection of the nose and sinuses in polyposis is probably underestimated, as supported by both clinical and experimental studies[16,17,23]. Sinus infection is likely to be an important predisposing factor in the formation of nasal polyps, which in turn may interfere with proper drainage and aeration of the sinus cavity, thus causing a vicious circle with sinus infection–polyposis. Clinically glucocorticosteroids have been shown to reduce polyps and local pathology together with inflammatory exudate and experimental studies have pointed towards an inhibitory effect on new polyp formation together with a reduced bacterial colonization[23,19]. Prolonged bacterial colonization may require periods of treatment with antibiotics before tissue pathology resolves and to prevent polyp formation. However, the pressure of selection towards more antibiotic resistant bacterial strains could make the long-term treatment ineffective and give overall ecological problems. Thus, the medical and surgical treatment of patients with nasal polyposis requires solid basic knowledge of the clinical behaviour of the different clinical entities of nasal polyposis to initiate treatment with glucocorticosteroids, combined with antibiotics or surgery and geared to progression and intensity variations of disease in each individual patient[24].

REFERENCES

1. Settipane G.A., Settipane R.A. Tetrad of nasal polyps, aspirin sensitivity, asthma and rhinosinusitis. In: Sinusitis. Pathophysiology and treatment, ed. H.M. Druce, Marcell Dekker. 227–246, 1994.

2. Busuttil A., More A.R., McSeveney D. Ultrastructure of the stroma of nasal polyps. Arch. Otolaryngol, 102: 589–595, 1976.

3. Petruson B., Hansson H-A., Petruson K. Insulinlike growth factor I immunoreactivity in nasal polyps. Arch Otolaryngol Head & Neck Surg. 114:1272–1275, 1988.

4. Dolovich J., Gauldie J., Ohtoshi T., Denburg J., Jordana M. Nasal polyps: local inductive microenvironment in the pathogenesis of the inflammation. In: Rhinitis and Asthma. Similarities and differences, eds. Niels Mygind, Ulf Pipkorn, Ronald Dahl, Munksgaard 233–241, 1989.

5. Sweet, J.M., Stevenson, D.D., Simon, R.A., Mathison, D.A. Long-term effects of aspirin desensitization—Treatment for aspirin-sensitive rhinosinusitis-asthma. J Allergy Clin Immunol. 85, 59–65, 1990.

6. Larsen K., Tos M. Clinical course of patients with primary nasal polyps. Acta Otolaryngol (Stockh) 114: 556–559, 1994.

7. Hartwig, S., Lindén, M., Laurent, C., Vargö, A-K, Lindqvist, N. Budesonide nasal spray as prophylactic

treatment after polypectomy. The Journal of Laryngology and Otology, 102:148–151, 1988.

8. Knutsson P.U., Brönnegård M., Marcus C., Stierna P. Regulation of glucocorticoid receptor mRNA in nasal mucosa by local administration of fluticasone and budesonide. J Allergy Clin Immunol, 96:1–8, 1996.

9. Dawes P., Bates G., Watson D., Lewis D., Lowe D., Drake-Lee A.B. The role of bacterial infection of the maxillary sinus in nasal polyps. Clin. Otolaryngol. 14: 447–450, 1989.

10. Gilbert J.G. Antroscopy in maxillary sinus disease associated with nasal polyposis. The Journal of Laryngology and Otology. 103:861–863, 1989.

11. Cuenant G., Stipon J.P., Plante-Longchamp G., Baudoin C., Guerrier Y. Efficacy of endonasal neomycin-tixocortol pivalate irrigation in the treatment of chronic allergic and bacterial sinusitis. ORL 48:226–232, 1986.

12. Calenoff E., McMahan J.T., Herzon G.D., Kern R.C., Ghadge G.D., Hanson D.G. Bacterial Allergy in nasal polyposis. Arch Otolaryngol. Head & Neck Surg., 119, 830–836, 1993.

13. Melén I., Lindahl L., Andréasson L., Rundcrantz H. Chronic maxillary sinusitis. Definition, diagnosis and relation to dental infections and nasal polyposis. Acta Otolaryngol. (Stockh) 101:320–327, 1986.

14. Stierna P., Jannert M. (eds) Current opinions on the pathogenesis of sinusitis. The importance of local inflammatory response and ostial patency. Proceedings of a Workshop, Lund, Sweden, August 27, 1993. Acta Otolaryngol (Stockh) Suppl. 515, 1–64, 1994.

15. Tos M. The pathogenetic theories on formation of nasal polyps. Am J Rhinology 4(2):51–56, 1990.

16. Norlander T., Fukami M., Westrin KM., Stierna P., Carlsöö B. Formation of mucosal polyps in the nasal and maxillary sinus cavity by infection. Otolaryngol. Head & Neck Surg. 109, 522–529, 1993.

17. Fukami M., Norlander T., Stierna P., Westrin KM., Carlsöö B., Nord C.E. Mucosal pathology of the nose and sinuses: A study in experimental maxillary sinusitis in rabbits induced by Streptococcus pneumoniae, Bacteroides fragilis and Staphylococcus aureus. Am J Rhinology, 7:125–132, 1993.

18. Norlander T., Westrin KM., Fukami M., Stierna P., Carlsöö B. Experimentally induced polyps in the sinus mucosa. Laryngoscope. 106; 196–203, 1996.

19. Norlander T., Hyun-Kwon S., Henriksson G., Westrin KM., Stierna P. The inhibition of sinus mucosal polyp formation in the rabbit by systemic treatment with betamethasone. Manuscript, 1995.

20. Infeld M.D., Brennan J.A., Davis P.B. Human fetal lung fibroblasts promote invasion of extracellular matrix by normal human tracheobronchial epithelial cells in vitro: A model of early airway gland development. Am J Respir Cell Mol Biol. 8:69 –76, 1993.

21. Hay E.D. Extracellular matrix alters epithelial differentiation. Current Opinion in Cell Biology, 5:1029–1035, 1993.

22. Larsen P.L., Tos M., Baer S. En block removal of the ethmoid and ostiomeatal complex in cadavers, with a practical application. Rhinology 32(2): 62–64, 1994.

23. Holmberg, K., Karlsson, G. Nasal polyps: surgery or pharmacological intervention? Eur Respir Rev., 4:20, 260–265, 1994.

24. Drake-Lee, A.B. The value of medical treatment in nasal polyps. Clin Otolaryngol, 16:237–239, 1991.

Chapter XVI

Allergic Fungal Sinusitis/Polyposis

John P. Bent, III, M.D., and Frederick A. Kuhn, M.D.

ABSTRACT

In the last decade the medical community has recognized allergic fungal sinusitis as a unique clinical entity strongly associated with nasal polyps. This chapter will review its differential diagnosis, clinical features, diagnosis, treatment, and prognosis. Appropriate management requires distinguishing allergic fungal sinusitis from other forms of chronic fungal and bacterial sinusitis. Surgical treatment initially results in dramatic improvement, and oral steroids help maintain postoperative success. However, recurrent disease eventually prevails, leaving a glaring need for improved medical treatment.

INTRODUCTION

Allergic fungal sinusitis (AFS) is a newly appreciated diagnosis, first described in the early 1980s. Over the last decade, it has come to be acknowledged as a significant cause of nasal polyposis and the most common form of fungal sinusitis in the United States. Although much has been learned about AFS since its discovery, it remains a mysterious and chronic condition for which there exists no effective long-term treatment.

In order to properly diagnose and treat AFS, the full spectrum of fungal sinusitis must be understood. Currently, most rhinologists recognize 4 types of fungal sinusitis: acute/fulminant (invasive), chronic/indolent (invasive), fungus ball, and allergic fungal sinusitis (AFS)[1-3]. This system can be broken down into 2 invasive and 2 non-invasive, or 1 acute and 3 chronic (Table 1). Other forms of fungal sinusitis may exist that have not yet been described. This chapter will outline the 4 recognized types of fungal sinusitis, highlighting the differences between each category. Emphasis will be placed on the pathophysiology, diagnosis, and treatment of AFS.

ACUTE/FULMINANT (INVASIVE) FUNGAL SINUSITIS

Fulminant (invasive) fungal sinusitis is the only form of acute fungal sinusitis. It occurs exclusively in diabetic or immunosuppressed patients, most typically among oncology or transplant patients. The patient generally presents with ischemic tissue in the paranasal region, but not with polyps. Fungal penetration progresses rapidly, within hours or days, destroying mucosa and bone while invading blood vessels, orbit, brain, and skin. Histologic exam demonstrates vascular occlusion and necrosis (Figure 1), and fungal cultures usually reveal Phycomycetes (*Mucor* or *Rhizopus*) or *Aspergillus* species. The term "mucormycosis", which describes acute fungal sinusitis caused by *Mucor*, frequently appears in the medical literature.

This condition requires emergency surgical attention. Necrotic tissue should be debrided until viable tissue is encountered, which may require orbital enucleation or craniotomy. The goal is to minimize the number of fungal organisms present, but complete fungal eradication is usually not possible with surgery alone. Adjuvent antifungal therapy with amphotericin B helps improve survival, but morbidity and mortality rates are quite high. Outcome does not appear to be dependent on whether the etiologic organism is *Mucor* or *Aspergillus*. Survival rates range from 20–75% and correlate with the control of underlying disease[4]. Aggressive correction of any metabolic or immune disorder is therefore of paramount importance. Diabetics tend to fare better than patients with more refractory systemic disorders, such as leukemia and chronic renal failure,[4] probably because diabetes can be more readily controlled.

HIV-related immunosuppression does not predispose patients to acute fungal sinusitis, but AIDS victims may

Table 1. Classification of Fungal Sinusitis

Acute:	acute fulminant	} invasive
Chronic:	chronic indolent	
	fungus ball	} non-invasive
	allergic fungal sinusitis	

be at risk for fungal sinusitis caused by *Pseudallescheria boydii*, *Cryptococcus*, or *Histoplasma*. [5]

CHRONIC/INDOLENT (INVASIVE) FUNGAL SINUSITIS

Chronic invasive fungal sinusitis features insidious symptomatology complicated by fungal penetration into tissue. It occurs in immunocompetent individuals who usually have a longstanding history of rhinosinusitis. The disease progresses slowly, producing chronic granulomatous inflammation and extension beyond sinus walls. Polyps may be present. It has been compared to a locally aggressive neoplasm[6]. Plasmocytes and eosinophils may be seen in sinus mucosa, a finding also seen in AFS. Many of these patients have allergic histories[7], making differentiation from AFS difficult. Fungi must be microscopically visualized within sinus tissue to dis-

tinguish this entity from the 2 non-invasive forms of fungal sinusitis.

Aspergillus species and members of the *Dematiaceous* family are the usual causative organisms. Chronic invasive fungal sinusitis is virtually endemic in some areas, such as Sudan[6] and northern India[7]. Reports of this disease have decreased significantly in the United States over the last decade. We have seen no cases since 1980, and believe that it is quite rare, certainly the least common of the fungal sinus infections.

When pathologic examination confirms fungal invasion, the physician is obligated to treat the patient aggressively. Complete surgical excision with wide exposure and generous bone removal is indicated. Extensive antifungal therapy, directed by *in vitro* fungal culture sensitivities, should also be utilized. Although recurrences commonly occur, some patients achieve cure[8], and the prognosis is much better than for acute fungal sinusitis.

FUNGAL BALL

Older names for this non-invasive form of chronic fungal sinusitis include mycetoma and aspergilloma. It affects immunocompetent, non-atopic patients and usually pro-

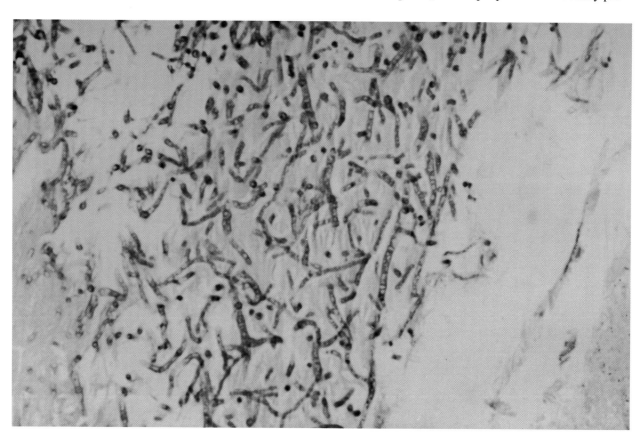

Figure 1. Hematoxylin and eosin stain from ischemic middle turbinate. Multiple fungal hyphae are seen in this necrotic tissue, consistent with acute fungal sinusitis.

duces either no symptoms or a mild sensation of pressure. The disease may involve any sinus, but usually occurs in a single sinus, most frequently the maxillary antrum. Bone erosion and mucosal invasion does not occur. Fungal proliferation produces a tangled and tightly packed mass with a clay-like appearance. The lack of sinus inflammation distinguishes this disorder from other forms of chronic fungal sinusitis.

The etiologic organism is almost always Aspergillus fumigatus.[9] Treatment consists of debridement of the fungus and sinus aeration; cure rates should approach 100%. In our recent review of 20 consecutive cases of chronic fungal sinusitis, 2 had fungus balls, equating to an incidence of 10%. This is unlike the European experience, where it appears to be the most common form of fungal sinusitis.[9]

ALLERGIC FUNGAL SINUSITIS

Historical Background

AFS was first appreciated in the early 1980s because of its histologic resemblance to allergic bronchopulmonary aspergillosis (ABPA). This connection was first appreciated in 1981 by Millar et al., who noted a similarity between the sinus contents removed from 5 chronic sinusitis patients and the typical pathologic appearance of ABPA.[10] Two years later, Katzenstein et al. independently made the same observation, stimulating a retrospective review of 119 chronic sinusitis surgical specimens in which they identified 7 patients (5.9%) with septate fungal hyphae scattered among necrotic eosinophils and amorphous mucin. They termed this condition "allergic *Aspergillus* sinusitis" based on the assumption that *Aspergillus* species were the causative organisms.[11] Gourley et al.'s retrospective review of 200 patients demonstrated a 7% prevalence of AFS among chronic sinusitis patients requiring surgery,[14] corroborating Katzenstein et al.'s study. No prospective data exists regarding true disease prevalence, but the 6–7% rate established in retrospective studies may be an underestimate. As it became apparent that *Dematiaceous* fungi, not *Aspergillus* species, were the primary etiologic agents, the name was changed to AFS.[12,13]

Clinical Characteristics

Warm humid climates, typified by the southeastern United States, seem to foster fungal proliferation. AFS patients are usually adolescents or young adults. We have now diagnosed over forty cases in the last 4 years, with an age range of 9 to 69 years, but have observed no sexual or ethnic predilection. Atopy and asthma have been present in most reported cases. Patients typically give a history of sinonasal polyposis, recurrent sinusitis, and multiple pre-

vious surgeries. Usually, the inflammation affects all paranasal sinuses but asymmetrically involves one side.

Computerized tomography (CT) scans have a characteristic appearance (Figure 2). Fungal elements release ferromagnetic elements (magnesium and calcium), creating a serpinginous area of high attenuation.[20] CT scans often demonstrate bone erosion and deviation of adjacent structures. Investigators have reported bone destruction ranging from 19%[27] to 80%[16] of AFS cases. Such a CT appearance in an allergic patient complaining of chronic sinus obstruction is highly suggestive of AFS. Magnetic resonance imaging (MRI) also has a characteristic appearance, as the ferromagnetic elements have a decreased signal intensity, leading to a hypointense T1 image and a markedly hypointense T2 image (Figures 3 and 4). Some surgeons recommend MRI as the optimal imaging method[21], but we believe that CT adequately displays AFS while providing superior bone definition.

Nasal endoscopy demonstrates a characteristic allergic mucus, which is thick and viscous, often stained brown, yellow, or green by bacterial superinfection or fungal material. Polyposis may be massive (Figure 5) and strikingly unilateral. Intraoperative findings include pockets of greenish-brown fungal concretions buried within polyps and allergic mucus. Often the allergic mucus and fungal debris become intermixed, resulting in a material often referred to as "machine oil", "pistachio pudding", or "peanut butter paste". (Figure 6)

Pathogenesis and Pathology

Histologic observation of the surgical specimen reveals a triad of eosinophilia, Charcot-Leyden crystals, and extramucosal hyphae. Charcot-Leyden crystals are simply a byproduct of necrotic eosinophils. (Figure 7) Hyphae can usually be seen with hematoxylin-eosin or potassium-hydroxide stains, and if necessary, special stains such as Gomori methenamine silver (GMS). The pathologist must examine sinus mucosa and bone to specifically exclude tissue invasion. The presence of fungi in the mucin but *not the tissue* of AFS patients differentiates AFS from chronic invasive fungal sinusitis. By definition fungal invasion *does not* occur in any case of AFS.

Prompt culturing of carefully collected fungal debris will usually reveal the etiologic organism. In our early experience with AFS, over 50% of our cases were culture negative. By selecting a specimen rich in fungal debris and rapidly placing it into culture media, yield increased to almost 100%. *Dematiaceous* fungi (phaehyphomycosis), which include *Curvularia*, *Bipolaris*, and *Alternaria* predominate, followed by *Aspergillus* species (Table 2). These are ubiquitous organisms with no potential for contagion. The particular fungal species has no apparent effect on disease manifestations, and at present has no clinical implications.

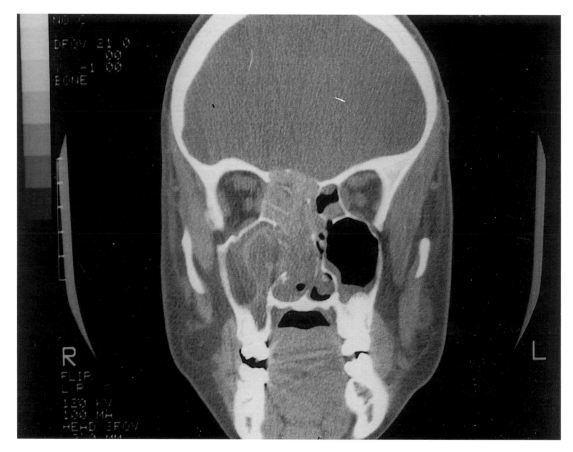

Figure 2. CT scan demonstrating unilateral *Curvularia* AFS affecting multiple right ethmoid sinuses. Expanding inspissated fungal debris has eroded the medial wall of the right maxillary sinus, the lamina papyracea, and the ethmoid roof, deviating the nasal septum to the left. The opacified sinuses display a heterogenous character.

Several retrospective studies have described an AFS-like syndrome, in which typically AFS features were seen in the absence of identifiable fungus.[14,15,22] When there is no suspicion of AFS, the surgeon will usually not submit mucus for pathologic exam or fungal culture. Therefore, retrospectively identified AFS-like syndromes probably represent AFS without preserved fungal elements rather than a distinct syndrome. We have no experience with an AFS-like case without a positive fungal stain. However, as suggested by Schwietz and Gourley, there may be an unrecognized, non-fungal antigen capable of producing clinical manifestations equivalent to AFS.[14]

The pathogenesis of AFS is incompletely understood. Presumably, fungi become entrapped in the sinuses of allergic individuals with ostiomeatal complex obstruction, extremely thick mucus, or a mucociliary clearance disorder. The ensuing immune response exacerbates the disease. Immunologists believe that both Type I (IgE mediated) and Type III (IgG mediated) immunity influence AFS, based on their proven association with ABPA. The AFS-ABPA association has been strengthened by si-

multaneous AFS and ABPA documented in the same patient.[24] Type I immunity has been clearly implicated in AFS based on skin testing, RAST, and total IgE elevations.[15,16] Brummund et al. demonstrated that the etiologic fungal antigen, when used in skin testing, prompted a dramatic Type I cutaneous response.[23] Manning et al. later reported 9 consecutive cases of AFS with elevated IgE specific to the fungal antigen.[17] Type III immune reactions, which involve antibody binding of antigen, result in potentially harmful circulating immune complexes. These immune complexes have been shown to contribute to ABPA, and although they have been more superficially studied in AFS, initial studies indicate their involvement.[23,24,25]

The distinction between AFS and the other 2 forms of chronic fungal sinusitis (indolent/invasive and fungus ball) is often blurred. The typical features of each fungal sinusitis category are summarized in Table 3. It is uncertain if these 3 diseases are simply stages along the same spectrum or unrelated disorders. Could all chronic fungal sinusitis begin as a fungus ball that eventually progresses

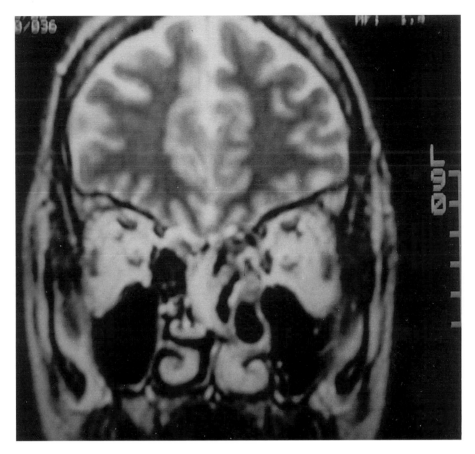

Figure 3. T2 weighted MRI of the same patient seen in Figure 4 showing the characteristic hypointense center.

to an allergic response in some and invasion in others? What permits chronic fungal sinusitis to progress to invasion in a small subset of patients? The fact that the same fungal organisms are cultured in each of the 3 different forms of chronic fungal sinusitis supports the notion that all the chronic fungal sinus disorders are in fact interrelated. AFS may be a continuation of fungus ball, different only by the presence or absence of an immune response to the fungal saprophyte. The immune response then generates an inflammatory reaction, resulting in nasal polyps, allergic mucus, and occasionally, bone erosion. Allphin et al. observed that in AFS "a spectrum of disease clearly exists ranging from mild allergic symptoms, polyps, and scant allergic mucin with few scattered hyphae, to an extreme atopic state with massive expansile disease that is non-invasive, but has the potential to destroy bone or cause facial deformity or eye changes."[12] We have also found this to be true, and wonder if the extension of the extremes described by Allphin might be fungus ball on the mild end and chronic invasive disease on the severe side. A report from Hawaii by Zieske et al.[19] described 4 patients with "allergic mucin" and fungal invasion, which perhaps represents the advanced end of the spectrum. Although no proof exists at present, it may be that unrecognized, submucosal fungal infection causes recurrence in AFS. However, our experience leads us to believe this is purely an allergic disease. The patients do no present with fever, leukocytosis, or other signs of infection. Furthermore, the successful response to steroids cannot be explained in the face of infection.

Before 1983 AFS cases were probably diagnosed as either bacterial sinusitis or chronic invasive fungal sinusitis. It is no coincidence that case reports of chronic invasive fungal sinusitis have dropped dramatically as AFS became better understood. Many older reports of so-called "invasive" disease were considered invasive based on bone destruction or proptosis (commonly seen in AFS), not histologic tissue invasion. As recently as 1988, Washburn et al. described a young man with *Bipolaris* sinusitis, eosinophilic mucus, bone erosion, and recurrent infections, but no mucosal invasion.[8] Although the authors believed the patient had chronic invasive fungal sinusitis, he probably suffered from AFS. Most likely, chronic invasive fungal sinusitis was over-diagnosed prior to the description of AFS, and the current paucity of chronic invasive disease reflects its true prevalence.

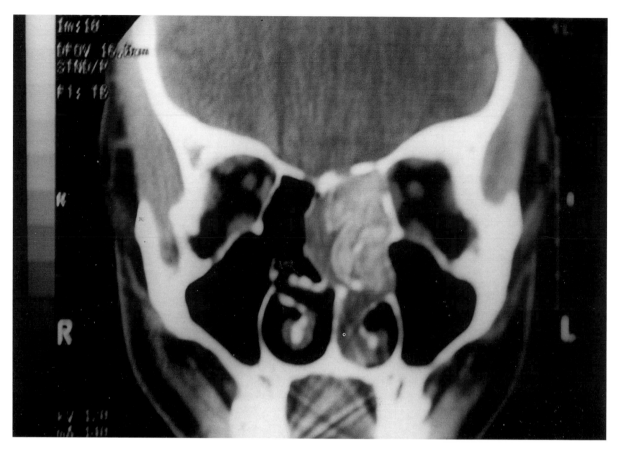

Figure 4. CT scan of left ethmoid AFS. Expanding inspissated fungal debris has caused deviation of the adjacent lamina papyracea and nasal septum. The heterogenous opacification typical of fungal sinusitis is present.

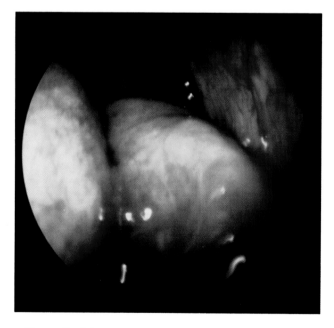

Figure 5. A large polyp originates from the right middle meatus and extends anterior to the middle turbinate.

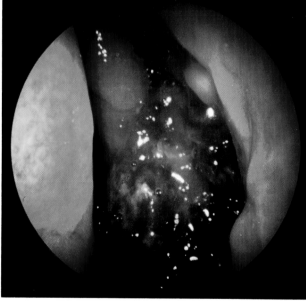

Figure 6. Fungal and mucoid concretions in left ethmoid cavity, consistent with recurrent allergic fungal sinusitis.

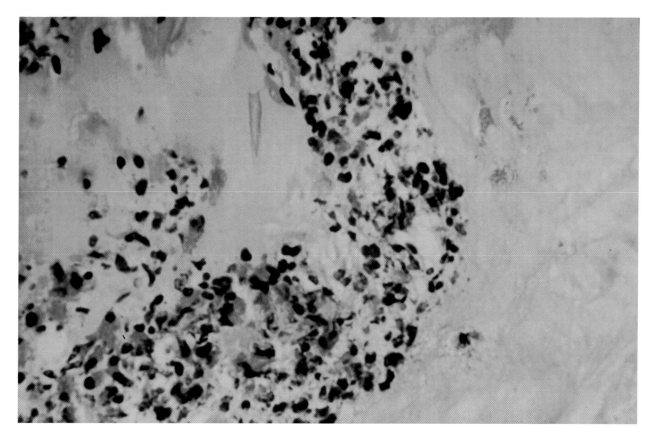

Figure 7. Allergic mucus with sheets of eosinophils. A Charcot-Leyden crystal, released by necrotic eosinophils, is seen near the center (arrow).

Table 2. AFS Culture Results (n=26)

Dematiaceous		18
Curvularia	10	
Alternaria	3	
Bipolaris	3	
Dreschlera	1	
Exserohilum	1	
Aspergillus		7
Penicillium		2
Cladosporium		1
Fusarium		1
Hyalinase		1
No Growth		4
Total		34*

*5 cultures grew 2 or 3 different fungi.

Diagnosis

Physicians must maintain an index of suspicion for AFS to avoid overlooking the diagnosis. It may be easily mistaken for chronic bacterial sinusitis or non-allergic fungal sinusitis, both of which have significantly different treatments and outcomes. Without an adequate aware-

ness the rhinologist will miss AFS and become frustrated by unexplained recurrences among "chronic sinusitis" patients. Alternatively, the recognition of extramucosal fungal hyphae may be mistaken for the potentially lethal acute fungal sinusitis, resulting in the inappropriate use of radical surgery or toxic intravenous antifungals. To clarify the diagnosis of AFS, we prospectively evaluated 15 consecutive patients with overt AFS (Table 4).[16] Type I hypersensitivity evidenced by a strong allergic history, positive skin tests, or elevated serum IgE levels was uniformly documented. Nasal polyps were also present in all patients. CT scans reliably showed the characteristic heterogeneous opacification of the involved sinuses. The typical histology was observed in all patients, although Charcot-Leyden crystals were not seen in 9 of 15 specimens. A history of asthma and unilateral predominance of sinus disease was seen in most but not all patients. Radiographic bone erosion appeared in 12 of 15 patients, but no tissue had evidence of fungal invasion. Not all patients had a positive fungal culture or peripheral eosinophilia, and none had a history of aspirin sensitivity. Because the following features were identified in all 15 patients, we proposed that they be established as criteria for the diagnosis of AFS: 1) type I hypersensitivity,

Table 3. Characteristics of Fungal Sinusitis

	Immune Status	Role of Fungus	Tissue Invasion	Sinuses Affected	Treatment	Polyps
Acute	compromised	pathogen	yes	one	radical debridement systemic antifungals	no
Indolent	competent	pathogen	yes	variable	complete excision systemic antifungals	maybe
Fungus Ball	competent nonatopic	saprophyte	no	one	debridement aeration	no
AFS	competent atopic	allergen	no	multiple unilateral	debridement aeration steroids ? immunotherapy ? topical antifungals	yes

2) nasal polyps, 3) a characteristic CT scan, 4) eosinophilic mucus without fungal invasion into sinus tissue, and 5) a positive fungal stain.[16] Post-operative patients pose a particularly challenging diagnostic dilemma, since early recurrences may lack polyps and classic CT abnormalities.

Treatment

Most otolaryngologists now understand what constitutes AFS, but this improved recognition has not translated into treatment advances. Most authorities concur that functional endoscopic sinus surgery (FESS) with complete removal of inspissated fungi and debris is indicated. The extent of surgery correlates with the amount of pathology. FESS allows preservation of all non-diseased tissue, and external or obliterative surgery is contraindicated in uncomplicated AFS. In any form of surgery, microscopic fungal contamination of the sinuses probably persists, and this may be the source of recurrent disease. Patients generally attain tremendous benefit from surgery, but unfortunately, the improvement is most often transient.

Steroids decrease the abnormal immune response, and are being used with increased frequency post-operatively.

Our recent retrospective analysis of 26 patients indicated that steroids effectively diminish inflammation and help maintain disease-free interval. However, disease recurred as steroids were weaned, and patients treated with steroids had no apparent outcome advantages with extended follow-up (mean follow-up = 12.5 months).[26] Despite the lack of data to support the efficacy of steroids, we still advocate their use post-operatively to prolong remissions. We recommend post-operative oral prednisone (0.4 –0.6 mg/kg/day), tapering 0.1 mg/kg/d every 4 days to 0.2 mg/kg/day. Patient symptoms and objective signs guide subsequent steroid titration. The proper length of steroid treatment is unknown. Alternate day prednisone at 0.5 mg/kg for three months, then taper should be considered. Some physicians reserve steroids for recurrent disease,[18] because of several well-known side effects, including premature epiphyseal closure in children, peptic ulcers, weight gain, moodiness, and immunosuppression (that could potentially lead to fungal invasion). Others argue that "understanding that AFS is a hypersensitivity reaction and not an invasive process lends support to the use of systemic steroids."[1] Our experience has been that all patients not treated with steroids will eventually recur. Pre-operative use of steroids also may be consid-

Table 4. Characteristics of AFS patients (n = 15)[16]

Common Traits (present in all patients)	Associated Traits (# patients)
Type I hypersensitivity nasal polyps CT scan eosinophilic mucus fungal stain	unilateral predominance (13) radiographic bone erosion (12) fungal culture (11) asthma (8) Charcot-Leyden crystals (6) eosinophils (6)

ered, but the potential benefits must be weighed against the known risks and lack of clinical experience. Essentially, steroids act by blunting the pathologic hypersensitivity to fungal antigens, but they do not permanently reverse the disease process, leaving a great need for other forms of therapy.

Topical steroids can be used for local immune modulation without risking systemic complications. However, they have not helped noticeably, possibly due to the spray entering the nose but not the sinuses. Systemic antifungals such as amphotericin B play no role in AFS. We have had anecdotal success with using less toxic systemic antifungal, such as itraconazole or ketoconazole, but they have generally been of no benefit. In theory, systemic antifungals should be ineffective against the fungi, which are located extramucosally, outside the range of the drug circulation. Thus in order to produce an effect, a systemic antifungal must be secreted in sinus mucus, a phenomenon that has not been supported and probably does not occur. More realistically, there may be a future role for topical antifungal drugs, which could hypothetically decrease antigen load. Our initial *in vitro* analysis of fungal susceptibilities indicates that the common AFS pathogens are sensitive to several antifungals available in irrigation solution[29].

Probably the most promising future AFS treatment is serial endpoint titration (SET), or allergy desensitization. Densensitizing patients to the fungal antigen that stimulates their abnormal Type I immune response has therapeutic potential. If fungi function as antigens and not infectious agents, then successful treatment will depend on cleansing each patient's sinuses of fungal antigens and modifying the pathological immune response. Most allergists express skepticism about desensitizing AFS patients, feeling that IgG blocking antibodies will be generated, aggravating the Type III immune contribution, and worsening the disease. We have anecdotal experience of SET producing successful results, but have not used it on a routine basis. Recent data presented by Mabry et al. exemplifies that immunotherapy may be both safe and effective: prospective study of 10 AFS patients treated with immunotherapy resulted in "a marked decrease in nasal crusting, a minimum amount of recurrent polypoid mucosa, and a lessened or absent requirement for steroids (systemic or topical) in the vast majority of these patients".[30] Given this preliminary information, further study of immunotherapy can be undertaken with greater earnest and confidence.

Prognosis

In 1986 Waxman et al. divided post-operative AFS patients into three categories: immediate recurrence (months), delayed recurrence (years), or disease free.[18]

Table 5. AFS Objective Staging and Results (>1 month follow-up; n = 24)[26]

Stage 0: no evidence of disease	4
Stage 1: mucosal edema/allergic mucin	1
Stage 2: polypoid edema/allergic mucin	7
Stage 3: polyps and fungal debris	12

They retrospectively studied 15 patients, of whom 2 were lost to follow-up and 5 had less than one year of follow-up. Most of their patients had immediate or delayed recurrence, but three individuals remained disease free for as long as 2 years post-operatively. Since they did not mention using an endoscopic exam, which often demonstrates early recurrence in the form of asymptomatic mucosal disease, their data probably portrays an unrealistically optimistic prognosis. Reports from other otolaryngologists have cited recurrence rates ranging from 32% (5 of 16)[14] to 100% (3 of 3).[24]

In order to objectively classify post-operative outcome, we proposed a subjective and objective staging system. Subjectively, patients classify themselves as improved, no change, or worse. Reviewing our results, 22 of 26 patients (84.6%) were improved, and none were worse (mean follow-up=12.5 months).[26] Objectively, endoscopic nasal examination permits staging into one of four objective categories (Table 5), ranging from Stage 0 (no evidence of disease) to Stage III (polyps and fungal debris present). Results from 24 patients seen beyond 1 month follow-up are displayed in Table 5.[26] Disease severity ranged from mild, asymptomatic inflammation to rapid recurrences featuring extraordinarily high serum IgE and immediate return of polyps. Physical findings tended to reflect more disease than patient's symptoms, and many patients who felt asymptomatic had endoscopic evidence of pathology. All patients followed beyond 12 months post-operatively developed objective evidence of recurrence, with the longest time to recurrence being 34 months.[28] We do not know if recurrence results from re-exposure to fungus or an immune reaction to persistent fungal antigens. With continued follow-up, we suspect that asymptomatic patients followed less than 12 months will eventually develop sinonasal complaints. Consequently, we follow patients with endoscopic exams every 1–3 months for at least 3 years.

Conclusions

A greater understanding exists regarding disease recognition and diagnosis of AFS. Although most patients can be helped tremendously with current management strategies, many questions persists about immunopathology and treatment. Hopefully, future research will deal with these issues and enable improved post-operative results.

BIBLIOGRAPHY

1. Ence, BK, Gourley, DS, Jorgensen, NL, Shagets, FW, Parsons, DS. Allergic fungal sinusitis. Am J Rhin 4 (5): 169 –78, 1990.

2. Goldstein MF, Atkins PC, Cogen FC, Kornstein MJ, Levine RS, Zweiman B. Allergic *Aspergillus* sinusitis. J All Clin Imm 76: 515–24, 1985.

3. Gourley, DS. Allergic fungal sinusitis. Insights Allergy 4 (1): 1–4, 1989.

4. Blitzer A, Lawson W. Fungal infections of the nose and paranasal sinuses. Otolaryngol Clin 26 (6): 1007–35, 1993.

5. Tami TA, Wawrose SF. Diseases of the nose and paranasal sinuses in the human immunodeficiency virus-infected population. Otolaryngol Clin 25 (6): 1199–1210, 1992.

6. Veress B, Malik OA, El Tayeb AA, El Daoud S, El Mahgoub S, El Hassan AM. Further observations on the primary paranasal aspergillus granuloma in the Sudan. Am J Trop Med Hyg 22: 765–72, 1973.

7. Chakrabarti A, Sharma SC, Chander J. Epidemiology and pathogenesis of a paranasal sinus mycosis. Otolaryngol Head Neck Surg 107: 745–750, 1992.

8. Washburn RG, Kennedey DW, Begley MG, Henderson, DK, Bennett, JE. Chronic fungal sinusitis in apparently normal hosts. Medicine 67: 231–47, 1988.

9. Stammberger H, Jakse R, Beaufort F. Aspergillosis of the paranasal sinuses. Ann Otol Rhinol Laryngol 94 (Suppl 119): 1–11, 1985.

10. Millar, JW, Johnston, A, Lamb, D. Allergic Aspergillosis of the maxillary sinuses. Thorax 36: 710, 1981.

11. Katzenstein, AA, Sale, SR, Greenberger, PA. Allergic Aspergillus sinusitis. A newly recognized form of sinusitis. J All Clin Imm 72: 89–93, 1983.

12. Allphin, AL, Strauss, M, Abdul-Karim, FW. Allergic fungal sinusitis: problems in diagnosis and treatment. Laryngoscope 101 (8): 815–20, 1991.

13. Manning, SC, Schaefer, SD, Close, LG, Vuitch, F. Culture-positive allergic fungal sinusitis. Arch Oto 117 (2): 174–8, 1991.

14. Schwietz, LA, Gourley, DS. Allergic fungal sinusitis. Allergy Proc 13 (1): 3–6, 1992.

15. Corey, JP. Fungal diseases of the sinuses. Otolaryngol Head Neck Surg 103: 1012–15, 1990.

16. Bent JP, Kuhn FA. The diagnosis of allergic fungal sinusitis. *Otol Head Neck Surg* 111: 580–88, 1994.

17. Manning SC, Mabry RL, Schaefer SD, Close LG. Evidence of IgE-mediated hypersensitivity in allergic fungal sinusitis. Laryngoscope 103: 717–21, 1993.

18. Waxman, JE, Spector, JG, Sale, SR, Katzenstein, AA. Allergic Aspergillus sinusitis: concepts in diagnosis and treatment of a new clinical entity. Laryngoscope 97: 261–66, 1987.

19. Zieske, LA, Kopke, RD, Hamill, R. Dermatiaceous fungal sinusitis. Otolaryngol Head Neck Surg 105 (4): 567–77, 1991.

20. Yoo, GH, Francis, HW, Zinreich, SJ. Imaging quiz case: non-invasive Aspergillus sinusitis. Arch Otol 119: 123–4, 1993.

21. Waitzman AA, Birt BD. Fungal sinusitis. J Otolaryngol 23 (4): 244–9, 1994.

22. Cody DT, Neel HB, Ferreiro JA, Roberts GD. Allergic fungal sinusitis: The Mayo Clinic experience. Laryngoscope 104: 1074 –79, 1994.

23. Brummond, W, Kurup, VP, Harris, GJ, et al. Allergic sino-orbital mycosis. A clinical and immunologic study. JAMA 256 (23): 3249–53, 1986.

24. Sher, TH, Schwartz, HJ. Allergic Aspergillus Sinusitis with concurrent Allergic Bronchopulmonary Aspergillus: a report of a case. *J All Clin Imm* 81 (5 Pt 1): 844–6, 1988.

25. Gourley, DS, Whisman, BA, Jorgensen, NL, et al. Allergic Bipolaris sinusitis: clinical and immunopathologic characteristics. J All Clin Imm 85: 583–91, 1990.

26. Kupferberg SB, Bent JP, Kuhn FA. The prognosis for allergic fungal sinusitis. Otolaryngol Head Neck Surg (in press).

27. Handley GH, Visscher DW, Katzenstein AA, Peters GE. Bone erosion in allergic fungal sinusitis. Am J Rhin 4: 149–53, 1990.

28. Kuhn FA, Fravel WJ, Wood AP et al. Allergic fungal sinusitis: a treatment protocal. Submitted to Am J Rhin, May 95.

29. Bent JP, Kuhn FA. Antifungal activity against allergic fungal sinusitis organisms. Laryngoscope (in press).

30. Mabry RL, Mabry CS. Immunotherapy for allergic fungal sinusitis: the second year. Presented at the 1996 Annual Meeting of the American Academy of Otolaryngologic Allergy (Washington, DC), September 26, 1996.

Chapter XVII

Nasal Polyps in Cystic Fibrosis

Peter M. G. Deane, M.D., and Robert H. Schwartz, M.D.

ABSTRACT

Cystic fibrosis (CF) is an autosomal recessive disease, the most common inherited lifeshortening disease of white children, caused by a defective mucosal chloride transport gene. The most severe manifestations are malabsorption and progressive obstructive pulmonary disease, but about one third of children and almost one half of affected adults suffer from multiple, bilateral nasal polyps. These patients also suffer from chronic pansinusitis. Common symptoms include nasal obstruction, rhinorrhea, anosmia and chronic cough. The etiology of the polyps is believed to be related to the chronic sinus inflammation and excessive epithelial sodium and water reabsorption. The histology of the nasal polyps from CF patients differs significantly from those of non-CF allergic rhinitis patients, with less tissue eosinophils and more lymphocytes and plasma cells. Also, the basement membrane is not thickened.

Treatment is based on degree of symptoms. Polyps may spontaneously regress. Smaller polyps may respond to topical nasal steroids. More significant and refractory polyps require surgery. Simple polypectomy is helpful but recurrence of the polyps is common. Ethmoidectomy and functional endoscopic sinus surgery carry the potential for higher perioperative morbidity, but also reduce postoperative symptoms and recurrence rate.

INTRODUCTION

Cystic fibrosis (CF, mucoviscidosis) is the most common life-shortening inherited disease of Caucasian children. Its incidence varies among different populations, ranging from one in 1700 live births in Northern Ireland to one in 7700 in Sweden. This implies a carrier frequency of about one in 20 to one in 40. It is rare in Asians and in African Blacks (less than one in 100,000). CF is lethal because of chronic bronchopulmonary infec-

tion and progressive lung destruction. However, in recent years, its prognosis has improved: in 1992 the proportion of adult (18 years and older) CF patients was 33%, a fourfold increase from 1969 (8%). The median age of survival in 1992 was 29.4 years, also a fourfold increase since 1969.

The familial nature of CF was first described by Fanconi in 1936. Long known to be an autosomal-recessive illness, CF was found in 1989 to be caused by a mutation of a normal gene on the long arm of chromosome 7[1-3]. The most common mutation occurring on approximately 70% of CF chromosomes is the ΔF508 which is a 3-bp deletion of the triplet CTT in exon 10 resulting in the deletion (delta, or Δ) of phenylalanine (F) at position 508 of the predicted protein[2]. The encoded protein is called the cystic fibrosis transmembrane regulator (CFTR). It forms the major chloride transport channel, with secretion stimulated by cyclic adenosine monophosphate. The CFTR protein is expressed on the lumenal surface of pancreatic and sweat gland epithelial cells and in submucosal glands and epithelium lining the airways. More than 300 mutations of the CF gene have been described[4]. Some genotypes cause less pancreatic disease[5]; others do not cause abnormal sweat chloride concentrations.[6,7] No particular genotype has been associated with nasal polyposis. It should be pointed out, however, that multiple nasal polyps may occur in children and adults who have sweat chloride concentrations in the normal range and yet have abnormal CF genotypes.[7]

CLINICAL FEATURES AND DIAGNOSIS

Because CF is a multisystem disease, there are many complicating features; nasal polyposis is one. (Table 1). The diagnostic hallmarks of CF are pancreatic enzyme deficiency with malabsorption, chronic progressive obstructive pulmonary disease, chronic pulmonary infection with *Staphylococcus aureus, Pseudomonas aeruginosa*

Table 1. Clinical Features and Complications of Cystic Fibrosis

Integument and external areas
1. Pallor
2. Failure to thrive
3. Purpura
4. Telangiectasia
5. Erythema nodosum
6. Digital clubbing
7. Protuberant abdomen
8. Emphasematous chest
9. Short stature
10. Delayed puberty
11. Cyanosis
12. Angular stomatitis
13. Salt crystals on face
14. Paronychia
15. Edema

Head
1. Sinusitis
2. Nasal polyposis
3. Optic neuritis
4. Nyctalopia
5. Enlarged submaxillary glands

Thorax and pulmonary system
1. Bronchiolitis
2. Bronchitis
3. Bronchiectasis
4. Pneumonia
5. *Staphylococcus* organisms in sputum
6. *Pseudomonas* organisms in sputum
7. Allergic bronchopulmonary aspergillosis
8. Pulmonary cysts and abscesses
9. Atelectasis
10. Pneumomediastinum
11. Pneumothorax
12. Massive hemoptysis
13. Botryomycosis
14. Pulmonary insufficiency
15. Pulmonary failure

Thorax and cardiac system
1. Pulmonary hypertension
2. Right ventricular hypertrophy
3. Cor pulmonale
4. Right ventricular failure
5. Myocardial fibrosis

Abdomen and gastrointestinal
1. Pancreatic enzyme deficiency
2. Steatorrhea
3. Azotorrhea
4. Pancreatitis
5. Meconium ileus
6. Intestinal atresia
7. Fecal impaction
8. Intussusception
9. Duodenitis and ulceration
10. Mucocele of appendix
11. Biliary cirrhosis of liver
12. Hepatomegaly
13. Splenomegaly
14. Portal hypertension
15. Esophageal varices
16. Ascites
17. Gallbladder stones
18. Pneumatosis intestinalis
19. Pneumatosis coli
20. Pseudomembranous colitis
21. Rectal prolapse
22. Inguinal hernia
23. Diabetes mellitus

Genitourinary system
1. Absence of vas deferens
2. Male sterility
3. Thick cervical mucus
4. Cervical polyps
5. Female decreased fertility

or both, and abnormal electrolyte loss in sweat. Confirmation of the diagnosis of CF requires two positive sweat tests, done on different days, according to methods approved by the Cystic Fibrosis Foundation Center Committee and Guidelines Subcommittee. A positive test result is defined by sweat chloride measurements in excess of 60 mmol/L in an adequate sample of sweat (a minimum of 75 mg collected on 2" × 2" gauze or filter paper or 15 μL collected in Macroduct coils during a 30-minute period). Repeated borderline measurements (40 to 60 mmol/L) require clinical correlation for diagnosis, preferably confirmed by DNA genotyping for the common and uncommon mutations. Most (98%) CF sweat chlorides fall between 60 mmol/L and 160 mmol/L[8]. Less than 2% are below 60 mmol/L. Diagnostic testing can be supplemented with genotyping in patients who appear on clinical grounds to have CF, but have normal sweat tests. Nasal polyps in CF can occur prior to pulmonary or gastrointestinal disease manifestations[9]. As nasal polyps from other causes are uncommon in childhood and CF can present in very mild forms, sweat tests (and if need be, genotypes) should be performed on children with unexplained nasal polyps. By contrast, among adults with nasal polyps who have not been diagnosed with CF, sodium sweat levels are normal[10].

GENETICS OF CYSTIC FIBROSIS

Our understanding of the etiology, pathophysiology, and genetics of CF has changed considerably since the orig-

Table 2. Selected Common and Uncommon Cystic Fibrosis Mutations

Mutation	Mutation Type	Location	Frequency USA*	Frequency World**
ΔF508	Inframe Deletion	Exon 10	82.1	67.2
G542X	Nonsense	Exon 11	3.5	3.4
G551D	Missense	Exon 11	3.4	2.4
N1303K	Missense	Exon 21	1.8	1.8
W1282X***	Nonsense	Exon 20	1.6	2.1
R553X	Nonsense	Exon 11	1.3	1.3
621+1G→T	Splice site	Intron 4	1.0	1.3
R117H****	Missense	Exon 4	0.7	0.8
3848(9)+10kbC→T*****	Splice site	Intron 19	0.6	1.4
1717-1G→A	Splice site	Intron 10	0.4	1.1
M1101K******	Missense	Exon 17b	Rare	Rare

* = Cystic Fibrosis Foundation, Patient Registry 1992 Annual Report, Bethesda, Maryland, October 1993.
** = CF Genetics Analysis Consortium (Tsui, 1992a)
*** = most common (60%) mutation in the CF Askenazi Jewish population of Israel
**** = associated with pancreatic sufficiency
***** = associated with normal sweat chloride concentration
****** = most common (69%) mutation among CF Hutterites of North America

inal pathologic description by Dorothy Anderson in 1938, and since the recognition of the sweat chloride reabsorption defect by Paul A. diSant'Agnese in 1953. In 1989, the CF gene was found on the long arm of chromosome 7[1-3]. The CF gene consists of about 250 kb of DNA containing 27 exons. The mRNA transcript contains about 6500 basepairs encoding a protein of 1480 amino acids. This protein is called the cystic fibrosis transmembrane regulator (CFTR). It forms the major electrochemical apparatus, a channel for Cl^- ion transport regulated by cyclic AMP. RNA transcripts of the CFTR gene are found in lung, pancreas, sweat gland, liver, nasal polyps, salivary glands, and colon. The CFTR protein is expressed on the apical surface of pancreatic and sweat gland epithelial cells and in submucosal glands lining the airways. The proposed functions of CFTR and the relationship of abnormal CFTRs to CF pathophysiology are described below[11].

More than 300 mutations of the CF gene have been described[5]. The most common mutation (ΔF508) consists of a three basepair **inframe deletion** in exon 10 at codon 508 resulting in a deletion (Δ) of phenylalanine (F). Other types of mutations include **missense** (substitution of a single amino acid), **nonsense** (premature termination leading to a nonfunctional CFTR), **frameshift** (deletions or additions of basepairs), and **splicing** (involving splice junctions) mutations (Table 2).

The ΔF508 mutation is present on about 67 percent of CF chromosomes worldwide (82% of CF patients in U.S.—1992 CF Foundation Patient Registry Annual Data Report). ΔF508 homozygotes and most Δ_{508} compound heterozygotes (Δ_{508} plus another mutation) usu-

ally have pancreatic insufficiency of early onset with markedly elevated sweat chloride concentrations. In one important study (n = 798 CF patients, The Cystic Fibrosis genotype-phenotype consortium, 1993), compound heterozygotes having the genotype R117H/ΔF$_{508}$ (n = 23) had lower sweat chloride concentrations (80+/−18 vs 108+/−14 mmol/L, P<0.001) than age-matched more common ΔF$_{508}$ homozygotes (n = 399). Also, they more often had pancreatic sufficiency (87 percent vs 4 percent, P<0.001). Meconium ileus was not seen in this group (n=23). This study of genotype-phenotype relationships has genetic counseling, therapeutic, and prognostic implications[5]. Patients with R117H/ΔF$_{508}$ can expect long-term pancreatic sufficiency. Those with other genotypes can expect early onset of pancreatic insufficiency. However, this first report found no statistically significant differences in the incidence of common features of CF such as pseudomonas colonization, nasal polyps, pancreatitis, diabetes mellitus, distal intestinal obstruction syndrome, rectal prolapse, cirrhosis, and gallbladder disease. Obviously, additional genetic and environmental factors influence the phenotypic expression of CF. Nutritional factors are probably of importance since other non-genetic studies[12] suggest that CF patients with pancreatic sufficiency have milder lung disease. Also, in one study[13], poor pulmonary clinical status of ΔF$_{508}$ homozygotes (n = 44) was associated with heavy exposure to tobacco smoke. The studies of genotypes and phenotypes continues.

There are differences in the frequency of various mutations among different national, ethnic, and racial groups. These variations need to be considered to allow precise carrier detection and prenatal diagnosis. The frequency of ΔF_{508} is found to be 65–80% in North American, British, Swiss and Dutch patients but only 51–58% in Spanish and Italian populations and 37% of black American patients. Among the French-Canadians in Saquenay-Lac St. Jean, Quebec province, the frequency is 56%[14]. The frequency of the ΔF_{508} mutation is only 22% in the Ashkenazi Jewish population in Jerusalem whereas the W1282X nonsense mutation is the most common (60% of CF chromosomes). The ΔF_{508} mutation accounts for only 31% of mutations in CF families representing the three endogamous subdivisions (Dariusleut, Lehrerleut, and Schmiedelut) of the Hutterite population of North America[15]. A rare missense mutation (M1101K) has been found on the other 69% of CF chromosomes[16]. These two mutations account for all of the CF mutations among Hutterites, making it possible to offer the Hutterites accurate carrier testing and genetic counseling of adults and early diagnosis and treatment of CF infants[17].

Further caution is needed if carrier screening and genetic counseling of populations other than at-risk families is to be undertaken because the less common mutations may account for phenotypic variations such as milder disease in CF patients with pancreatic sufficiency, less severe CF in black persons, and other very mild forms of the disease. These associations are only beginning to be identified and understood. For example, in a group of 23 non-CF patients with congenital absence of the vas deferens, 11 were heterozygous for the ΔF_{508} mutation[18]. Among patients with congenital absence of the vas deferens without unilateral renal agenesis the frequency of the R117H mutation of exon 4 was found to be high (4 of 18). These unrelated patients in their thirties had normal chest films and FEV1s. Their sweat chloride values were elevated (62 to 90 mmol/L).

STRUCTURE AND FUNCTION OF THE CYSTIC FIBROSIS TRANSMEMBRANE REGULATOR (CFTR)—RELATIONSHIP TO THE PATHOGENESIS OF CF

CF is caused by mutations in the cystic fibrosis transmembrane conductance regulator (CFTR) gene; its product has been shown to be a cAMP-regulated chloride channel. The CFTR structure consists of 12 membrane-spanning regions (transmembrane domains—TM1 to TM12) two ATP-binding domains (nucleotide binding folds—NBF1 and NBF2), and a regulatory domain (R-domain). Perturbation of CFTR's normal structure results in abnormal transport of chloride ions across sweat duct epithelial cells and across mucosal surface epithelial cells. In the sweat gland there is abnormal reabsorption

of chloride and sodium, accounting for the elevation of these ions in sweat, providing the genetic pathophysiologic basis for the diagnostic sweat test. At the respiratory, pancreatic and hepatic organ levels, there is a block in chloride channel transport to the luminal surface of epithelial cells, resulting in a decrease in sodium and water transport to the mucus sol layer. A dehydrated thickened viscous mucus impairs mucociliary clearance and contributes to obstruction of bronchioles, bronchi, pancreatic ducts, and bile canaliculi. In the respiratory tract, mucus viscosity is increased even more by large amounts of DNA from the neutrophilic response to infection and to a lesser extent by exopolysaccharides from infecting mucoid strains of *Pseudomonas aeruginosa*.

There are at least four mechanisms by which mutations disrupt CFTR function. Their elucidation and enumeration will have implications for understanding the many phenotypic variations in CF and for developing therapeutic strategies to correct different degrees of CFTR dysfunction. Class I mutations (defective production) produce no CFTR protein; Class II (defective protein processing) results in defective trafficking of CFTR protein from the endoplasmic reticulum to the Golgi where normally it would be glycosylated and then move to the plasma membrane[19]; Class III have defective regulation at the nucleotide binding folds; Class IV mutants have defective conduction through the CFTR chloride channel. Defective trafficking (Class II mutation) accounts for 60% to 80% of the CF alleles (ΔF_{508}). Therapeutic strategies (Table 3) currently include gene therapy to restore normal CFTR structure and function[20] and pharmacologic therapy to correct abnormal CFTR function[21].

EPIDEMIOLOGY AND CLINICAL FEATURES OF CF NASAL POLYPS

The first description of "polypoid degeneration of the nasal mucosa" in CF was made by Lurie[22]. Nasal polyps are uncommon in the general childhood population. The incidence of nasal polyposis in children with CF is 7 to 32 percent[23–25] and increases during adolescence until in adults it reaches 44 to 48 percent[26,27]. Most polyps are seen in patients who are already diagnosed with CF.[28] Gender does not play a significant role. The great majority of patients have multiple and bilateral polyps[25,29]. Polyps have been reported in children as young as 18 months[30], and detection may be limited by the ability of young children to tolerate nasal examination. Fiberoptic rhinoscopy should facilitate detections of polyps in all CF patients.

The most common symptom of the polyps is obstruction of airflow, in about two-thirds of affected patients[25,31]. Rhinorrhea is almost as prevalent; about 40%

Table 3. Approaches to Cystic Fibrosis Therapy

Abnormality	Solution	Approach
Abnormal CF gene ⇓	Provide normal gene	Gene therapy
Abnormal CFTR protein ⇓ ⇓	Provide normal protein Activate mutant form	Protein therapy ?
Abnormal salt transport ⇓ ⇓	Block sodium ion uptake Increase chloride ion efflux	Amiloride ATP/UTP
Viscid pancreatic duct mucus Abnormal respiratory mucus ⇓	Replace enzymes Decrease viscosity	Oral pancreatic enzymes DNAase (Pulmozyme)
Impaired clearance ⇓ ⇓	Augment ciliary action	Chest percussion
Pseudomonas infection ⇓ ⇓ ⇓	Reduce bacterial count Prevent colonization	Antibiotics Hyperimmune globulin Pseudomonas vaccines
Inflammatory response ⇓ ⇓	Decrease host reaction	Glucocorticosteroids Other mediator inhibitors (Ibuprofen) Alpha-1-antitrypsin
Bronchiectasis	Replace irreversibly damaged lung	Lung transplantation

Adapted from: Collins FS. Cystic fibrosis: Molecular biology and therapeutic implications. Science 1992; 256: 774–779.[11]

have chronic mouth-breathing and less than 10% epistaxis. Other problems patients report include anosmia, chronic cough and throat clearing, bad breath and foul taste in the mouth. The post nasal drip is prominent in the mornings, and causes frequent morning coughing and gagging. The gagging is a particular problem for younger children[32].

Most of the polyps originate from the ethmoid and maxillary sinuses. Often the multiple polyps press the middle turbinate against the septum, which may then deviate to the side with a smaller mass of polyps[28]. Polyps may also protrude posterior to the choanae[30] or out the front of the nose. Polypoid change can be seen within the sinuses themselves, and on the middle and inferior turbinates. In one study of 84 CF patients, children and adults, each of whom had fiberoptic rhinoscopy performed, polyps were seen protruding from the middle meatus in 45%; no other site of polyp origin was described[33].

The polyps form in the setting of the chronic sinus disease which occurs in CF due to the patients' impaired mucociliary flow. Not only is their mucus more viscid due to abnormal mucosal ion transport, but some patients go on to develop ciliary microtubular defects as well[34]. Al-

most all patients have their paranasal sinuses opacified on plain sinus films[35] or on computed tomographic scan[33]. The frontal and sphenoid sinuses usually form but never aerate. At surgery the sinuses are found to be filled with purulent mucus, often thick, pasty and foul smelling; the organisms most often cultured are *Staphylococcus aureus, Pseudomonas aeruginosa* and normal flora[30,28]. Diagnosis of acute sinusitis depends on the presence of fever, facial pain and sinus tenderness; once the sinuses have opacified, medical therapy will not clear them. Mucoceles and pyoceles may form, and erode the sinus wall into the orbit or anterior cranial fossa; sinus surgery is then indicated, as it would be in any patient. The persistent chronic sinus disease may cause widening of the ethmoid air cells of the growing child[30]. This in turn may cause widening and flattening of the nasal bridge, which alters the child's facial appearance[23,25]. Either through chronic pressure or because of osteitis, the lamina papyracea and the medial bony wall of the maxillary antrum may also be destroyed[30,9] or protrude medially and partially obstruct the nasal cavity[33].

Ear disease is no more of a problem for a child with CF than for other children. The incidence of otitis media and impaired hearing is consistent with that of the general population[32,24].

THE NATURE OF THE POLYPS

The reason for polyp formation in cystic fibrosis remains unknown, but some clues are available. The role of allergy in polyp formation has been studied; the histology of the nasal mucosa and polyps has been examined. Based on this, some conclusions may be drawn.

Atopy does not seem to play a significant role in polyp formation. The incidence of atopy in patients with polyps is not greater than that found in the general population[36,25]. Many CF patients have nasal stuffiness and wheezing; but in most, these symptoms are due to their underlying disorder, not allergic rhinitis or extrinsic asthma. Moreover, the definition of "atopy" varies among studies, from seasonal nasal symptoms alone to positive traditional allergy skin tests. Immediate wheal and flare skin test reactions can be demonstrated in 25 to 50 percent of patients with CF, but the development of these immune phenomena does not imply a pathogenic significance. When "atopy" was defined as positive immediate skin test reactions to at least five allergens, we found 46% of CF patients to be atopic[37]. Significantly more severely affected (63%) were atopic compared to a healthier group of CF patients (30%). Skin test positivity correlated well with *Pseudomonas aeruginosa* colonization of the respiratory tract, which in turn was associated with more severe pulmonary disease[38,39]. When CF patients were studied for aspirin sensitivity, which is associated with an "intrinsic" form of airway disease, no association was found[40]. In fact, one nonsteroidal antiinflammatory drug (NSAID), ibuprophen has been used successfully to lessen the pulmonary inflammatory reaction in CF patients[41]. A study of the nasal response to exercise challenge in CF patients likewise found no significant results[42].

The polyps themselves have been studied to attempt to define their etiology. Early studies focussed on the mucous glands in the polyps, but ultimately their number, shape and size has not been found to differ from those of polyps associated with other diseases[43,44]. More recent work by several groups has found significant differences in the histology of the polyps. Associated with whatever illness, polyps are noted to be covered with pseudostratified columnar epithelium, with foci of squamous metaplasia in areas of high airflow and turbulence. However, both Oppenheimer and Rosenstein[45] (1979) and our group[46] found that extensive hyaline thickening of the basement membrane of polyp mucosa seen in patients with allergic or aspirin-sensitive rhinitis or chronic sinusitis (not associated with CF) was not seen in polyps from CF patients. The nature of the inflammatory infil-

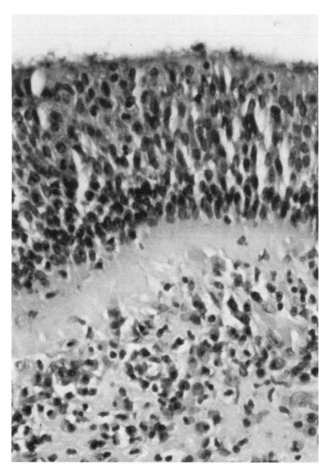

Figure 1. (Original magnification 20×) Polyp from a non-CF patient with sinusitis. Note the irregular and thickened basement membrane, with a subepithelial infiltrate dense with eosinophils. (Courtesy Dr. Fadi Hatem.)

trate in the polyp differs as well. Polyps associated with allergic or aspirin-sensitive rhinitis have a significantly more eosinophilic infiltrate than those of CF patients. The CF polyps (whether the patients had a coexisting allergic disease or not) had low tissue eosinophil counts and elevated numbers of lymphocytes and plasma cells. (See Figure 1 and Figure 2). Henderson and Chi[47] (1992) used morphometric analysis to demonstrate that, compared to polyps from atopic or aspirin-sensitive patients, CF nasal polyps contained significantly greater numbers of lymphocytes, plasma cells, endothelial cells and mast cells. The increased numbers of endothelial cells suggest that the CF polyps are more vascular than other polyps. Not only were there more mast cells in the CF polyps, they were significantly more degranulated, which suggests spontaneous mast cell activation in the CF polyps—the same polyps which have a relative dearth of eosinophils. They did not characterize the mast cells into T or TC subtypes. Oppenheimer and Rosenstein[45] noted a third characteristic of CF polyps, acid mucopolysac-

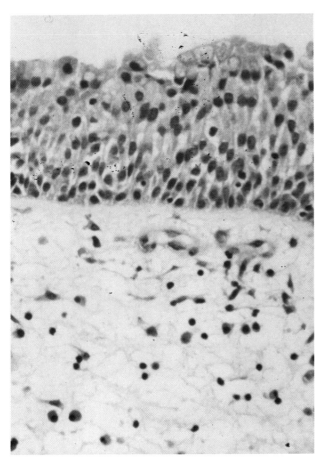

Figure 2. (Original magnification 20×) Polyp from a CF patient. Note the thin basement membrane, with a subepithelial chronic inflammatory infiltrate and scant eosinophils. (Courtesy Dr. Fadi Hatem.)

charides predominating in the glands and mucus blanket. We were unable to confirm this.

Another piece of the puzzle may be provided by physiology studies of the nasal mucosa. Normally, sodium is reabsorbed across the nasal mucosa through specific channels, while chloride is secreted by the CFTR protein. In CF patients, not only is the CFTR channel defective, but sodium channel permeability is increased[48]. The result is sodium hyperabsortion across the mucosa. Chloride and water passively follow. This has a number of effects. First, removal of significant amounts of water from the mucus dehydrates it; this leads to increased mucus viscosity. Second, because sodium concentration in the lumenal mucus is so low, the usual negative transepithelial electrical gradient is greatly increased: from about -20 mV to about -50 mV. This difference is not merely statistically significant. There is essentially no overlap among patient groups: CF patients' nasal mucosa have consistently had higher gradients than normal controls or primary ciliary dyskinesia patients[49,50]. This dif-

ferences has been used to diagnose CF in patients with normal sweat tests, who subsequently had the diagnosis confirmed with genotype analysis[7]. We know that inflammatory, mast cell-derived mediators such as histamine, prostaglandins and leukotrienes increase the chloride permeability of human nasal epithelial cells. Together, increased sodium reabsorption and increased chloride permeability would promote electrolyte and water reabsorption into the nasal submucosa, leading to edema and polyp formation[51].

One hypothesis, then, for the formation of nasal polyps in CF would be this: in the setting of a mucosal barrier which is predisposed to edema formation, chronic inflammation caused by persistent sinusitis leads to submucosal tissue proliferation, edema, then prolapse—which we see as nasal polyps.

MANAGEMENT

The mere presence of polyps does not mean that they require a physician's management. Only when a patient becomes adequately symptomatic is intervention required. This is an important principle in dealing with a problem such as nasal polyposis in CF, which we can ameliorate but not cure.

Medical management of the polyps benefits many patients. Antihistamines and decongestants are said, not surprisingly, to provide "transient symptomatic relief"[25]. In that same study it was reported that among patients with symptomatic polyps, about 40% of patients had clearance of their polyps and associated symptoms with medical management only. (The others went on to surgery.) Topical nasal steroids have been known since the 1960's to cause some polyp shrinkage[23,30]. Topical beclomethasone decreases nasal mucosal thickening, the size of smaller polyps and symptoms due to polyps. Larger polyps do not respond. Thus, topical nasal steroids may also play an important role in preventing recurrences after polypectomy[52,53].

Surgery for nasal polyps is the second most common class of operations performed on CF patients, less common only than laparotomies for meconium ileus[54]. General anesthesia presents an increased risk in CF patients due to their obstructive lung disease, and bleeding can be a problem in the malabsorbing patient with inadequate vitamin K levels. Nonetheless, a long experience with upper airway surgery in CF patients exists. Most patients do well if they have been followed closely as outpatients; with use of modern surgical techniques, little blood is lost and surgery can often be performed on a same-day basis[55,56]. The simplest procedure, and the one most commonly performed, is polypectomy. This provides satisfactory relief of nasal obstructive symptoms, but symptomatic recurrence occurs in about 60% of patients within 18 months[54,28]. A variety of more aggressive procedures have been combined with polypectomy: ethmoidectomy, Caldwell-Luc antrostomies and more recently functional endoscopic sinus surgery (FESS). Good evidence exists to suggest that nasal antral windows by themselves are not helpful in treating chronic sinusitis in any group of children[57]. Caldwell-Luc procedures have also fallen from favor. However, since the late 1980's, evidence has accumulated to support the belief that intranasal ethmoidectomy and FESS decrease polyp recurrence. Any cause of blockage of the ostiomeatal complex through which the frontal, maxillary and ethmoid sinuses drain predisposes to sinusitis. Enhancing the drainage of these sinuses should decrease local inflammation, and therefore polyp recurrence. Crockett et al. (1987)[28] found that any sinus procedure decreased the polyp recurrence rate to 35% over a number of years, and other studies are consistent with this[30,54,58]. FESS in particular has been well tolerated by patients and provides good symptomatic relief[31].

Amiloride is a drug which blocks epithelial sodium channels. Currently physicians prescribe it for use by mouth as a sodium sparing diuretic. When applied to respiratory mucosa it blocks sodium reabsorption, which causes the overlying mucus blanket to retain chloride and water[59]. For the CF patient, this might markedly reduce mucus viscosity and subepithelial edema. Whether topical nasal amiloride would affect nasal polyps is unknown.

A treatment for CF which has received much attention, both scholarly and popular, has been gene therapy. If functional CFTR genes could be placed into the patients' mucosal cells, the disease process could be halted or averted. Adenovirus modified to carry CFTR has been used experimentally to place the gene into the mucosa of the lower airway. CFTR has likewise been placed into CF nasal polyp mucosal cells with good expression *in vitro* and temporary normalization of patients' transepithelial electrical membrane gradients *in vivo*[60,59]. If the gene could be permanently transfected into patients' upper airways, this might truly cure their upper airway disease.

REFERENCES

1. Kerem E, Rommens JM, Buchanan JA and Riorden JR. Identification of the cystic fibrosis gene: genetic analysis. Science 245: 1073–1080 (1989).

2. Riordan JR, Rommens JM, Kerem B and Buchanan JA. Identification of the cystic fibrosis gene: cloning and characterization of complementary DNA. Science 245: 1066–1073 (1989).

3. Rommens JM, Iannuzzi MC, Kerem B, and Riordan JA. Identification of the cystic fibrosis gene: chromosome walking and jumping. Science 245:1059–1065 (1989).

4. Tsui, L-C. The cystic fibrosis transmembrane conductance regulator gene. Am J Respir Crit Care Med 151:547 –553 (1995).

5. Tsui, L-C. Mutations and sequence variations detected in the cystic fibrosis transmembrane regulator (CFTR) gene: a report from the cystic fibrosis genetic analysis consortium. Human Mutation 1:197–203 (1992).

6. Highsmith WE, Burch LH, Zhou Z, Olsen JC, Boat TE, Spock A, Gorvoy JD, Quittell L, Friedman KJ, Silverman LM, Boucher RC and Knowles MR. A novel mutation in the cystic fibrosis gene in patients with pulmonary disease but normal sweat chloride concentrations. New Engl J Med 331:974–980 (1994).

7. Stewart B, Zabner J, Shuber AP, Walsh MJ and McCray PB Jr. Normal sweat chloride values do not exclude the diagnosis of cystic fibrosis. Am J Resp Crit Care Med 151:899–903 (1995).

8. FitzSimmons SC. The changing epidemiology of cystic fibrosis. J Pediatr 122:1–9 (1993).

9. Wiatrak BJ, Myer CM III and Cotton RT. Cystic fibrosis presenting with sinus disease in children. AJDC 147:258–260 (1993).

10. Levine MI, Green RL, and Rodnan J. Sweat sodium levels in adults with nasal polyps. Ann All 58:377–378 (1987).

11. Collins FS. Cystic fibrosis: molecular biology and therapeutic implications. Science 256:774–779 (1992).

12. Gaskin K, Gurwitz D, Durie P, Corey M, Levison H, Forstner G. Improved respiratory prognosis in patients with cystic fibrosis with normal fat absorption. J Pediatr 100:857–862 (1982)

13. Campbell PW, Parker RA, Roberts BT, Krishnamani MRS, and Phillips JA. Association of poor clinical status and heavy exposure to tobacco smoke in patients with cystic fibrosis who are homozygous for the F508 deletion. J Pediatr 1992;120:261 –264.

14. Rosen R, Schwartz RH, Hilman BC, Stanislovitis P, Horn GT, Klinger K, Daigneault J, De Braekeleer M, Kerem B, Tsui L-C, Fujiwara TM, and Morgan K: Cystic fibrosis mutations in North American populations of French ancestry: Analysis of Quebec French-Canadian and Louisiana Acadian Families. Am J Hum Genet 47:606–610 (1990).

15. Fujiwara TM, Morgan K, Schwartz RH, Doherty RA, Miller SR, Klinger K, Stanislovitis P, Stuart N, and Watkins PC. Genealogical analysis of cystic fibrosis families and chromosome 7q RFLP haplotypes in the Hutterite Brethren, Am. J Hum Genet 44:327–337 (1989).

16. Zielenski J, Fujiwara TM, Markiewicz D, Paradis AJ, Anacleto I, Richards B, Schwartz RH, Klinger KW, Tsui, L-C, and Morgan K. Identification of the M1101K mutation in the cystic fibrosis transmembrane conductance regulator (CFTR) gene and complete detection of cystic fibrosis mutations in the Hutterite population. Am J Hum Genet 52:609–615 (1993).

17. Miller SR, Schwartz RH. Attitudes toward genetic testing of Amish, Mennonite, and Hutterite families with cystic fibrosis. Am. J. Public Health 82:236–242 (1992).

18. Gervais R, Dumer V, Rigot J-M, Lafitte J-J, Roussel. High frequency of thee R117H cystic fibrosis mutation in pa-

tients with congenital absence of the vas deferens. N Engl J Med 1993; 328:446–447.

19. Yang Y, Engelhardt JF, Wilson JM. Ultrastructural localization of variant forms of cystic fibrosis transmembrane conductance regulator in human bronchial epithelia of xenografts. Am J Respir Cell Mol Biol 11:7–15 (1994).

20. Olsen JC, Johnson LG, Stutts MJ, Sarkadi B, Yankaskas JR, Swanstrom R, Boucher RC. Correction of the apical membrane chloride permeability defect in polarized cystic fibrosis airway epithelia following retroviral-mediated gene transfer. Human Gene Therapy 3:253–266 (1992).

21. Knowles MR, Clarke LL, Boucher RC. Activation by extracellular nucleotides of chloride secretion in the airway epithelia of patients with cystic fibrosis. N Engl J Med 325:533–638 (1991).

22. Lurie MH. Cystic fibrosis of the pancreas and nasal mucosa. Ann Otorhinolaryngol 68:478–486 (1959).

23. Shwachman H, Kulczycki LL, Mueller HL and Flake CG. Nasal polyposis in patients with cystic fibrosis. Pediatrics 30:389–401 (1962).

24. Bak-Pedersen K and Larsen PK. Inflammatory middle ear disease in patients with cystic fibrosis. Acta Otolaryngol Suppl 360:138–140 (1979).

25. Stern RC, Boat TF, Wood RE, Matthews LRW and Doershuk CF. Treatment and prognosis of nasal polyps in cystic fibrosis. AJDC 136:1067–1070 (1982).

26. Sant'Agnese PAD and Davis PB. Cystic fibrosis in adults. Am J Med 66:121–132 (1979).

27. Kerrebijn JDF, Poublon RML and Overbeek SE. Nasal and paranasal disease in adult cystic fibrosis patients. Eur Resp J 5:1239–1242 (1992).

28. Crockett DM, McGill TJ, Healy GB, Friedman EM and Salkeld LJ. Nasal and paranasal sinus surgery in children with cystic fibrosis. Ann Oto Rhinol Laryngol 96:367–372 (1987).

29. David TJ. Nasal polyposis, opaque paranasal sinuses and usually normal hearing: the otorhinolaryngological features of cystic fibrosis. J Royal Soc Med Suppl 79:23–26 (1992).

30. Jaffe BF, Strome M, Khaw K-T and Shwachman H. Nasal polypectomy and sinus surgery for cystic fibrosis—a 10 year review. Otolaryngol Clin N Amer 10:81–90 (1977).

31. Jones JW, Parsons DS and Cuyler JP. The results of functional endoscopic sinus (FES) surgery on the symptoms of patients with cystic fibrosis. Int J Ped Otorhinolaryngol 28:25–32 (1993).

32. Neely JG, Harrison GM, Greenberg SD and Presberg H. The otolaryngologic aspects of cystic fibrosis. Trans Am Acad Ophth Otol 76:313–324 (1972).

33. Brihaye P, Clement PAR, Dab I and Desprechin B. Pathological changes of the lateral nasal wall in patients with cystic fibrosis (mucoviscidosis). Int J Ped Otorhinolaryngol 28:141–147 (1994).

34. Carson JL, Collier AM, Fernald GW and Hu SS. Microtubular discontinuities as acquired ciliary defects in airway epithelium of patients with chronic respiratory diseases. Ultrastruct Path 18:327–332 (1994).

35. Gharib R, Allen RP, Joos HA and Bravo LR. Paranasal sinuses in cystic fibrosis: incidence of roentgen abnormalities. AJDC 108:499–502 (1964).

36. Schramm VL and Effron MZ. Nasal polyps in children. Laryngoscope 90:1488–1495 (1980).

37. Nelson LA, Callerame ML and Schwartz RH. Aspergillosis and atopy in cystic fibrosis. Am Rev Resp Dis 130:863–873 (1979).

38. Warner JO, Taylor BW, Norman AP and Soothill JF. Association of cystic fibrosis with allergy. Arch Dis Childhood 51:507–511 (1976).

39. Wilmott RW. The relationship between atopy and cystic fibrosis. Clin Rev All 9:29–46 (1991).

40. Noritake D, Hen J and Dolan TF. Effects of aspirin on pulmonary function in patients with cystic fibrosis. Cystic Fibrosis Club Abstracts, 22nd Annual Meeting. San Francisco, CA. 22:144 (1981).

41. Konstan MW, Byard PJ, Hoppel CL, and Davis PB. Effect of high dose-ibuprofen in patients with cystic fibrosis. N Engl J Med 322:848–854 (1995).

42. Strohl KP, Arnold JL, Decker MJ, Hoekje PL, Doershuk CF and Stern RC. The nasal response to exercise in patients with cystic fibrosis. Rhinology 4:241–248 (1992).

43. Magid SL, Smith CC and Dolowitz DA. Nasal mucosa in pancreatic cystic fibrosis. Arch Otolaryngol 86:106–110 (1967).

44. Tos M, Mogensen C and Thomsen J. Nasal polyps in cystic fibrosis. J Laryngol Oto 91:827–835 (1977).

45. Oppenheimer EA and Rosenstein BJ. Differential pathology of nasal polyps in cystic fibrosis and atopy. Lab Invest 40:445–449 (1979).

46. Miller CH, Hatem F, Metlay LA, Schwartz RH and Hengerer AS. Can histologic criteria of nasal polyps be used to screen for cystic fibrosis? Pediatr Asthma All Immunol 8:51–56 (1994).

47. Henderson WR Jr and Chi EY. Degranulation of cystic fibrosis nasal polyp mast cells. J Path 166:395–404 (1992).

48. Chinet TC, Fullton JM, Yankaskas JR, Boucher RC and Stutts MJ. Mechanism of sodium hyperabsorption in cultured cystic fibrosis nasal epithelium: a patch clamp study. Am J Physiol (Cell Physiol) 266:C1061–C1068 (1994).

49. Knowles M, Gatzy J and Boucher R. Increased bioelectric potential difference across respiratory epithelia in cystic fibrosis. New Engl J Med 305:1489–1495 (1981).

50. Alton EWFW, Hay JG, Munro C and Geddes DM. Measurement of nasal potential difference in adult cystic fibrosis, Young's syndrome and bronchiectasis. Thorax 42:815–817 (1987).

51. Bernstein JM and Yankaskas JR. Increased ion transport in cultured nasal polyp epithelial cells. Arch Otolaryngol Head Neck Surg 120:993–996 (1994).

52. Canciani M and Mastella G. Efficacy of beclomethasone nasal drops, administered in the Moffat's position for nasal polyposis. Acta Paediatr Scand 77:612–613 (1988).

53. Donaldson JD and Gillespie CT. Observations on the efficacy of intranasal beclomethasone dipropionate in cystic fibrosis patients. J Otolaryngol 17:43–45 (1988).

54. Cepero R, Smith RJH, Catlin FI, Bressler KL, Furuta GT and Shandera KC. Cystic fibrosis—an otolaryngologic perspective. Otolaryngol Head Neck Surg 97:356–360 (1987).

55. Reilly JS, Kenna MA, Stool SE and Bluestone CD. Nasal surgery in children with cystic fibrosis: complications and risk management. Laryngoscope 95:1491–1493 (1985).

56. Duplechain JK, White JA and Miller RH. Pediatric sinusitis: the role of endoscopic sinus surgery in cystic fibrosis and other forms of sinonasal disease. Arch Otolaryngol Head Neck Surg 117:422–426 (1991).

57. Muntz HR and Lusk RP. Nasal antral windows in children: a retrospective study. Laryngoscope 100:643–646 (1990).

58. Clement PAR and Brihaye P. Resultaten van ethmoidectomieen bij kinderen met mucoviscidosis. Acta Otorhinolaryngologica Belg 48:17–22 (1994).

59. Zabner J, Couture LA, Gregory RJ, Graham SM, Smith AE and Welsh MJ. Adenovirus-mediated gene transfer transiently corrects the chloride transport defect in nasal epithelia of patients with cystic fibrosis. Cell 75:207–216 (1993).

60. Flotte TR, Afione SA, Conrad C, McGrath SA, Solow R, Oka H, Zeitlin PL, Guggino WB and Carter BJ. Stable in vivo expression of the cystic fibrosis transmembrane conductance regulator with an adeno-associated virus vector. Proc Natl Acad Sci USA 90:10613–10617 (1993).

Medical Management

Niels Mygind, M.D., and Torben Lildholdt, M.D., Ph.D.

ABSTRACT

The objectives of medical management of nasal polyposis are (1) to eliminate nasal polyps and rhinitis symptoms, (2) to re-establish nasal breathing and olfaction, and (3) to prevent recurrence of nasal polyps. Whilst antibiotics are used for infectious complications of nasal polyposis, only glucocorticosteroids (steroids) have a proven effect on the symptoms and signs of nasal polyps. Topically applied steroids is the therapeutic modality which has been best studied in controlled trials. It reduces rhinitis symptoms, improves nasal breathing, reduces the size of polyps and the recurrence rate, but it has a negligible effect on the sense of smell and on any sinus pathology. Topical steroids can, as long-term therapy, be used alone in mild cases, or combined with systemic steroids/surgery in severe cases. Systemic steroids, which are less well studied, have an effect on all types of symptoms and pathology, including the sense of smell. This type of treatment, which can serve as a 'medical polypectomy', is only used for short-term improvement due to the risk of adverse effects. Individualized management of nasal polyposis may use long-term topical steroids, short-term systemic steroids, as well as surgery, in various combinations. Exactly how these therapies, which differ in their control of various symptoms, are optimally combined is not yet well established.

INTRODUCTION

This chapter deals with glucocorticosteroids (steroids) which are the only type of drugs with proven efficacy in the disease, nasal polyposis. Antibiotics and vasoconstrictors are used for infectious complications. Antibiotics are not discussed further as their use follows the general principles for treatment of infections of the nose and paranasal sinuses. Topical vasoconstrictors are only used for short periods due to the risks of rebound congestion in this chronic disease.

OBJECTIVES OF TREATMENT

In discussing and comparing different types of therapy it may be useful to define the objectives for the management. As there has been in recent years improvements in both medical and surgical treatment it seems justified to aim high and try to obtain freedom from symptoms and normal nasal function (Table 1). The requirements of the ideal treatment are summarized in Table 2. In the evaluation of the various therapeutic principles, it is a major problem that a clinically relevant staging of the disease has not been established.

MECHANISMS OF STEROID EFFECT

The introduction of modern steroid sprays was followed by a series of studies which have shed light on the effect of glucocorticoids on various aspects of the inflammatory reaction in the airway mucosa[1]. These drugs have a multifactorial effect initiated by their binding to a specific cytoplasmic glucocorticoid receptor. Within hours the drug-receptor complex modifies gene transcription and induces a change of protein synthesis in the cell. This is responsible for the clinical effect which, within days, becomes manifest when treating polyposis. The number of glucocorticoid receptors is reduced by glucocorticoid administration,[2] but studies have not indicated any development of tachyphylaxis to therapy in nasal polyposis[3,4] or in other airway diseases.

Langerhans' Cells

A study of the nasal mucosa in allergic rhinitis has shown an increased number of antigen-presenting Langerhans' cells and a normalizing effect of topical steroid therapy.[5]

Table 1. Objectives of Treatment
of Nasal Polyposis

1. Elimination of nasal polyps or considerable reduction of their size.
2. Re-establishment of open nasal airway and nasal breathing.
3. Freedom from rhinitis symptoms.
4. Normal sense of smell.
5. Prevention of recurrence of nasal polyps.
6. NOT necessarily elimination of sinus pathology.

Table 2. Requirements of the Ideal Treatment

1. High patient compliance (no pain or discomfort, low cost, short duration of treatment and long-lasting effect).
2. No risk of serious adverse effects.
3. No change in normal nasal structure and function.

The role of Langerhans' cells in nasal polyposis has not been studied.

T Lymphocytes and Cytokines

There is accumulating evidence that the inflammatory reaction in asthma,[6] allergic rhinitis and nasal polyposis[7,8] is, at least in part, driven by T lymphocytes and their humoral products, cytokines. As T-cell kinetics, activation, and cytokine production are highly sensitive to steroids,[6,8] it seems likely that an important part of the clinical benefit from this type of treatment is due to a damping effect on T-cell function.

Kanai et al[8] have shown that topical steroids, reduce the number of lymphocytes, total T cells (CD3+), T helper cells (CD4+) and T effector cells (CD8+) in nasal polyp tissue.

Steroids may not only inhibit the synthesis of cytokines from lymphocytes but also from alternative sources such as epithelial cells.[8] The findings of cytokine production in nasal polyps and their possible role in the pathogenesis of polyposis has recently been reviewed by Jordana et al.[9] This group has advanced the hypothesis of nasal polyposis as a self-perpetuating inflammatory reaction caused by tissue-derived growth factors and cytokines[7] in an inductive microenvironment.

Mast Cells

Although polyp fluids have high histamine levels[10] the role of the mast cell in nasal polyposis is unclear.[11] Prolonged topical steroid treatment in the airways reduces the number of mast cells at the epithelial surface in asthma and allergic rhinitis. Following topical steroid therapy in nasal polyposis, a reduced number of mast

cells was found in one study,[12] while another study failed to show a significant drug effect.[8]

Eosinophils

There is influx, accumulation and activation of eosinophils in polyp tissue. Topical steroids reduce the total number of eosinophils in polyps[13,14] and, to a greater degree, the number of activated cells[8] in polyp tissue. The activation or perpetuation of activated eosinophils at tissue sites is, at least in part, a Th2 lymphocyte-driven process. Because this is dependant upon processes that occur locally,[7] intranasal steroids seem to be a logical choice for therapy.

Blood Vessels

A property of the vasculature which may play an important pathogenic role in nasal polyposis is the 'leakiness' of the vessels.[15] Not only cells, but also several active plasma components, such as bradykinin, leak into the nasal mucosa and polyps tissue.[16] In inflammatory diseases steroid treatment, having no direct effect on blood vessels, indirectly reduces microvascular leakage due to inhibition of the formation of mediators and cytokines.[17] The finding of a reduced level of albumin in nasal secretions following topical steroid treatment for nasal polyposis[18] is evidence of an anti-exudative effect of this type of therapy.

TOPICAL STEROID TREATMENT

Responsiveness to Topical Steroids

Intranasal steroids are, by far, the most well documented type of treatment for nasal polyposis. There are at least 13 placebo-controlled studies and they have all shown a significant effect. However, it is evident that nasal steroids do not solve all problems for a number of patients with nasal polyposis. This is understandable considering the limited distribution of an intranasal spray as compared to the extensive involvement of nasal and paranasal mucous membranes in this disease.

Some patients with nasal polyps apparently do not respond to topical steroids, which may be for two reasons. First, the disease may be genuinely unresponsive to glucocorticoids. This may apply to cystic fibrosis, primary ciliary dyskinesia and other diseases, characterized by local infiltration with neutrophils and not eosinophils.[18] Second, the disease can temporarily be unresponsive to topical steroids due to a purulent infection or due to inadequate intranasal distribution of the steroid spray in a blocked nose. An initial negative result with topical therapy, however, does not preclude a beneficial effect from systemic steroid treatment and followed by subsequent topical therapy.[4]

Disappearance of Nasal Polyps

The results of controlled studies will be discussed according to the objectives of treatment advanced in Table 1.

Disappearance of nasal polyps is an obvious goal for therapy. A considerable reduction of polyp size may be sufficient to render some patients symptom-free, but even small polyps in the upper part of the nose may compromise ostiomeatal function and reduce the sense of smell.

A rhinoscopic judgement of polyp size, made by different investigators and at different time points, is not reliable as a semiquantitative parameter unless well-defined criteria of polyp size are used, for example, distance in millimeters between the lowest polyp and the nasal floor. Johansen et al[19] defined three degrees of nasal polyposis dependent upon whether the largest polyp is above the upper edge of the inferior turbinate, between the upper and lower, or beneath the lower edge. Using these criteria, Johansen et al[19] found a clear reduction in polyp score during treatment with budesonide (Fig. 1), while Lildholdt et al[20] found a decrease in the mean polyp size in 52% of budesonide treated patients compared with 21% in the placebo group.

While Chalton et al,[21] using nose drops of betamethasone, found disappearance of polyps in 9 of 15 patients, as compared to 2 of 15 in a placebo group, Drettner et al,[22] using beclomethasone dipropionate aerosol, stated that 'polyps never disappear completely'. Probably the severity of the disease differed between the two studies, but it is also a possibility that the application of drops is more efficient in reaching the upper part of the nose than is the spraying of an aerosol from a pressurized canister.

Nasal Airway and Breathing

Nasal breathing is the least that therapy should provide, but a patent airway is not necessarily a normal airway. Pressure from long-standing nasal polyps may have changed the normal narrow cavity to a wide tube in the lower part of the nose.

The patient's evaluation of the symptom of nasal blockage is subjective. In one study blockage decreased 25% in the placebo group and 65% in the active group.[23] Added use of an objective and quantitative measure of nasal patency is valuable in clinical trials. Controlled studies have shown increased nasal patency during active therapy, measured by nasal peak flow[19,20,23,24] (Fig. 2) and by rhinomanometry.[25] Acoustic rhinometry has only been used in a pilot study of systemic steroids.[26]

No attempts have been made, in controlled studies, (1) to relate steroid-induced changes in nasal patency to normal values, (2) to evaluate whether patients have nasal breathing at day and at night, (3) to judge whether the configuration of nasal cavity is normal or abnormal, e.g. by measuring the distance between the medial and the lateral wall, or (4) to evaluate quality of life during treatment.

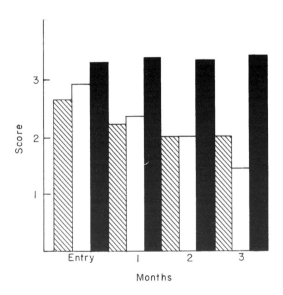

Figure 1. Mean polyp score in 86 patients before and after 3 months of treatment with budesonide aerosol 400 μg/day (hatched bars), budesonide aqua 400 μg/day (white bars) or placebo (black bars). From Johansen LV, Illum P, Kristensen S, Winther L, Petersen SV, Synnerstad B. The effect of budesonide (Rhinocort©) in the treatment of small and medium sized nasal polyps. Clin Otolaryngol 1993;18:524-7. Ref. 19

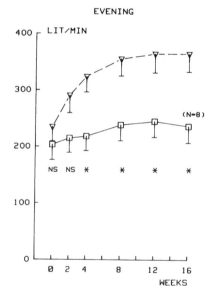

Figure 2. Effect of nasal steroid on nasal peak flow (mean and SEM; *p < 0.05; squares, placebo; triangles, budesonide). From Holopainen E, Grahne B, Malmberg H, Mäkinen J, Lindqvist N. Budesonide in the treatment of nasal polyposis. Eur J Respir Dis 1982;63 (suppl 122):221-8. Ref. 24

Rhinitis Symptoms

While all studies have shown an effect on nasal blockage, the effect on sneezing and secretion has varied, probably because many patients predominantly suffer from blockage with little sneezing and rhinorrhoea. The overall symptom reduction is about 50%[19,24,27] (Fig. 3). It seems likely, but not proven, that topical steroids are more effective in small and medium-sized polyps than in large polyps which significantly block the nasal airway.

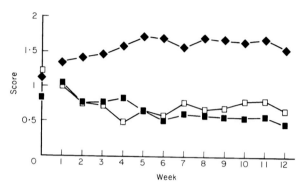

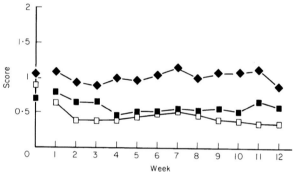

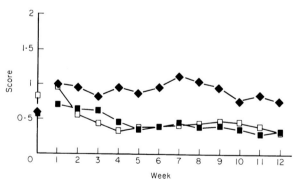

Figure 3. Effect of nasal steroid as the only treatment. Nasal mean symptom scores in 86 patients treated with budesonide aqua (open squares), budesonide aerosol (filled squares) or placebo (filled diamonds). Upper figure, blocked nose. Central figure, runny nose. Lower figure, sneezing. From Johansen LV, Illum P, Kristensen S, Winther L, Petersen SV, Synnerstad B. The effect of budesonide (Rhinocort©) in the treatment of small and medium sized nasal polyps. Clin Otolaryngol 1993; 18:524-7. Ref. 19

Two open studies of 1-year topical treatment have shown that the anti-rhinitis effect is maintained and that symptoms only slowly recur when the treatment is discontinued.[3,4] Although steroids do not cure the disease long-term, therapy may break some vicious circles and have a long-lasting efficacy especially in mild cases.

Sense of Smell

Loss of the sense of smell, and with that 'taste', caused by polyp obstruction of the upper part of the nasal cavity, is a very annoying symptom for most patients. Clinical experience indicates that the effect of topical steroids, in contrast to systemic administration, is poor, but, unfortunately, controlled studies have paid little attention to this symptom. Lildholdt et al,[20] using a semiquantitative test of smell, found that budesonide powder (400 or 800 μg/day) caused an improvement in 80% and 71% of actively treated patients but also in 45% of placebo treated patients (difference not significant).

Recurrence of Polyps

Although small polyps may become invisible during topical therapy they may not be completely eliminated from the upper part of the nasal cavity which is not reached by a nasal aerosol or spray. Even systemic steroids or radical surgery will not, as a rule, eliminate all polypoid tissue in the nose. Thus, the reappearance of polyps which can be identified by rhinoscopy and are symptomatic, is, strictly speaking, a more correct description than recurrence of polyps.

Dingsør et al[28] performed polypectomy and then treated with flunisolide spray (200 μg/day) or placebo for 12 months. At the end of the treatment period polyps were more frequent and larger in the placebo group than in the flunisolide group (p = 0.03). Karlsson & Rundcrantz[29] found it necessary to perform 4 revision repolypectomies during a 30 month period in 20 patients treated with beclomethasone dipropionate aerosol (200 μg/day) as compared to 14 polypectomies in a control group (Fig. 4).

Virolainen & Puhakka[30] undertook radical ethmoidectomy and reexamined patients after aerosol treatment for 12 months. Nasal polyps were absent, judged by rhinoscopy, in 54% of patients treated with beclomethasone dipropionate (400 μ g/day) as compared to 13% in the placebo group.

Whilst the reappearance of nasal polyps can be prevented in some cases, the frequency of relapses is merely reduced in others, which are probably characterized by ongoing inflammation in the nasal and paranasal mucosa.

Sinus Pathology

In Table 1 normalization of all sinus pathology has not been included as a goal for treatment. This is because it is an unrealistic goal in most patients, and because it may

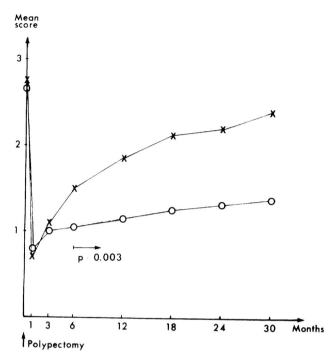

Figure 4. Mean nasal symptom scores before and after polypectomy in 20 patients receiving long-term therapy with beclomethasone dipropionate (open circles) and in 20 untreated patients (crosses). From Karlsson G, Rundcrantz H. A randomized trial of intranasal beclomethasone dipropionate after polypectomy. Rhinology 1982;20:144-8. Ref. 29

not be necessary, as patients can be symptom-free in spite of clouding of paranasal sinuses on X-ray or CT scan. However, ostial obstruction can cause sinus symptoms, increase the frequency of purulent episodes and, rarely, result in a serious infectious complication.

Dingsør et al[28] found no statistically significant difference with regard to sinus X-ray findings between 18 patients treated with flunisolide 200 μg/day and 19 treated with placebo for 12 months.

Drug, Spray, Dosage

Placebo-controlled studies have been performed with beclomethasone dipropionate (five), flunisolide (two) and budesonide (five), but these molecules have not been compared with each other in nasal polyposis.

Few studies have compared different types of intranasal drug administration. A pressurized aerosol was compared with a simple powder delivery system for beclomethasone dipropionate without any difference in efficacy.[12] There was a tendency of a better effect of budesonide delivered from an aqueous pump spray as compared to a pressurized aerosol[19] (Fig. 1).

With regard to dosage, one study has shown equal efficacy of 400 and 800 μg budesonide delivered as a powder from a multidose device.[4]

SYSTEMIC STEROID TREATMENT

Investigation of systemic steroids in the treatment of rhinitis in general and in polyposis in particular has been insufficient. In hay fever there is one placebo-controlled study showing efficacy of a depot-injection of methylprednisolone (80 mg).[31] Another hay fever study compared a depot-injection of betamethasone (14 mg) with oral prednisolone (7.5 mg/day for 3 weeks), showing equal efficacy.[32] Oral steroids have, to our knowledge, not been compared with placebo in any rhinitis or polyposis study.

There are three studies describing the effect of systemic steroids in nasal polyposis. Lildholdt et al,[33] in their first study, randomized 53 patients to either surgical removal of visible polyps with a snare or a depot-injection of steroid (betamethasone 14 mg, corresponding to about 100 mg prednisolone). All patients continued with topical steroid (beclomethasone aerosol, 400 μg/day) for 12 months. Both regimens caused substantial and equal increase in nasal expiratory peak flow and the improvement was maintained during the 1-year observation period (Fig. 5). The sense of smell improved significantly in the systemic steroid group at 2 weeks but the effect was not maintained at 2-12 months during topical therapy.

In a second study of 124 patients, Lildholdt et al[4] randomized 33 patients, who failed to respond to the initial treatment with topical steroid (budesonide powder 400 or 800 μg/day), to treatment with systemic steroid (depot-injection of 14 mg betamethasone) or polypectomy with

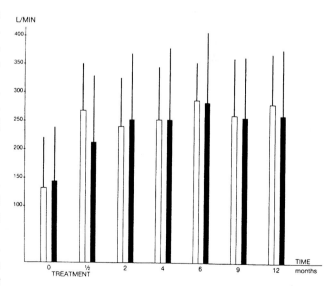

Figure 5. Mean nasal peak flow (+SD) in 53 patients treated with beclomethasone dipropionate following an initial depot-injection of steroid (betamethasone 14 mg) (white bars) or polypectomy with a snare (black bars). From Lildholdt T, Fogstrup J, Gammelgaard N, Kortholm B, Ulsøe C. Surgical versus medical treatment of nasal polyps. Acta Otolaryngol (Stockh) 1988;105:140-3. Ref. 33

Mean score

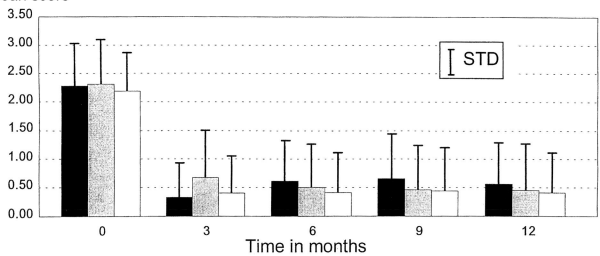

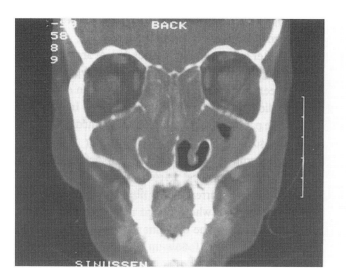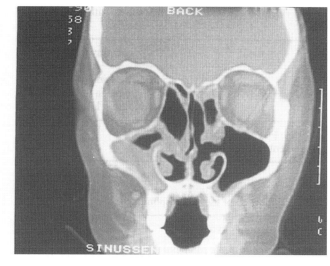

Figure 6. Scores for nasal blockage (mean+SD) in 119 patients treated with topical steroid (budesonide powder 400 or 800 μg/day) for 12 months. Initially all patients were treated with budesonide for one month. Those who were 'responders' (85 of 119) continued on topical therapy only (white bars), while those who were 'non-responders' (34 of 119) also received either systemic steroid (betamethasone 114 mg as a depot-injection) (gray bars) or polypectomy (black bars). From Lildholdt T et al. (1996).

a snare. After one year of continuous topical therapy there was no difference between the two groups with regard to any symptomatic parameter (Fig. 6). The authors found that only 15% of all patients did not respond satisfactory to the treatment given and needed surgery. They concluded that "the primary treatment of nasal polyps should be systemic and local steroids."

Van Camp & Clement[34] gave 25 patients with massive nasal polyposis a large dosage of oral prednisolone (60

mg/day for 4 days and then tapered off with 5 mg daily, giving a total dose of 570 mg). These investigators found that there was a considerable reduction in the frequency of all symptoms, in particular nasal obstruction, and the sense of smell improved. Nasal polyps became invisible at rhinoscopy in 10 of 25 patients. Half of the patients (13 of 25) showed improvement judged by a CT scan of the sinuses (Fig. 7). Although these 13 patients, called "responders", continued on topical steroids, "there was a

Figure 7. Example of CT-scan before (left) and after (right) treatment with oral steroid in 15 days (total 570 mg of prednisolone) in a 'responder'. From van Camp P, Clement PAR. Results of oral steroid treatment in nasal polyposis. Rhinology 1994;32:5-9. Ref.34

strong tendency of recurrence within five months after successful oral steroid therapy which made surgical intervention inevitable". Only one of the initial 25 patients succeeded in avoiding endoscopic sinus surgery after a 9 month observation period. The authors concluded that "systemic steroid treatment should be reserved for those cases that require surgery". They emphasize that surgery can be considerably facilitated by preoperative systemic steroid therapy.

Medical treatment of nasal polyposis has recently been described in two excellent reviews by Drake-Lee[35] and by Holmberg & Karlsson,[36] as well as in a short 'Position Statement on Nasal Polyps'.[37]

DISCUSSION

Topical Steroids

It is definitely proven that topical steroid treatment can reduce polyp size and associated nasal symptoms. Treatment after polypectomy significantly reduces the number of recurrences, which is especially valuable in patients who have previously been subjected to frequent polypectomies.

While topical steroids can usually completely control the symptoms of allergic rhinitis, nasal polyposis, involving the entire nasal and paranasal mucosa, is more difficult to control exclusively by topical medication.

When polyps are large, polypectomy or short-term systemic steroids will improve the intranasal distribution of the topical steroid. This therapy can be necessary in order to open a blocked nose, for example, when the patient catches a cold or gets a bacterial sinusitis resulting in a temporary failure of topical therapy.

There is reason to use topical steroids in many patients with nasal polyposis with the possible exception of patients without rhinitis symptoms who have polyps removed for the first time.[38] Some of the unselected patients who present in the otorhinolaryngologist's office with nasal polyps for the first time probably experience a short symptomatic episode and may be relieved by a single polypectomy.[39]

The following are indications for starting topical steroid treatment: (1) daily rhinitis symptoms, (2) repeated polypectomies, (3) severe disease with massive involvement of the mucous membrane in nose and paranasal sinuses, (4) blood eosinophilia, (5) asthma (6) intolerance to acetylsalicylic acid and other NSAIDs,[39,40] (7) patient's preference for medical therapy. In moderately severe disease topical steroids may be used in 3-6 months periods, while patients with severe disease may benefit from constant daily treatment for as long as the disease persists.

Systemic Steroids

Although systemic steroid treatment has not been studied in placebo-controlled trials there is no doubt that it is highly effective. Rhinitis symptoms and polyp size are reduced, and, in contrast to topical steroids, there is some effect on the sense of smell as well as an effect on the paranasal sinuses. A short course of systemic steroids is equally effective to polypectomy with a snare.[4,33] In severe disease, requiring endoscopic ethmoidectomy, preoperative use of systemic steroids will facilitate surgery.[34]

Only a single course of systemic steroids has been used in published studies. However, the authors believe that some patients with severe recurrent polyposis may benefit from repeated use of short-term systemic steroids but there has been, at present, no analysis of the pro's et con's of this management. If, for example, a depot-injection (methylprednisolone 80 mg or betamethasone 14 mg) is given no more frequently than every 3 months, it will correspond to 1-2 mg prednisolone a day. Adverse effects from this therapy cannot be expected to be severe and may, in some patients with severe disease and anosmia, be outweighed by increased quality of life.

CONCLUSION

Topical steroid therapy has a well established role in the management of nasal polyposis as efficacy has been proven by a series of controlled studies and clinical experience and biopsy studies[41] have indicated that the therapy is safe.

Although recent studies have shown systemic steroids to be as efficient as polypectomy their role has not yet been defined and they are not widely used for nasal polyposis. The potential benefit of repeated short-term therapy in severe disease has not been explored.

In order to reach the objectives advanced in Table 1, therapy with long-term topical and short-term systemic steroids should be combined in a treatment plan that is tailored for each individual patient. As the goal cannot be reached in all patients, further studies of combined use of steroids and surgery, are warranted in order to improve our management of this annoying disease.

The medical therapy approaches the requirements of the ideal treatment (Table 2) but patient compliance is crucial. Accordingly, the individualized therapy must be based on a high level of information. Otherwise many patients object to daily spraying and to the use of systemic steroids, even for short periods of time.

REFERENCES

1. Mygind N. Glucocortico-steroids and rhinitis. Allergy 1993;48:476–90.

2. Knutson U, Stjärna P, Marcus C, Carlstedt-Duke J, Carlström k, Brönnegård M. Effects of intranasal glucocorticoids on endogenous glucocorticoid peripheral and central function. Endocrinology 1995; 144:301–310.

3. Pedersen CB, Mygind N, Sørensen H, Prytz S. Long-term treatment of nasal polyps with beclomethasone dipropionate aerosol. Acta Otolaryngol (Stockh) 1976;82: 256–9.

4. Lildholdt T, Rundcrantz H, Bende M, Larsen K. Glucocorticoid treatment for nasal polyps. A study of budesonide powder and depot-steroid injection. Allergy 1995;50: 204–209.

5. Fokkens WJ, Godthelp T, Holm AF, Mulder PGH, Vroom TM, Rijntjes E. The effect of nasal corticosteroid spray on Langerhans cells in the nasal mucosa. Allergy 1995;50: 204–209.

6. Kay AB. Asthma and inflammation. J Allergy Clin Immunol 1991;87:893–910.

7. Dolovich J, Gauldie J, Ohtoshi T, Denburg J, Jordana M. Nasal polyps: local inductive microenvironment in the pathogenesis of the inflammation. In: Mygind N, Pipkorn U, Dahl R, eds. Rhinitis and asthma: similarities and differences. Copenhagen: Munksgaard, 1990:233–41.

8. Kanai N, Denburg J, Jordana M, Dolovich J. Nasal polyp inflammation. Effect of topical nasal steroid. Am J Respir Crit Care Med 1994;150:1094–100.

9. Jordana M, Dolovich J, Ohno I, Finotto S, Denburg J. Nasal polyposis: a model for chronic inflammation. In: Busse WW, Holgate ST, eds. Asthma and rhinitis. Boston: Blackwell Scientific Publications, 1995:156–64.

10. Drake-Lee AB, McLaughlan P. Clinical symptoms, free histamine and IgE in patients with nasal polyps. Int Arch Allergy Appl Immunol 1982;69:268–71.

11. Mygind N. Editorial. Nasal polyposis. J Allergy Clin Immunol 1990;86:827–9.

12. Toft A, Wihl J-Å, Toxman J, Mygind N. Double blind comparison between beclomethasone dipropionate as aerosol and as powder in patients with nasal polyposis. Clin Allergy 1982;12:391–401.

13. Sørensen H, Mygind N, Pedersen CB, Prytz S. Long-term treatment of nasal polyps with beclomethasone dipropionate aerosol. Acta Otolaryngol (Stockh) 1976;82:260–2.

14. Klemi PJ, Virolainen E, Puhakka H. The effect of intranasal beclomethasone dipropionate on the nasal mucosa. Rhinology 1980;18:19–24.

15. Cauna N, Hinderer K, Manzethi G, Swanson E. Fine structure of nasal polyps. Ann Oto Rhinol Laryngol 1992;81:41–58.

16. Baumgarten CR, Togias A, Naclerio RM, Norman PS, Lichtenstein LM, Proud D. Kininogens are generated following nasal challenge with allergen in allergic individuals but not in non-allergic individuals. J Clin Invest 1985;76:191–7.

17. Svensson C, Klementsson H, Andersson M, Pipkorn U, Alkner U, Persson CG. Glucocorticoid-induced attenuation of mucosal exudation of fibrinogen and bradykinins in seasonal allergic rhinitis. Allergy 1994;49:177–83.

18. Sørensen H, Mygind N, Tygstrup I, Flensborg EW. Histology of nasal polyps of different etiology. Rhinology 1977;15:121–128.

19. Johnasen LV, Illum P, Kristensen S, Winther L, Petersen SV, Synnerstad B. The effect of budesonide (Rhinocort) in the treatment of small and medium sized nasal polyps. Clin Otolaryngol 1993;18:524–7.

20. Lildholdt T, Rundcrantz H, Lindqvist N. Efficacy of topical corticosteroid powder for nasal polyps: a double-blind, placebo-controlled study of budesonide. Clin Otolaryngol 1995;20:26–30.

21. Chalton R, Mackay I, Wilson R, Cole P. Double blind placebo controlled trial of betamethasone nasal drops for nasal polyposis. Br Med J 1985;291:788.

22. Drettner B, Ebbesen A, Nilsson M. Prophylactic treatment with flunisolide after polypectomy. Rhinology 1982;20:149–58.

23. Rhuno J, Andersson B, Denburg J et al. A double-blind comparison of intranasal budesonide with placebo for nasal polyposis. J Allergy Clin Immunol 1990;86:946–53.

24. Holopainen E, Grahne B, Malmberg H, Mäkinen J, Lindqvist N. Budesonide in the treatment of nasal polyposis. Eur J Respir Dis 1982;63(suppl 122):221–8.

25. Deuschl H, Drettner B. Nasal polyps treated with beclomethasone dipropionate aerosol. Rhinology 1977;15: 17–23.

26. Elbrønd O, Felding JU, Gustavsen KM. Acoustic rhinometry used as a method to monitor the effect of intramuscular injection of steroid in the treatment of nasal polyps. J Laryngol Otol 1991;105:178–80.

27. Mygind N, Pedersen CB, Prytz S, Sørensen H. Treatment of nasal polyps with intranasal beclomethasone dipropionate aerosol. Clin Allergy 1975;5:159–64.

28. Dingsör G, Kramer J, Olsholt R, Södersström T. Flunisolide nasal spray 0.025% in the prophylactic treatment of nasal polyposis after polypectomy. A randomized double-blind parallel, placebo-controlled study. Rhinology 1985;23:49–58.

29. Karlsson G, Rundcrantz H. A randomized trial of intranasal beclomethasone dipropionate after polypectomy. Rhinology 1982;20:144–8.

30. Virolainen E, Puhakka H. The effect of intranasal beclomethasone dipropionate on the recurrence of nasal polyps after ethmoidectomy. Rhinology 1980;18:9–18.

31. Borum P, Grønborg H, Mygind N. Seasonal allergic rhinitis and depot injection of a corticosteroid. Allergy 1987; 42:26–32.

32. Laursen LC, Faurschou P, Pals H, Svendsen UG, Weeke B. Intramuscular betamethasone dipropionate vs. oral prednisolone in hay fever. Allergy 1987;42:168–72.

33. Lildholdt T, Fogstrup J, Gammelgaard N, Kortholm B, Ulsøe C. Surgical versus medical treatment of nasal polyps. Acta Otolaryngol (Stockh) 1988;105:140–3.

34. van Camp P, Clement PAR. Results of oral steroid treatment in nasal polyposis. Rhinology 1994;32:5–9.

35. Drake-Lee AB. Medical treatment of nasal polyps. Rhinology 1994;32:1–4.

36. Holmberg K, Karlsson G. Nasal polyps: surgery or pharmacological intervention? Eur Respir Rev 1994;4: 20:260–5.

37. Lildholdt T. Position statement on nasal polyps. Rhinology 1994;32:126.

38. Hartwig S, Linden M, Laurent C, Vargo A-K, Lindqvist N. Budesonide nasal spray as prophylactic treatment after polypectomy (A double blind clinical trial). J Laryngol Otol 1988;102:148–51.

39, Larsen K, Tos M. Polypectomy frequency in primary and recurrent nasal polyposis. Acta Otolaryngol (Stockh) 1994;114:556–9.

40. Jäntti-Alanko S, Holopainen E, Malmberg H. Recurrence of nasal polyps after surgical treatment. Rhinology 1989;(suppl 8):59–64.

41. Mygind N, Sörensen H, Pedersen CB. The nasal mucosa during long-term treatment with beclomethasone dipropionate aerosol. A light and scanning electron microscope study of nasal polyps. Acta Otolaryngol (Stockh) 1978;85:437–43.

Chapter XIX

Surgical Treatment—Nasal Polyps

Valerie J. Lund, M.S., F.R.C.S.

ABSTRACT

For most patients the management of nasal polyps comprises a combination of medical and surgical therapies. Surgical intervention ranges from the most conservative intranasal polypectomy performed with a snare to radical external fronto-ethmo-sphenoidectomy. There is a significant paucity in the literature of well constructed trials considering the various surgical approaches and/or comparing them to medication, but of the operations available, a clearance performed under endoscopic control is felt by many surgeons to offer the best results in the long-term. However, even with the most meticulous surgery it is difficult to replace polypoid sinonasal mucosa with one of macroscopic normality by surgical interference. As a consequence, surgical success must be measured in subjective symptomatic improvement, objective measurement of clinical change, the duration of symptom-free interval and possible improvement of related disorders such as asthma.

INTRODUCTION

Many people would agree that nasal polyposis represents a spectrum of disease whose primary treatment is medical but in which surgery may play a part. As a consequence, surgical procedures have ranged from the most conservative intranasal polypectomy performed with a snare, to radical external fronto-ethmo-sphenoidectomy. No one surgical approach has proved entirely curative and patients frequently undergo repeated procedures during the course of a life-time combined with long term medication. It is clear from the foregoing chapters that the aetiology of this condition is complex and may be multifactorial. This may in part explain the variation in therapeutic success experienced with a particular surgical procedure or by an individual surgeon.

Even with the most meticulous surgery it is most difficult to replace a polypoid sinonasal lining with one of macroscopic normality by surgical interference. Consequently, surgical success must be measured in subjective symptomatic improvement, objective measurement of clinical change, the duration of the symptom-free interval and possible improvement in related disorders such as asthma.

BIOPSY, HISTOPATHOLOGY AND MICROBIOLOGY

The long list of differential diagnosis (p. 91–94) mean that clinicians should always be alert to the possibility of a more sinister pathology presenting as "simple" nasal polyposis. Whilst alarm bells may be rung by a unilateral lesion or especially one which is fleshy in appearance, one should not ignore the possibility that neoplasia can present as bilateral disease or co-exist with polypoid change. Consequently an assumption cannot be made that polyps are benign until tissue has been submitted for histology. This should be done sooner rather than later in all patient presenting with the condition. Similarly all tissue removed at formal polypectomy should be sent to the pathologist. Inverted papilloma can certainly occur in association with non-neoplastic polyposis, and malignant tumours such as mucinous adenocarcinoma can affect the ethmoids bilaterally and masquerade as a more benign condition. If thick inspissated greeny brown secretion is encountered in association with polyps, the possibility of a fungal infection should immediately be suspected and it is often the histopathologist rather than his microbiological colleague who will confirm the diagnosis by specific staining for fungal hyphae.

OPERATIONS

Intranasal Polypectomy

This procedure which has been available since the Middle Ages (p. 7) may be performed under local or general anaesthetic and is generally performed using a snare which may be either cutting or avulsing. The latter is considered less safe by many surgeons, particularly for revision procedures as it relies upon tearing tissue in close proximity to important structures such as the orbit. In the past intranasal polypectomy was performed with the minimum of imaging, using headlight illumination but clearly visualization can be improved by fibre-optic illumination via a self-retaining speculum, by use of a binocular microscope or with a rigid Hopkin's endoscopic rod. The operation is generally a conservative procedure removing polyps from within the nasal cavity though, inevitably in revision procedures, portions of the middle turbinate and/or anterior ethmoid may be intentionally or inadvertently removed.

Intranasal Ethmoidectomy

Mosher is credited in 1913 with the first description of an intranasal ethmoidectomy based on careful anatomical studies.[1] By 1929 he concluded, that theoretically the operation was easy but in practice it had proven to be one of the easiest operations with which to kill the patient[2]. This was largely due to the possibility of entering the anterior cranial fossa due to poor visualization during the surgery. However, large series by Eichel 1972[3] and Freedman and Kern in 1979[4] considered patients mainly treated for polyposis in whom the overall complication rate was extremely low.

Transantral Ethmoidectomy

This procedure described by Jansen in 1902[5] and Horgan in 1926[6] approaches the ethmoids via a Caldwell Luc which renders most anterior and posterior cells largely inaccessible unless combined with an intranasal approach. It thus offers the worst of both worlds and although it was described for removal of nasal polyps, has little to recommend it.

Caldwell Luc Approach

The Caldwell Luc operation[7,8] was primarily designed for the treatment of chronic maxillary sinusitis. However it has been utilized for the removal of generalized polypoid disease, for fungal sinusitis and for the removal of antrochoanal polyps. The main elements of a Caldwell Luc approach: anterior maxillary fenestration, complete mucosal removal, and inferior meatal antrostomy may be modified and tailored to the individual patient, thus avoiding some of the complications commonly associated with this procedure. Damage to the infra-orbital nerve resulting in paraesthesia or neuralgia and damage to the anterior superior alveolar nerve supply to the dentition, have been encountered in up to 41% of patients[9]. Limited anterior fenestration performed precisely with a drill, the use of an endoscope, preservation of less diseased mucosa particularly in the vicinity of the infra-orbital nerve and the fashioning of a middle meatal

antrostomy have all been suggested as methods of limiting morbidity[10]. Under these circumstances the operation may have a role in recurrent allergic fungal polyposis or a recurrent antrochoanal polyp.

External Fronto-ethmo-sphenoidectomy

A number of surgeons are associated with external approaches to the sinuses, perhaps the best known of whom are Lynch and Howarth, both describing their operations in 1921[11,12]. Their names are attached to this approach although Patterson, who is now associated with the inferior incision in the naso-jugal fold also described a superior approach, albeit it eighteen years later[13]. These procedures have been advocated by some surgeons for recurrent polyposis and for other conditions associated with nasal polyps such as fronto-ethmoidal mucocoeles in 10% of which polyps may play an aetiological role[14].

These operations are associated with a number of complications, notably related to the incision and the orbit. In 6% of patients undergoing a Lynch Howarth procedure, webbing of the incision may occur[15], though such problems are rarely encountered with the Patterson approach. Persistent diplopia may also occur with the superior incision in up to one third of cases unless a specific attempt is made to re-attach periosteum in the region of the trochlea[16]. Epiphora is a common, though rarely permanent, sequelae of the Patterson's operation due to almost inevitable bruising of the naso-lacrimal duct. In addition, paraesthesia in the distribution of the supra-trochlear, supra-orbital and infra-orbital nerves may be encountered with these operations.

Endoscopic Polypectomy and Ethmoidectomy

Removal of polyps under endoscopic control, aided by the anatomical knowledge derived from CT scanning has greatly enhanced the precise and meticulous removal of disease. Thus all grades of surgery may be performed from simple polypectomy to radical clearance of the entire sinus system, dependent upon the extent of the disease process. Other limiting factors will be technical problems due to anatomic variation, intra-operative bleeding and the experience or philosophical stance of the surgeon. However, whatever the circumstances, endoscopic polypectomy cannot qualify as a 'functional' operation in the sense in which the term was originally coined.

COMPLICATIONS

By their very nature polyps arise in close proximity to the orbit and anterior cranial fossa. Complications due to penetration of these adjacent structures can occur during any type of surgical procedure for nasal polyposis and the surgery of nasal polyposis has always been a potent

Table 1. Complications of Ethmoidal Surgery

	No.	Death	Blindness	Orbital haematoma	Meningitis	CSF rhinorrhoea	Nasolacrimal duct damage	Haemorrhage
Intranasal ethmoidectomy Freedman & Kern[4]	1000	0	0.4%	0.1%	0.1%	0.1%	0.1%	1.2%
Functional endoscopic ethmoidectomy Wigand[37]	600	0	0	0	0.5%	0.3%	0.5%	0
Stammberger[40]	4000	0	0	0	0.2%	0	0	0
External ethmoidectomy Harrison & Lund[41]	350	0	0	0	0	0.3%	0.6%	0

source of medical litigation. Many patients have undergone previous surgical procedures which have altered the anatomical landmarks, there is frequently bleeding and the polyps themselves can thin the bone of the skull base and lamina papyracea. However with all sinus surgery, an understanding of the anatomy and pathology will minimize this risk. The incidence of serious complications in major surgical series is minimal. (Table 1).

PRE- AND POST-OPERATIVE CARE

The range of medical strategies used for the pre- and post-operative management of patients will vary enormously from surgeon to surgeon. Many surgeons use a regular intra-nasal steroid preparation up to the time of surgery, irrespective of which procedure is undertaken. In the case of an endoscopic approach some have advocated a short course of oral steroids (dexamethasone 12 mgms for three days, 8mgms for three days and 4mgms for three days) as long as there are no other medical contraindications and this is usually administered for three to four weeks prior to admission. Similarly parenteral injection of synthetic ACTH (Synacthen, 1mgm intramuscularly, two injections given 48 hours apart) will stimulate endogenous cortisol production. Both strategies will reduce the size of the polyps and facilitate an endoscopic removal.

As the aetiology of polyposis is more often unknown, there is a significant chance of recurrence following all forms of surgery and most patients are encouraged to continue with regular intra-nasal steroids in the long term, often interspersed with additional courses of parenteral steroids as required.

WHEN TO OPERATE

In contradistinction to the need for histological diagnosis, therapeutic excision of nasal polyps is generally un-

dertaken after failure of medical treatment. This would usually be encompassed by three to four months of adequate medication, though in cases of gross polyposis the situation may be beyond medical intervention and surgery will be undertaken *ab initio*. The younger the age at which nasal polyps present, the greater the incidence of ethmoidal expansion and hypertelorism[17], so it is important that pre-emptive surgery should be considered in such individuals.

OBJECTIVE ASSESSMENT [18]

The following tests may be used in the objective assessment of nasal polyposis and therapeutic response.

Airway

a. Peak Nasal Expiratory or Inspiratory Flow Rate
This technique, which uses a oral peak flowmeter, has the advantage of being inexpensive, quick, and easy to perform; it is useful for repeated examinations and compares well with rhinomanometry[19] (Fig. 1). Of the two methods, forced inspiration is preferred although it can produce significant vestibular collapse. However, this can be a useful diagnostic test, with a range of 80-220L/min for an adult Caucasian male. In the presence of significant nasal obstruction, forced expiration inflates the eustachian tubes which the patient may find distressing, and discourages maximum expiratory effort. It also may produce an unpleasant amount of mucus blown into the mask. The technique is dependent on pulmonary capacity, and it is necessary to do peak oral expiration to obtain values independent of pulmonary function.

b. Rhinomanometry
Rhinomanometry attempts to measure nasal airway resistance by making a quantitative measurement of nasal flow and pressure. It employs the principle that air will flow only through a tube when there is a pressure

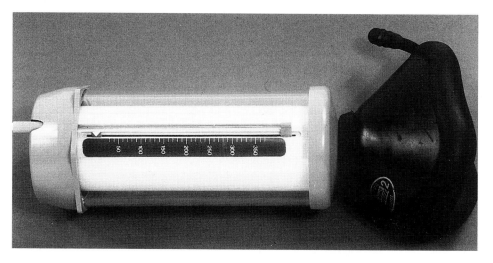

Figure 1. Photograph showing peak flow meter modified for nasal use.

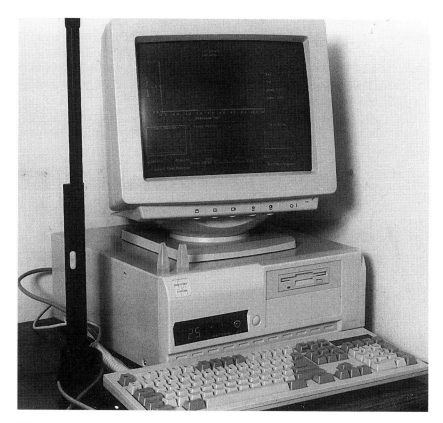

Figure 2. Photograph of Hood acoustic rhinometer.

differential, passing from areas of high to low pressure. This differential is created by respiratory effort altering pressure in the postnasal space relative to external atmospheric pressure, resulting in air flow in and out of the nasal cavities. To resolve the complex mathematics, the European Committee for Standardization of Rhinomanometry in 1984 selected the formula $R = \Delta p/v$ at a fixed pressure of 150 Pa, which has been widely accepted[20]. This standardization has allowed comparison of results not hitherto possible and the production of normal ranges, taking into account such factors as size, height, and age. Ideally, however, each individual clinician should produce a set of normal ranges for the population he or she treats.

Rhinomanometry can be performed by active or passive techniques and by anterior or posterior approaches, of which the active is the most widely used, being the most physiologic. In the anterior active technique pressure is recorded in one nostril while the patient breathes through the other. This is done using a catheter connected in an airtight fashion with adhesive tape, while flow is measured through the other open nasal cavity. Care must be taken not to distort the nostril. A transparent face mask is used incorporating a linear pneumatachograph, connected to an amplifier and recorder and the resistance at a fixed pressure of 150 Pa is expressed in SI units (pressure:pascals, flow:cm^3 X sec^{-1}).

The machine needs at least 30 minutes to warm up and should be regularly calibrated. The patient should be seated comfortably, in a pleasant ambient temperature and preferably having taken no physical exercise for 30 minutes before testing. Rhinomanometry should be undertaken both before and after decongesting the nose to reduce the effect of the nasal cycle and to indicate the reversibility of obstruction. Children as young as 4 years old have been tested, and with an experienced technician, it is reasonably easy to perform. The technique can be time consuming, however, and both nasal cavities must be tested separately. There are a number of circumstances when it cannot be used, such as in the presence of septal perforations and when one or both cavities are totally obstructed. Nor can it accurately assess a specific lesion of the nasal cavity.

In posterior active rhinomanometry, pharyngeal pressure is measured by a catheter inserted into the mouth, around which the lips are closed. Flow through both cavities can be simultaneously measured, although it is possible by plugging one nasal cavity to measure each separately. The technique is essentially noninvasive and theoretically less likely to distort the nasal cavities, although in practice this should not be a problem with the anterior technique. Its main disadvantage is the inability of between 17% and 25% of patients to relax the soft palate, and some patients cannot resist the temptation to suck the tube[21,22].

The essential difficulty with active rhinomanometry is that of reproducibility of results. There have been errors of up to 20% to 25% reported in rhinomanometry repeated within 15 minutes, and there may be a day to day variation of 50% so the patient may not even be able to act as his or her own control[23,24]. Subjective nasal sensation of air flow correlates poorly with objective nasal resistance[25], and these problems of accuracy, reproducibility, and cost-effectiveness have limited the popularity of this technique, particularly in the office setting.

c. Acoustic Rhinometry

In this technique, an audible sound pulse (150 to 10,000 Hz) generated either electronically or by a spark passes

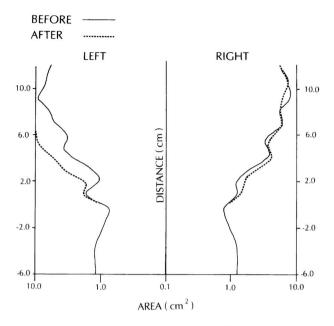

Figure 3. Tracing from Hood acoustic rhinometer.

down a tube into the nasal cavity where it is reflected by local changes in acoustic impedance owing to variations cross-sectional area with distance. It is possible to determine the size of the change in cross-sectional area the function of distance from the nostril, and from this a total volume can be derived[26] (Fig. 3). Thus acoustic rhinometry measures topography not airflow but provides important clinically relevant information. Nose pieces with different diameters and shapes are available, and it is important that these fit the nostril tightly but without deformation of the vestibule. As the technique takes a split second to perform, many measurements may be taken and averaged to obtain the most accurate signal. However the individual coefficient of variation is small and the technique very reproducible[27]. The technique again is performed before and after decongestion and the information it provides is especially pertinent to the surgeon, allowing accurate sequential quantification of the abnormality and the individual's response to treatment, be it medical or surgical[28,29,30].

The technique has already been used in the assessment of nasal polyps treated medically[31] and the speed, ease and reproducibility of technique will undoubtedly ensure its future use in both the clinical and research setting.

d. Respiratory Function Tests

Many patients with nasal polyps are also asthmatic and it is worth performing serial oral peak flows on anyone in whom this is suspected. This can be done using a daily record card with full respiratory function tests performed as required.

Olfaction

Quantitative Olfactory Test

a. University of Pennsylvania Smell Identification Tests.
"Scratch and sniff" tests using patches impregnated with microencapsulated odorants are available[32]. The patient is forced to choose between a number of options after scratching the patch to release the odour. The results take into account answers guessed correctly and deliberately given incorrectly.

b. Olfactory Thresholds. Estimation of olfactory thresholds may be established by presentation of serial dilutions of pure odorant such as pm-carbinol[33]. The patient is presented with two bottles, one containing only the diluent solution as the control, the other, the odorant, in progressively increasing or decreasing concentrations. Each is sniffed in turn. The point is reached at which the patient cannot distinguish between the control and test bottle, which indicates the minimum detectable odour.

RESULTS

In the absence of randomized placebo controlled trials, it is very difficult to compare the success rates of the various surgical procedures described for nasal polyposis. It has also been assumed that concomitant medical conditions such as asthma and aspirin sensitivity may adversely affect results, though this has not necessarily proved to be the case[34]. Surgical success in pre-endoscopic studies relied upon the subjective assessment by the patient and frequently lacked long-term follow-up. However, on this basis a surgical success (with no further surgery) has been reported at between 62% and 75% for intra-nasal ethmoidectomy[3,35,36] compared with 82% for 220 cases undergoing endoscopic removal and responding to a post-operative questionnaire with variable length of follow-up[37]. Patients undergoing conventional snare polypectomy are most likely to get recurrent symptoms and are sometimes offered external surgery after multiple polypectomies. It is of interest, however, to consider 10 patients who had 20 year follow-up following external fronto-ethmoidectomy, who had had between 2 and 10 intranasal polypectomies performed prior to the external surgery[38]. The average interval between each intra-nasal polypectomy was 23 months whilst the average interval between external ethmoidectomy and the next polypectomy was 73 months (p => 0.05). However, the most interesting finding is that 8 out of the 10 patients nevertheless required further polypectomies despite radical external surgery.

The role of endoscopic surgery in significantly lengthening the symptom-free interval will be discussed in other chapters but the following observations may be made on 300 individuals who underwent endoscopic polypectomy and were available for assessment at six months[39]. Eighty per cent of this group consider themselves significantly improved and 9% asymptomatic which is comparable to the results in patients with chronic rhinosinusitis. Those individuals with asthma (81 cases {aspirin sensitivity in 19}) did not appear to do worse than the group as a whole, with 94% cured or improved. However, as expected a subgroup of patients with nasal polyps and cystic fibrosis did less well (54% cured or improved) with dramatic recurrence occurring in those individuals undergoing heart/lung transplantation for which they received cyclosporin (10 cases). Clearly in the longer term symptomatic recurrence may be anticipated, though the judicious use of regular medication may significantly lengthen the symptom free interval.

REFERENCES

1. Mosher HP. The applied anatomy and intranasal surgery of the ethmoidal labyrinth. Laryngoscope 1913, 23: 881–901.
2. Mosher HP. The applied anatomy of the ethmoidal labyrinth. Ann Otol Rhinol Laryngol 1929, 38: 869–901.
3. Eichel BS. The intranasal ethmoidectomy procedure: historical, technical and clinical considerations. Laryngoscope 1972, 82: 1806–1821.
4. Freedman HM, Kern EB. Complications of intranasal ethmoidectomy: a review of 1000 consecutive operations. Laryngoscope 1979, 89: 421–434.
5. Jansen A. Die Killian'sche Radical-Operation Chronischer Stirnhohleneiterungen. Ohren Nasen Kehlkopfheil 1902, 56: 11–112.
6. Horgan JB. The surgical approach to the ethmoidal cell system. J Laryngol Otol 1926, 41: 510–521.
7. Caldwell GW. Disease of the accessory sinuses of the nose and an improved method of treatment for suppuration of the maxillary antrum. NY Med J 1893, 58: 526–528.
8. Luc H. Une nouvelle methode operatoire pour le cure radicale et rapide de l'empyeme chronique du sinus maxil-

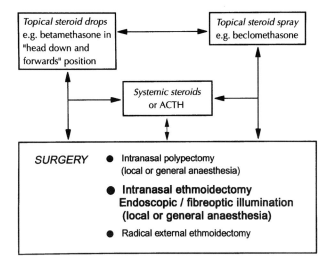

Figure 4. Algorithm of polyp management.

laire. Archives internationales de laryngologie, d'otologie et de rhinologie 1897, 10: 273–285.

9. Pentilla MA, Rautiainen MEP, Pukander JS, Karma PH. Endoscopic versus Caldwell-Luc approach in chronic maxillary sinusitis: Comparison of symptoms at one-year follow-up. Rhinology 1994, 32: 161–165.

10. Maybury RL. The case for the Caldwell-Luc procedure. Am J Rhinology 1994, 8: 311–315.

11. Lynch RC. The technique of a radical frontal sinus operation which has given me the best results. Laryngoscope 1921, 31: 1–5.

12. Howarth W. A radical frontal sinus operation. J Laryngol Otol 1921, 38: 341–343.

13. Patterson N. External operations on the frontal and ethmoidal sinuses. J Laryngol Otol 1939, 54: 235–244.

14. Lund VJ. Anatomical considerations in the aetiology of fronto-ethmoidal mucocoeles. Rhinology 1987, 25: 83–88.

15. Rubin JR, Lund VJ & Salmon BS. Fronto-ethmoidectomy in the treatment of mucoceles—a neglected operation. Archives of Otolaryngology 1985. 112: 434–436.

16. Lund VJ, Rolfe M. Ophthalmic considerations in fronto-ethmoidal mucocoeles. Journal of Laryngology and Otology 1989. 103: 667–669.

17. Lund VJ & Lloyd G. Radiological changes associated with benign nasal polyps. Journal of Laryngology and Otology 1983. 97:503–510 (Abstracted for International Synopses).

18. Lund VJ. Office evaluation of nasal obstruction. The Otolaryngologic Clinics of North America 1992. 25: 803–816.

19. Holmstrom M, Scadding GK, Lund VJ. The assessment of nasal obstruction: A comparison between rhinomanomerty and nasal inspiratory peak flow. Rhinology 1990. 28: 191–196.

20. Clement PAR. Committee report on standardization of rhinomanometry. Rhinology 1984. 22: 151–155.

21. Foxen EHM, Preston TD, Lack JA. The assessment of nasal airflow: A review of past and present methods. J Laryngol Otol, 1971. 85: 811–825.

22. Mygind N, Johnson NJ, Thomsen J. Intranasal allergen challenge during corticosteroid treatment. Clin Allergy 1977. 7: 69–74.

23. Hasegawa M, Kern EB, O'Brien PC. Dynamic changes of nasal resistance. Ann Otol Rhinol Laryngol, 1979. 88: 66–71.

24. Kumlien J, Schiratski H. Methodology aspects of rhinomanometry. Rhinology, 1979. 17: 107–114.

25. Jones AS, Willatt DJ, Durham LM. Nasal airflow: Resistance and sensation. J Laryngol Otol, 1989. 103: 909–911.

26. Hilberg O, Jackson AC, Swift DL, Pedersen OF. Acoustic rhinometry: Evaluation of nasal cavity geometry by acoustic deflection. J Appl Physiol 1989. 66: 295–303.

27. Fisher E, Lund VJ, Scadding GK. Acoustic rhinometry in rhinological practice. Proc Roy Soc Med, 1994. 87: 411–413.

28. Grymer LF, Hilberg O, Elbrond O, Pedersen OF. Acoustic rhinometry: Evaluation of the nasal cavity with septal deviations, before and after septoplasty. Laryngoscope, 1989. 99: 1180–1187.

29. Hilberg O, Grymer LF, Pedersen OF, Elbrond O. Turbinate hypertrophy. Arch Otolaryngol Head Neck Surg, 1990. 116: 283–289.

30. Lenders H, Pirsig W. Diagnostic values of acoustic rhinometry: Patients with allergic and vasomotor rhinitis compared with normal controls. Rhinology, 1990. 28: 5–16.

31. Elbrond O, Felding JU, Gustavesen KM. Acoustic rhinometry used as a method to monitor the effect of intramuscular injection of steroid in the treatment of nasal polyps. J Laryngol Otol, 1991. 105: 178–180.

32. Doty RL, Shaman P & Dann M. Development of the University of Pennsylvania Smell Identification Test: A standardized microencapsulated test of olfactory function. Physiol Behav, 1984. 32: 489–502.

33. Amoore JE. Odors standards in squeeze bottle kits for matching quality and intensity. Wat Sci Tech 1992. 25: 1–6.

34. Kennedy DW. Prognostic Factors, Outcomes and staging in Ethmoid sinus surgery. The Laryngoscope, 1992. 102 (suppl 57): 1–18.

35. Dixon F. The clinical significance of anatomical arrangement of the paranasal sinuses. Ann Otol Rhinol Laryngol, 1958. 67: 736–741.

36. Simonton K. The comprehensive surgical treatment of nasal polyposis. Trans Am Acad Opthal Otolaryngol 1958, 65: 75–81.

37. Wigand ME, Hosemann W. Microsurgical treatment of recurrent nasal polyposis. Rhinology 1989, Suppl 8: 25–30.

38. Tos M, Drake-Lee A, Lund VJ, Stammberger H. Treatment of nasal polyps-medication or surgery. Rhinology 1989, Suppl 8: 45–49.

39. Lund VJ, Mackay IS. Outcome assessment of endoscopic sinus surgery. proceedings of the Royal Society of Medicine 1994. 87: 70–72.

40. Stammberger H. Headaches and sinus disease: the endoscopic approach. Ann Otol Rhinol Laryngol, 1988. 97 (suppl 134): 1–23.

41. Lund VJ. Surgery of the ethmoids — past, present and future: a review. J Roy Soc Med, 1990. 83: 451–455.

Chapter XX

Rhinoscopic Surgery

Heinz Stammberger, M.D.

ABSTRACT

Over the last two decades, a considerable change has taken place in the surgical approach to nasal polyposis. With the advent of the endoscope as a diagnostic tool, better visualization and the ability to "view around the corner" has enabled not only for earlier detection, but for less traumatic and more precise surgical treatment of diseases presenting with nasal polyps. The concept of Functional Endoscopic Sinus Surgery (FESS) offers individualized surgery according to the respective patient's disease. Routine radical surgical approaches can be avoided with good functional results. In a stepwise fashion, after exact diagnosis, diseased compartments of the ethmoids are approached and—depending on the extend of the disease—maxillary, frontal and sphenoid sinuses opened via their natural ostia. Care is taken not to denude bone, but leave peripheral mucosa in all operated cavities. Rarely, middle turbinates need to be resected.

Patients with nasal polyposis histologically dominated by dense eosinophilic infiltration as present in Aspirin Intolerance, Allergic Fungal Sinusitis and many asthmatics, require a more aggressive approach and in many instances a combined therapy with corticosteroids. In these cases, extensive aftercare and follow-up is required by the physician and a good compliance by the patient to preserve the good postoperative result and to prevent regrowth of polyps. Massive scarring, postoperative osteoneogenesis and disease processes far laterally in the frontal and—rarely—the maxillary sinuses especially after previous external surgery, may present limitations to an exclusive endoscopic approach.

ENDOSCOPIC DIAGNOSIS AND THE FESS-CONCEPT

In the late 1960's and early 1970's Professor Messerklinger from Graz/Austria developed a technique of systematic endoscopic investigation of the lateral nasal wall which clearly demonstrated, that most infections of the paranasal sinuses are **rhinogenic.** Diseases usually spread to the large sinuses via the clefts and spaces of the lateral nasal wall. The narrow clefts of the ostiomeatal unit hold a key role for the normal physiology and pathophysiology of the entire paranasal sinus system. The clefts of especially the anterior ethmoid are "prechambers" for the frontal and maxillary sinuses with regard to ventilation and drainage. Embryologically, the frontal and maxillary sinus develop from the anterior ethmoid to which they remain connected via very complex "bottle necks". In addition, a considerable number of anatomical variants may narrow these prechambers on the lateral nasal wall and predispose to recurrent infections.

The combination of endoscopic diagnosis with modern imaging techniques, especially computed tomography over the last years has proven the ideal combination and in many parts of the world today is seen as "the standard of care" for the diagnoses of nasal and sinus diseases.

As a consequence, an endoscopic–surgical concept resulted from the diagnostic findings of Messerklinger, aimed at the diseased areas of the lateral nasal wall primarily. It was fascinating to see how after relatively circumscribed surgical procedures in these key areas even massive mucosal changes in the secondary larger sinuses normalised with time, without having been touched to any degree. As a consequence this endoscopic concept for cases of chronic rhinosinusitis (CRS) replaced the more radical external approaches of the time.

With growing experience and the development of special instrumentation, today even cases of massive diffuse polyposis, affecting all sinuses, can be approached endoscopically. In the extreme, a total sphenoethmoidectomy can be performed and the frontal sinuses opened and drained as well. Even under these circumstances, all anatomical landmarks such as the middle turbinate can be preserved and mucosa left in situ covering all the walls of the surgical cavity without significant areas of bone being exposed. This has resulted in shortened periods of recovery and normalization of the mucosa.

The mechanical concept of stenoses and contact areas in the lateral nasal wall by no means explains all pathological processes, especially not diffuse polyposis. But even in this case, the primary manifestations can be found in the ostiomeatal unit.

THE LOCATION OF NASAL POLYPS—AN ENDOSCOPIC VIEW

Endoscopic experience demonstrates that with rare exceptions most polyps which are visible in the nasal cavity arise from the ostiomeatal complex. As shown in Table 1, the origin of polyps in two hundred consecutive patients studied at our department clearly showed sites of preference.

It is important to realize, that in more than 30% of all our patients, polyps were only discovered after endoscopes were introduced **into** the middle nasal meatus allowing a view into the frontal recess, the retro- and suprabullar recess and the space between the ethmoidal bulla and the turbinate. All these polyps would have gone unrecognized during anterior rhinoscopy and even microscopic investigation.

Polyps visible between the nasal septum and the middle and/or superior turbinates usually originate either from the olfactory ridge—a rare feature with the exception of eosinophil-dominated diffuse polyposis—contact areas between the middle and/or superior turbinates and the nasal septum, from the posterior ethmoid and superior nasal meatus or, rarely, from the sphenoethmoidal recess.

Table 1: Origination of Polyps in 200 Consecutive Patients*

Primary sinuses affected	
80%	Uncinate-turbinate-infundibulum
65%	Face of bulla-hiatus-infundibulum
48%	Frontal recess
42%	"Turbinate sinus"
30%	Inside bulla
28%	Supra-/retrobullar recess
27%	Posterior ethmoidal sinus (superior meatus)
15%	Middle turbinate
Secondary sinuses affected	
65%	Maxillary sinus
23%	Frontal sinus
15%	Sphenoid sinus

*modified from H. Stammberger: 'FESS' (1991) B.C. Decker, Philadelphia

Polyps therefore predominantely originate from the clefts of the anterior ethmoid, where they may be hidden for an individually variable period, undetectable by the naked eye, but already causing symptoms such as a pressure sensation feeling and—subjectively—nasal obstruction. It is the endoscopist's impression, that in a "cascade effect" the disease may start to spread through the entire ethmoid, nasal cavity and into the secondary larger sinuses.

"CLASSIFICATION" OF POLYPS

For clinical and practical surgical processes, it helps to classify polyps into different groups. Each "group" of polyps may necessitate a different surgical approach and/or additional medical therapy.

I. Antrochoanal polyps
II. Large isolated polyps
III. Polyps associated with CRS (non eosinophil-dominated)
IV. Polyps associated with CRS (eosinophil-dominated) (Diffuse Polyposis in Aspirin Intolerance, Allergic Fungal CRS, and Asthma-patients)
V. Polyps associated with specific diseases (cystic fibrosis, malignancies)

Before individual approaches for the different kinds of polyps are described, the basic surgical steps and principles of FESS are briefly reviewed.

FESS—SURGICAL STEPS

With the FESS-concept, surgical procedures that were aimed directly at the large paranasal sinuses in previous years, today aim for the "prechambers" of the latter in the lateral nasal wall: the ostiomeatal complex, the key areas of the ethmoidal infundibulum and the frontal recess. Basically this is true for "removal" of nasal polyps, especially if these are associated with chronic rhinosinusitis. Surgery is more extensive and aggressive, when dealing with eosinophil-dominated polyps, but even then preserves the peripheral mucosa and the anatomical landmarks.

A variety of anatomical variants may complicate the anatomy of the lateral nasal wall and in the ostiomeatal unit. It is important to realize that none of those variants is a pathologic process **per se.** However, as combinations of variants may narrow the clefts of the ostiomeatal unit and cause contact areas and stenoses, we have to see them as factors predisposing to recurrent infections, some of which accompany nasal polyps. The differentiation between an anatomical variant as an incidental or a causative factor of CRS or polyposis may be extremely difficult in an individual case.

Table 2. Frequent Anatomical Variants Found in CRS and Polyp-patients

Variant	Significance
Septal deviations, spurs, crests	Narrowing common and/or middle nasal meatus, contact areas
Agger nasi-cell	Depending on degree of pneumatisation, narrowing frontal recess
Uncinate process	Bent laterally, contacting with lamina papyracea, causing atelectatic infundibulum (typical for the three grades of hypoplastic maxillary sinus). Medially bent, curved medially and anteriorly, contacting with the middle turbinate. Extending posteriorly, contacting with the bulla, occluding the hiatus semilunaris and the infundibulum.
Middle turbinate	Pneumatised (Concha bullosa), paradoxical curvature.
Ethmoidal bulla	Oversized due to extreme pneumatisation, totally filling the middle nasal meatus. Contact area with middle turbinate. Overlapping hiatus semilunaris. Narrowing the frontal recess. Pressing middle turbinate against the septum. Pneumatising anteriorly (even out of the middle meatus).
Haller's cells	Narrowing the ethmoidal infundibulum and/or the maxillary sinus ostium from above and posteriorly by pneumatising floor of orbit.

The most frequent variants considered important for CRS are listed in Table 2.

Surgical Technique—Preparation of the Nasal Mucosa

Regardless of whether the procedure is planned under local or general anaesthesia, the nasal mucosa must be carefully pretreated, trying to achieve good vasoconstriction and topical anaesthesia. For procedures under local we use cotton swaps soaked in a mixture of 4–5 parts of 2% Pontocain mixed with 1 part of Adrenalin (1:1000). The cottonoids are well squeezed before being inserted into the middle meatus, around the middle turbinate and onto all mucosal areas that can be reached, especially the posterior end of the middle turbinate near the sphenopalatine foramen. At the front, the nasal cavity is loosely filled with these cottonoids. In patients being operated under general anaesthesia, the cottonoids are soaked in Adrenalin (1:1000) only and squeezed out before being inserted.

The pledges stay in situ for at least 10 minutes and are then removed. A local anaesthetic with vasoconstrictor is applied under the mucosa of the uncinate process and into the anterior insertion of the middle turbinate near the agger nasi region. This especially blocks the final branches of both anterior ethmoidal artery and nerve. Usually 1 to 1.5 ml of this submucosal infiltration with 1% Lidocain with Epinephrine 1:200.000 are sufficient. Caution should be used with patients with cardiovascular disease.

Surgical Technique—Positioning the Patient and the Surgeon

The surgical steps presented in this chapter do not present routine steps which are performed in each and every pa-

tient. Here, the *possibilities of the technique* are demonstrated first. The basic principle always is an individualized surgical approach, adapted to the situation of the respective patient. The surgeon usually sits on the right side of the patient, with his/her knees under the patient's shoulders. The arms of the surgeon should be supported to allow for precise manipulation in a comfortable position. The same care should be used for each surgical step as in ear surgery. There is no need to use any self-retaining specula. With an endoscopic approach the elasticity of the nostrils can be used to reach even the remotest corners of the nose and sinuses. We perform all steps of the procedure strictly under endoscopic control. We do not recommend removing anterior masses of polyps using the headlight as this usually creates lesions of important structures at the entrance to the middle meatus resulting in bleeding and impaired anatomical orientation. In cases of massive polyposis usually significant polypoid masses can be removed with the first surgical step of resecting the uncinate process.

Utmost care should be applied with each manipulation: No lesion should occur to the intact mucosal surfaces especially at the entrance to the middle meatus to avoid postoperative scarring and stenoses.

Surgical Technique—Individual Steps

As in most cases the pathologic changes and polyps can be found in the key areas of the anterior ethmoid, the first surgical step is usually the resection of the uncinate process. This procedure, sometimes labelled "infundibulotomy", removes the medial wall of the ethmoidal infundibulum and thus opens the latter. The uncinate process is incised with a sickle scalpel or a Freer's elevator 2–3 mm posteriorly to its insertion on the lateral nasal wall. The knife should not penetrate into the infundibulum more than 1–2 mm and must then be placed **absolutely** parallel to the lateral nasal wall. Especially in a narrow or almost atelectatic infundibulum penetration through the lamina papyracea into the orbit can thus be avoided. In an anteriorly convex line the incision is taken down and posteriorly and then up and superiorly. If the insertion of the uncinate to the lateral nasal wall cannot be identified, the process should be resected in small strips from posteriorly to anteriorly or with a backbiting forceps. The uncinate process is then luxated medially and resected with a Blakesley forceps. Rotating movement with the instrument is best to avoid tearing of the mucosa. There is usually a free view now onto the anterior face of the ethmoidal bulla and polyps originating from this and/or between its medial wall and the middle turbinate. Should the frontal recess be diseased without involving the ethmoidal bulla (a relatively rare event) the surgeon can change from a 0 to 30 degree lens now and approach the frontal sinus through the frontal recess. If however the posterior ethmoid and/or sphenoid sinus are diseased, we would recommend to approach these first and as a last step of the procedure return to the frontal recess.

To resect the ethmoidal bulla, its anterior wall is carefully opened at its infero-medial aspect. Even if the lumen appears to be normal, the medial wall of the bulla should be resected to avoid leaving polyps behind between the latter and the middle turbinate. Depending on the anatomical situation, a suprabullar recess can be present above and a retrobullar recess behind the ethmoidal bulla. In both spaces, frequently polyps can be encountered. It has to be remembered that the superior wall of the suprabullar recess is the roof of the ethmoid, and the posterior wall of the retrobullar recess the ground lamella of the middle turbinate. This ground lamella must be perforated to reach the posterior ethmoid and superior meatus. Depending on the individual pathology, polyps from the posterior ethmoid can be removed now. With all these manipulations, extreme care must be taken, to always leave mucosa behind, covering the walls of the surgical cavity: i. e. laterally on the lamina papyracea of the orbit, superiorly on the roof of the ethmoid, medially on the middle turbinate. For this, careful handling of the instruments is mandatory. To avoid stripping off the mucosa, cutting punch forceps can be advantageous. The lamina papyracea of the orbit here can be extremely thin and even have dehiscences. If Onodi-cells are present and have developed laterally and/or superiorly to the sphenoid, the optic tubercle and even the optic nerve itself may be clearly prominent here. This situation should always be considered in cases of massive polyps in the region. In rare cases, even the internal carotid artery can be exposed in such an Onodi-cell. The surgeon should always keep in mind, that in the presence of Onodi-cells the

anterior wall of the sphenoid sinus must be sought *medially and inferiorly* via a transethmoidal route.

The sphenoid sinus basically can be approached by two routes: an extension of the route described above, transethmoidally that is or—in cases of isolated diseases of the sphenoid—by a direct route through the sphenoethmoidal recess. For this, the approach is between the nasal septum and the middle turbinate. For the transethmoidal route the anterior wall of the sphenoid sinus is carefully pressed in with a delicate curette medially and inferiorly. In no case sharp, cutting or punching instruments should be used unless the lumen of the sphenoid sinus has clearly been identified. Then, depending on the individual pathology, the perforation in the anterior wall of the sphenoid may be enlarged and the natural ostium incorporated. For this, circular cutting punches are ideal instruments. They allow one to enlarge the perforation to all direction without rotation of the handle of the instrument. Due to the blunt "head" of the punch accidental lesion to the surroundings can be avoided. Inside the sphenoid sinus no cutting or punching instruments should be used unless the surgeon has clearly identified the course of the internal carotid artery and the optic nerve.

All of the surgical steps described up to now can usually be performed without partial or total resection of the middle or superior turbinates. Thus, the functional anatomy can be preserved in most of the cases.

If required, the surgeon now can follow the skull base anteriorly and explore the frontal recess. For this, the insertion of the ground lamella of the middle turbinate at the skull base again is identified and the latter followed from the back to the front. Here, the anterior ethmoidal artery is encountered which may have a bony mesentery of up to 5 mm between its bony canal and skull base. Care must be taken not to strip mucosa totally off the bones of the skull base.

Surgery for polypoid disease of the frontal recess is by far the greatest challenge with regards to anatomical knowledge and surgical skills. Basically, there are three anatomical structures possibly narrowing the frontal recess and with this, the way to the frontal sinus, predisposing to persistence of infections, edema or polyps in this area: The uncinate process, the ethmoidal bulla and cells of the agger nasi. Especially combinations of anatomical variants of the structures together with a paradoxically curved middle turbinate or a Concha bullosa of the latter can present as a significant technical challenge. If anatomical orientation is obscured by scarring from previous operations and polyps are embedded in those scars, it can become extremely difficult to find the way to the frontal sinus. Yet with a careful and diligent approach in most cases more aggressive procedures—like using a drill to create a so-called "median drainage" can be avoided.

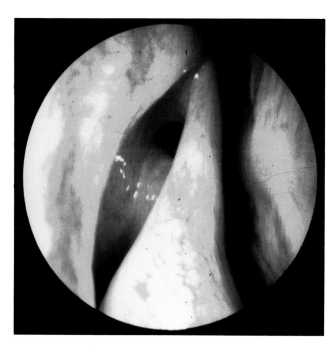

Figure 1 Endoscopic view into a middle nasal meatus on the right: A small polypoid lesion is visible between the uncinate process and the middle turbinate, which had not been discovered by anterior rhinoscopy.

If a large agger nasi cell—usually pneumatised from the frontal recess itself—develops from antero-inferiorly to postero-superiorly, it may narrow the frontal recess with its superior thin bony shell like "the cap of an egg". In a similar fashion the ethmoidal bulla or another anterior ethmoidal air cell may grow from postero-inferiorly to antero-superiorly occluding the frontal recess with its "egg cap" as well. The uncinate process with a recessus terminalis may have the same effect, if the latter is well developed and reaches superiorly. The "blind sack" of the terminal recess then occludes the frontal recess and this may impede ventilation and drainage of the frontal sinus.

The surgeon must be familiar with these variants and their combinations, if unnecessary radical approaches—and with that trauma—of the frontal recess is to be avoided. Specially modified instruments allow precise surgery in this area. If after resection of the uncinate process and bulla no free view through the frontal recess into the frontal sinus ostium can be achieved, then with a curved curette the "cap of the egg" must be identified extremely carefully and removed together with its diseased mucosa. In the case of a large Agger nasi-cell this must be done *from dorsally*. The instrument must be inserted between skull base and the thin shell of bone and the latter downfractured, away from skull base. In the case of an enlarged ethmoidal bulla the way to the frontal sinus ostium usually can be found between the respective bone shell and the middle turbinate. This holds true for a ter-

minal recess of the ethmoidal infundibulum as well. In this case, the instrument must be inserted between the skull base and the bone shell coming from *medially* i.e. between the middle turbinate and "the egg cap".

With delicate upbiting forceps and/or upbiting circular cutting punch bone fragments can be carefully removed without stripping the mucosa in this area. After exposure of the frontal sinus ostium, polyps can be removed out of the frontal sinus. Under no circumstances should the entire mucosa in the vicinity of the frontal sinus ostium be removed as this will induce scar formation and restenosis.

The enlargement of the natural ostium of the maxillary sinus is *not a routine step* of the surgical procedure. Only if pathologic changes inside the maxillary sinus present or polyps are encountered in the vicinity of the ostium, is the latter enlarged. After identification of the ostium, with the backwards cutting or a downwards cutting forcep the ostium can be enlarged anteriorly and posteriorly. Care should be taken not to injure the naso-lacrimal sac by cutting too far anteriorly. If there are accessory ostia in the nasal fontanelles, these should in any case be connected to the natural ostium to avoid a circular transport of mucosa postoperatively. If the ostium has been enlarged, under guidance of a 30 or 70 degree lens, pathologic processes like cysts and polyps can be removed with suitable instruments from inside the sinus. Again, care should be taken that the entire mucosa is not stripped from the maxillary sinus.

If a concha bullosa of the middle turbinate is present and if it is diseased, its lateral lamella is resected. For this, a local anesthetic with vasoconstrictor is infiltrated submucosally and scalpel the conchal air cell opened with a sickle. The maneuver must be performed taking care not to fracture the insertion of the middle turbinate. With scissors the lumen of the cell is opened and the lateral lamella removed with forceps. Frequently, polypoid changes of the mucosa inside a concha bullosa may be encountered. Here too, care should be taken not to strip the entire mucosa off the remaining medial lamella of the concha bullosa. If pneumatisation reaches far posteriorly toward the dorsal end of the turbinate, branches of the sphenopalatine artery maybe encountered.

Fess and Septal Deviation

Septal spurs and crests can be removed without difficulty during an endoscopic procedure: The mucosa is incised longitudinally and flaps created. Then the crest or spur is removed and the flaps folded back. The endoscopic procedure then continues as scheduled. If in a case of massive polyposis a complete septal correction is needed, we will first perform the endoscopic sinus surgery on the wider side of the nose, then perform the septal correction from a hemitransfixtion incision from

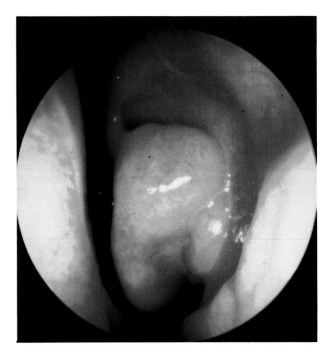

Figure 2 Concha bullosa of the middle turbinate on the left side, bulging into the lateral nasal wall, contacting the uncinate process. From the contact area edema has started to form a small polypoid lesion. Topical therapy with corticosteroids improved the aspect, but not the symptoms: Whenever steroid therapy was stopped, the lesion recurred. Surgical resection of the lateral lamella of the Concha bullosa eliminating the contact area took care of the problem without any further need for topical steroids.

that side and continue the endoscopic procedure on the previously narrower side of the nose.

Termination of the Surgical Procedure

We do not routinely use any packing. The normally minimal diffuse mucosal oozing usually ceases at the end of the procedure. Sometimes resorbable material like Sorbacel® can loosely be applied or Merocel® sponges inserted for 24 hours.

Choosing Endoscopes and Instruments

The majority of the surgical procedure is performed using a 4 mm, 0 degree lens. This is the only endoscope allowing a direct forward view which we consider of utmost importance. Surgery with deflected lenses requires significant training and experience. Only after important landmarks have been identified, would we switch to a 30 degree lens for special procedures inside the larger sinuses. For following skull base from posteriorly to anteriorly and manipulation in the frontal recess we usually prefer a 30 degree lens and very rarely use a 70 degree lens.

The instruments used should be delicate and appropriate. Their size should be chosen to allow their introduction into the middle meatus without creating a lesion of the middle turbinate. In some cases of diffuse polyposis and increased diffuse bleeding, Blakesley forceps with integrated suction channels can be helpful. However, we do not use these instruments on a routine basis. Cutting punch forceps can be of great help for *special indications,* especially for scars following previous surgery or if thicker pieces of bone have to be removed. We would not recommend routine use of these instruments however and they especially should be used with extreme care in the vicinity of the sphenoid sinus and ethmoidal roof.

APPROACHES FOR DIFFERENT KINDS OF POLYPS

The Antrochoanal Polyp

This is usually a unilateral lesion originating with a cystic portion from the posterior wall of the maxillary sinus, in most cases filling the sinus completely. There may be one large cyst or a septated one, and sometimes polypoid elements can be found inside the maxillary sinus. Apart from the relatively small area of origin of the cystic portion, the remainder of the maxillary sinus mucosal is usually normal. On its stalk, the antrochoanal polyp reaches into the middle nasal meatus, from where the solid portion may extend all the way to the choana, the nasopharynx and even appear behind the free margin of the soft palate in the oropharynx. In our patients there were only 12% where the stalk of an antrochoanal polyp reached through the natural ostium of the maxillary sinus.

Antrochoanal polyps are an ideal indication for endoscopic surgery. Care must be taken to completely remove the cystic portion, otherwise disease is bound to recur. Surgically, it is usually enough to resect the uncinate process (sometimes even this is not required), enlarge the accessory ostium into the natural ostium to resect the solid portion. If this too large to be removed through the nostril, it can be pushed back into the nasopharynx and removed transorally under endoscopic vision. Then, the cystic portion must be removed from the maxillary sinus together with the mucosa of its origin. If this proves to be too difficult to be achieved through the enlarged ostium in the middle meatus, a trocar can be inserted through the canine fossa into the maxillary sinus and under endoscopic vision the origin of the cystic portion be "shaved off" the posterior wall.

Large Isolated Polyps

These are usually unilateral lesions of sometimes significant size. In the anterior ethmoid they originate from contact areas between the uncinate process and the mid-

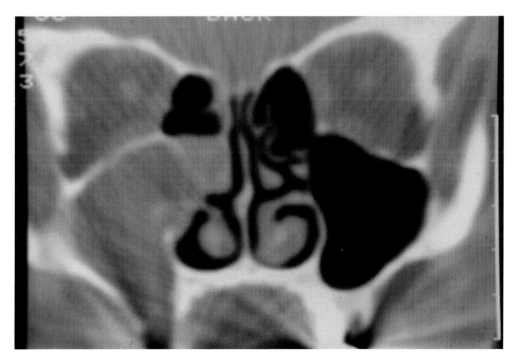

Figure 3 Typical CT-aspect of an antrochoanal polyp, the cystic lesion of which completely fills the right maxillary sinus.

dle turbinate or the uncinate process and the ethmoidal bulla. They may reach down all the way to the floor of the nose, or back into the choana. Isolated large polyps may originate from the sphenoethmoidal recess apparently without any contact areas here. The reason for their existence

remains unclear. Histologically, sometimes glandular-tubular structures are present, but not a constant feature in our own cases. Eosinophils are extremely rare.

Their therapy clearly is surgical which can ideally be performed endoscopically: The polyp is removed at its insertion, if required together with the underlying contact area. There is no need for any (partial or total) ethmoidectomy in most cases. After careful removal the recurrence rate is minimal. Topical corticosteroids usually do not have any significant effect and are not required postoperatively.

Polyps Associated with CRS (Non-eosinophil-dominated)

This kind of polyposis is usually encountered bilaterally and is the most frequent one associated with CRS. The edema leading to polyp formation usually starts at contact areas in the ostiomeatal unit, where polyps may gain a considerable size before the larger sinuses become effected. Anatomical variants narrowing the ostiomeatal complex can be found in a high percentage of these patients who have usually suffered from CRS for many months or even years, before they are seen first by an

ENT-doctor. Therapy is clearly surgical, **if** antibiotics and/or a relevant local therapy have failed to solve the problems. Topical corticosteroids can improve the situation, but usually do not provide a complete solution. Even if the polyps should shrink somewhat and retract into the middle meatus (and thus be not visible in anterior rhinoscopy or microscopic investigation) the symptoms of CRS will continue and/or increase again after topical corticosteroid therapy has been stopped. Depending on the extent of the disease, the classical steps of FESS can be performed in an individually adapted fashion for each patient. Rarely surgery *inside* the maxillary and/or frontal sinus are required here. FESS here gives its best results, with even considerable mucosal thickening in the larger sinuses normalising within a few weeks, in many cases without having been touched themselves. In these group III polyps, the findings of the CT-scans should not be overinterpreted especially with regards to frontal, maxillary and sphenoid sinus. In a very high percentage of even total opacification of the sinuses mentioned, retention of mucus is the underlying problem rather than significant mucosal swelling or polyp formation. Especially with frontal sinus opacification it is usually enough to remove disease from the frontal recess and expose the frontal sinus ostium. An active enlargement of the latter or even manipulations inside the frontal sinus are only rarely required.

Histologically, eosinophils may be present among other cells, but they do not dominate the histological picture.

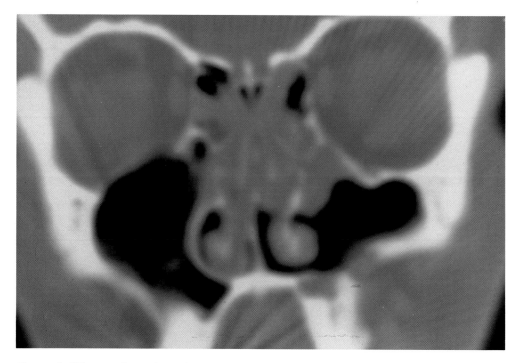

Figure 4 CT-scan of a patient after fenestration and Caldwell-Luc surgery to her left maxillary sinus: The mucosa of the latter has improved, the underlying disease in the ostiomeatal unit however was not improved and symptoms therefore persisted.

Polyps Associated with CRS, Eosinophil-dominated

This disease histologically is characterised by dense eosinophilic infiltrates in the mucosa and polyps. Electronmicroscopically and with immunhistochemical staining it can be demonstrated, that the eosinophils are degranulated and have released certain mediators into the tissue. Frequently, hyperreactivity of the lower airways is associated with this type of polyposis, regardless of their extent. The degree of hyperreactivity can be very variable and reach up to severe bronchial asthma. On the CT-scans of the sinuses, the generally bilateral opacification can be staged I–IV, I indicating a moderate opacification of the ostiomeatal complex, IV the total opacification of all sinuses with almost no air visible in the sinus system ("white-out"). Endoscopically, bilateral diffuse polyposis is found and in the extreme cases, the entire visible mucosa of the lateral nasal wall appears to be polypoid. Interestingly, polyps almost never originate from the inferior nasal turbinate or the septum, with the exception of contact areas and from scars or lesions after previous surgery.

Therapy aims to remove the massive polyps either surgically or with corticosteroids and to prevent the immigration of eosinophils and release of noxious and harmful mediators again. Semantically speaking, there are no true "recurrences" in this group of polyps, regrowth of polyps almost always is the result of *persistent underlying disease.*

The most effective medical therapy is with topical and/or systemic corticosteroids (see previous chapters). Not only can polyps sometimes significally shrink in size, or in less extensive cases be made to disappear completely, but the repeated influx of eosinophils can be partially or totally blocked and the cycle of "recurrence" thus interfered with.

In massive cases of eosinophil-dominated rhinosinusitis a combined approach appears to be the therapy of choice: After preceding topical and/or systemic corticosteroids therapy the polyp masses are endoscopically debulked. In these cases the approach is considerably more aggressive than in non eosinophil-dominated CRS. But even here almost always anatomical landmarks like the middle turbinate can be preserved. Maxillary and sphenoid sinus are entered and polyp masses and inspissated mucus removed. Here too, care should be taken not to denude bone, as this will lead to considerable granulations, and possibly infections (osteitis) with prolonged postoperative healing. The entrance to the frontal sinus is especially prone to stenoses if attacked in too radical a fashion. Under no circumstances should the mucosa be circularly removed at the level of the ostium or bone exposed.

Postoperatively continuous or interval therapy with topical corticosteroids is of the utmost importance to prevent regrowth of polyps.

Based on the underlying dominance of eosinophils and the accompanying hyperreactivity of the airways the fol-

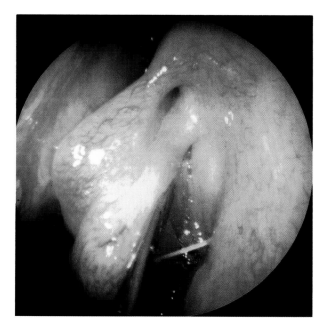

Figure 5a Endoscopic view into a middle nasal meatus on the left, demonstrating large polyps originating from a contact area between the superior aspect of the uncinate process and the middle turbinate as well as the anterior face of the ethmoidal bulla.

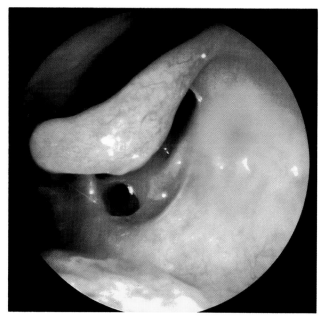

Figure 5b Aspect 3 months after endoscopic surgery, demonstrating a normal mucosa in a free middle meatus.

lowing diseases associated with nasal polyposis can also be clinically counted into group IV: Diffuse polyposis associated with aspirin intolerance, and allergic fungal rhinosinusitis. In our hospital, between 10 and 15% of all patients undergoing sinus surgery per year are patients with allergic fungal sinusitis which usually presents as a diffuse polyposis as well. Here apart from relatively aggressive removal of polyps for which sphenoethmoidectomy with preservation of the peripheral mucosa is required, the thick almost rubber-like mucus with the fungal masses must be carefully removed as well.

Nasal Polyps Associated with Specific Diseases

Primarily, cystic fibrosis must be mentioned. In these patients, with a genetically determined disease, surgical approach and corticosteroids can improve the situation, but do not provide a permanent cure. In our patients we have the impression, that the mucosal changes affect the maxillary sinuses more than the ethmoids at least in the early stages in children, resulting in mucocele-like formations with mucus or pus not only in the sinus and/or cell cavities, but in intramucosal retention cysts or abscesses. The endoscopic surgical approach is as for diffuse polyposis i.e. trying to debulk the diseased mucosa and remove the polyps but preserve the anatomical landmarks. Especially in these patients, more radical approaches (Caldwell-Luc procedures, turbinate resection) have not given any better results than the less traumatic endoscopic approach.

Sometimes non-invasive, non-allergic (saprophytic) mycotic diseases of paranasal sinuses may be associated with polyp formation. After surgical removal of the fungal material (the mycetoma) from the respective sinus and establishing good ventilation and drainage via the natural pathways, there is usually no need for any specific follow-up medication.

Sometimes malignant lesions of the nose, sinuses and nasopharynx are hidden behind "signal polyps," emphasizing the need to submit all tissue to histology and to remain suspicious of any unilateral lesion.

ENDOSCOPIC SURGERY WITH THE "SHAVER" ("MICRO-DEBRIDER", "HUMMER")

An ideal instrument to remove massive polyps is the so called "shaver". This instrument was primarily used in arthroscopy: Mucosa and polyps are aspirated into a suction channel and cut by a blade oscillating in this channel. The material removed can be collected in a filtration device and sent for histological examination. Larger polyps can be cut at their origin and removed with forceps and thus examined histologically. With different cutting blades and configurations of the "shavers head" thin bony segments like the uncinate process may be removed in individual cases as well. This instrument is especially well suited to remove polyps and diseased mucosa off the middle turbinate and the medial wall of

173

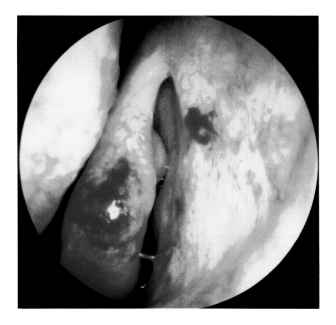

Figure 6a Endoscopic aspect of an allegedly small polyp (following topical corticosteroid therapy with persisting symptoms) prior to surgery.

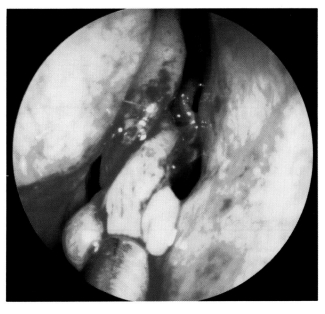

Figure 6b After resection of the uncinate process, masses of polyps are encountered in the infundibulum ethmoidale and the ostiomeatal unit.

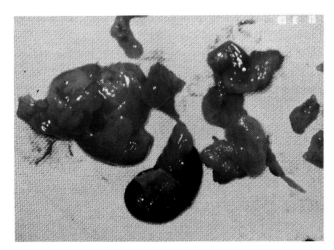

Figure 6c Polyps removed from the left side of the patient, note the small fragments of bone from the uncinate process and the ethmoidal bulla, which where removed as they held the origin of the polyps.

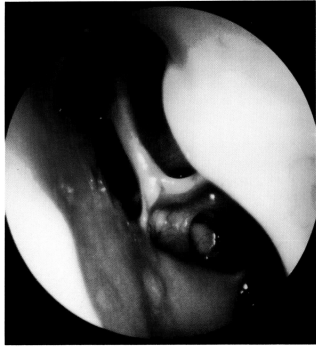

Figure 6d Endoscopic view (30 degree lens) one year postoperatively into the frontal recess and frontal sinus with normal mucosa.

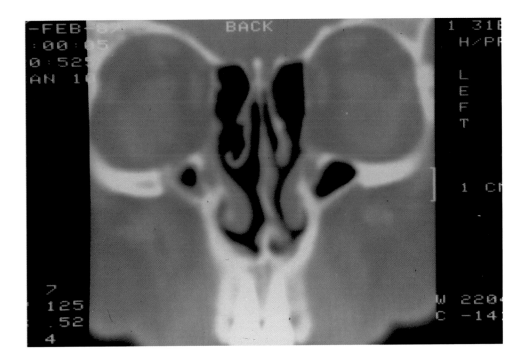

Figure 6e CT-cut through the anterior ethmoid one year postoperatively demonstrating normalised mucosa in the area.

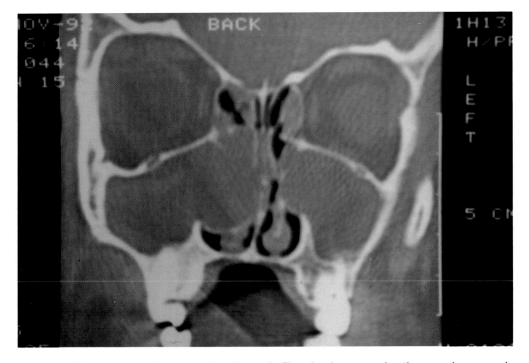

Figure 7 CT-scan of an eight year old with cystic fibrosis, demonstrating the pseudo-mucocele like aspect of the disease in the maxillary sinus. The ethmoids are affected to a significant lesser degree.

the orbit without removing the mucosa periosteum or exposing bone. Care must be taken however not to apply too much pressure on the underlying tissue as all soft tissue once sucked into the channel is cut. With correct handling accidental lesions of vital structures can be readily avoided. As suction is constantly applied, blood is simultaneously aspirated and allows for a clear surgical field. Frequent changes of instruments can largely be avoided. Though moderately angled suction channels and blades are available, "working around the corner" cannot yet be achieved with the instruments presently on the market nor can the thicker bony fragments be removed. Working with the Shaver therefore cannot be seen as a substitute for a careful endoscopic surgery. When exploring the sinuses, especially the frontal recess and working along the skull base, or inside the maxillary and sphenoid sinus individual instruments are still required. In many cases of diffuse polyposis and especially revision operations however, the Shaver must be seen as an extremely helpful and mucosal-preserving new tool.

CONCLUSIONS

From the rhino surgeon's point of view, "nasal polyps" do not appear to be one entity. The polyp manifestations presented in groups I-III are ideal indications for an endonasal endoscopic approach and have a very low recurrence rate. The larger paranasal sinuses only rarely have to be operated on in these cases, regardless of their degree of opacification. The sinus mucosa has a high potential for normalisation and recovery in these cases. Type IV, dominated by eosinophils on the light- and electron-microscopy, is in its early stages an indication for corticosteroid therapy. If this alone is not enough to control not only the polyps but also the accompanying chronic rhinosinusitis, a combined approach with endoscopic surgery and at least topical corticosteroids is the therapy of choice. The surgical approach is usually more aggressive. All larger paranasal sinuses can be readily reached endoscopically. Even when masses of polyps must be debulked in these cases, a peripheral layer of mucosa should always be preserved. No areas of bone should be exposed, especially not in the vicinity of the maxillary and frontal sinus ostia. The surgeon must inform the patient in these cases of the importance of postoperative topical corticosteroid therapy which will be required for varying intervals. As a rule endoscopic follow-up therefore is mandatory in these cases to detect the early stages of nasal mucosa change before the patient becomes symptomatic. Minimal amounts of topical corticosteroids may be enough in these situations to bring the appearance of the mucosa back to normal. Thus revision surgery for "recurrent" polyps can be avoided in many patients.

With today's possibilities of endonasal surgical procedures under microscopic and even more under endoscopic guidance, indications for external approaches have become rare. Even in cases of massive polyps and revision surgery important structures like the middle turbinate can be preserved in most cases and good nasal function preserved. External approaches are used almost exclusively for complications or revision operations in very special, tricky cases. In our patients, external approaches are used almost exclusively in these rare cases of frontal sinus problems, when the frontal recess is massively scarred or new bone formation does not allow an approach through the frontal recess, or if disease processes are encountered extremely far laterally in frontal and maxillary sinuses, especially in those, who have been previously operated by an external approach.

Chapter XXI

Outcome and Complications of Surgical Treatment

Maurice Roth, M.D., and David W. Kennedy, M.D.

ABSTRACT

Until a cure is found for sino-naso polyposis, surgical therapy will continue to play an important role in the overall management of this disorder. Overall results show that at least 85% of patients report marked improvement in nasal obstruction, congestion, and facial pain related to concurrent chronic sinusitis. Nasal drainage also improves in most cases. Improvement in associated asthma is less clear. Poorer prognosis is directly associated with greater extent of initial disease. Results are usually short term if patients do not receive concurrent medical therapy along with close observation. The use of the endoscope allows for greater precision in diagnosis and management and can be used as an effective tool when combined with medical therapy for the long term treatment of polyposis.

There is no evidence that endoscopic sinus surgery has decreased the overall complication rate from surgical therapy although most major centers with good endoscopic experience report less than 1% risk of major complications. Avoidance of complications is best achieved through careful preoperative planning including comprehensive nasal endoscopy, computed tomography, and aggressive pre-operative medical management. Endoscopic surgical experience including the recognition and treatment of surgical complications is essential for all surgeons engaged in the treatment of sino-nasal polyposis.

OUTCOME

The introduction of the endoscope to the field of rhinology has added a new dimension to the evaluation and documentation of outcome related to sinus surgery[1]. Endoscopic evaluation provides an objective means of assessing the paranasal sinuses independent of clinical symptoms. Recurrent polyps, focal areas of osteitis, and localized areas of inflammation can be detected and recorded. In addition, these areas can be addressed medically or surgically before the patient develops localized clinical symptoms.

In conjunction with comprehensive nasal endoscopy, computed tomography (CT) has greatly improved the evaluation of patients with sino-nasal polyposis[2]. Skull base erosion from expanded polyp lesions can be detected as well as new bone growth formation or focal areas of osteitis. CT can also be used to evaluate the extent of disease.

Unfortunately, endoscopic findings frequently do not correlate with clinical symptoms[3,4]. Until their relationship is fully determined, surgical results can be divided into improvements in clinical symptoms and endoscopic improvement within the sinus cavities. The most common clinical symptoms evaluated include: obstruction, congestion, facial pain, and post-nasal drainage. Improvement in associated asthma has also been evaluated. Finally, surgical outcome in the area of the frontal recess is critical since persistent disease or scarring within this region leads to recalcitrant to treat chronic frontal sinusitis.

There have been multiple publications regarding outcomes research related to the surgical treatment of sino-nasal polyposis (Table 1). Most authors either combined clinical symptoms into an overall measure or simply asked the patients to rate their general improvement. Most studies were unable to stage patients thus making their conclusions less reliable. In addition, few studies followed standardized medical regimens during the perioperative period. If patients received more aggressive medical therapy in the post-operative period, the degree to which surgical therapy was responsible for the marked improvements stated becomes less clear. The

Table 1. Outcome Studies Involving Sino-nasal Polyps

Author Reference	Stage	Patients	Outcome Measured	Medical Treatment	Length	Post-Op Care	Outcome
				Endoscopic Sinus Surgery			
Gaskins 5	3 Stages Based on Extent	50 R	Endoscopic Findings	Not Stated	11.5 mo.	Not Stated	Overall 88% Improvement, worsened with extent of disease
Stammberger & Posawetz 6	Extent of Polyposis	256 R	Symptoms and Endoscopic Findings	Not Stated	8 mo.–10 yrs.	Endoscopic as Needed	prognosis worse with diffuse polyposis
Wigand & Hosemann 7	"Massive" Polyps	220 R	Symptoms and Endoscopic Findings	Not Stated	Not Stated	Not Stated	Overall 82% Improvement 19% Recurrent Polyps
Lund & Mackay 8	Diffuse Polyposis	305 R	Symptoms	Antibiotics nasal steroids oral steroids	6 mo.	Weekly until Healed	Overall 87% Improvement
Jankowski et al 9	None	50R	Symptoms and Endoscopic Findings	Pre-operative Systemic Corticosteroids	12–34 mo. M=18 mo.	Not Stated	72% Improved 40% Endoscopic Resolution
Kennedy 10	50% Diffuse 50% Middle Meatal	71 P&R	Symptoms & Endoscopic Findings	Antibiotics Nasal Steroids	18 mo.	Debridement Weekly until Healed	98% Improved 24% Normal mucosa with diffuse polyposis
Levine 12	5 Groups Based Upon Location & Extent	131 R	Symptoms	Prednisone 40mg/day 7 days pre-op	12–42 mo. M=17 mo.	Debridement weekly if Crusting	88% Improved
May et al. 15	None	117 R	Symptoms	Not Stated	6–48 mo.	Not Stated	Overall 71% Improved, worse with allergy or asthma

Intranasal Ethmoidectomy

				Oral Steroids, Antibiotics			
Faugere 13 et al	None	144P	Symptoms Polyp Recurrence	Not Stated	Up to 5 yrs.	Not Stated	82% Initial Improvement
Sogg 14	35 without Allergy 41 with Allergy	76 R	Presence of Polyps or Purulence	Not Stated	Up to 6 yrs.	Not Stated	83% Controlled, Worse prognosis with allergy
Friedman 16 & Katsantonis	193 without Asthma 164 with Asthma	357 R	Recurrence of Hyperplastic Disease	Not Stated	6 mo.–8 yrs. M=31 mo.	Not Stated	92% Required less steroids to control asthma
Lawson 19	24 Diffuse Polyps 29 Polyps & Asthma	53 R	Presence of Hyperplasia, Patent Antrostomy	Not Stated	2–14 yrs. M=42 mo.	Not Stated	83% Controlled with diffuse polyposis, 48% Controlled with asthma

R=Retrospective, P=Prospective, M=Mean

Table 2. Gaskin Staging System Separated for Sino-nasal Polyposis

Stage I,	N=3 :	Localized <10% of the sinus space
Stage II,	N=28:	limited, 10–50% of the sinus/nasal cavities
Stage III,	N=19:	Sino-nasal polyposis filling >50%

widest variation in outcome studies relates to the intensity of post-operative care. Very few studies outlined the extent of post-operative debridements as well as continued endoscopic findings. At this time, endoscopic evaluation provides the best objective measurement of long term surgical outcome.

Gaskins retrospectively evaluated 303 consecutive patients over a one year period[5]. The mean follow-up period was 11.5 months. Patients were staged based upon pre-operative endoscopic findings and CT assessment of the paranasal sinuses (Table 2). Overall most patients reported symptomatic relief following surgery. Endoscopic outcome was also reported (Table 3). Peri-operative medical therapy and post-operative surgical debridement were not outlined.

Stammberger and Posawetz reviewed 500 patients with chronic rhinosinusitis in whom 256 suffered from polyposis[6]. Sixty four of these patients had diffuse polyposis. They found that patients with diffuse polyposis along with associated generalized mucosal hyper-reactivity had a poorer outcome in terms of symptomatic and endoscopic improvement than those patients with specific anatomic variations resulting in rhinosinusitis. Post-operative results were not improved with more radical surgical procedures and patients seemed to have greater suffering with open sinus procedures.

Wigand and Hosemann evaluated 220 patients with polyposis and found that 82% of patients reported overall improvement[7]. However, a normal mucosal lining was found in only 52% of patients after surgery. Eighteen percent of patients actually developed recurrent polyps while the remaining 34% had hyperplastic mucosa. The authors highlight the divergence between subjective complaints and endoscopic findings discussed earlier.

Lund and Mackay retrospectively evaluated 650 patients which included 331 patients with chronic rhino-sinusitis and 305 patients with polyposis[8]. They found no

Table 3. Normal Endoscopic Outcome by Stage from Gaskins Review

Stage I:	100%
Stage II:	75%
Stage III:	32%

difference in results between these two groups up to 6 months post-surgery. Nasal obstruction improved in 92% of patients, headache and facial pain in 85%, and post-nasal discharge in 78%. However, only 10% of patients who complained of nasal discharge reported resolution of this symptom.

Jankowski et al evaluated 50 patients with sino-nasal polyposis using questionnaires, and endoscopic examinations[9]. Follow up time ranged from 12 to 34 months with a mean of 18 months. Post-operative CT scans were also obtained. Ninety six percent of patients remained on topical nasal steroids during the follow up period. Post-operative endoscopic care was not defined. Two week post-operative CT revealed that most patients had undergone an incomplete ethmoidectomy. Thirty four percent of patients complained of some degree of nasal obstruction at 18 months. In addition, 32% of patients reported continued post-nasal drainage at 18 months. Less than 10% of patients showed resolution of mucosal disease at 18 months. The authors point out the need for continued medical therapy in these patients.

Kennedy reported the results of a detailed comprehensive study involving 120 patients aimed at determining prognostic factors related to the treatment of chronic inflammatory sinus disease[10]. These factors included: prior ethmoid surgery, allergy, aspirin sensitivity, asthma, presence of extra-mucosal fungal sinusitis, and extent of disease. Of the 120 patients evaluated, 37 had middle meatal polyps and 34 suffered from diffuse polyposis. Post-operative care was clearly outlined and included frequent debridements until the cavities were healed. Medical therapy included post-operative antibiotics, topical nasal steroids, and oral steroids titrated to the post-operative endoscopic exam. Eighty five percent of patients reported marked overall symptomatic improvement while 13% claimed mild improvement up to 51 months post-surgery. Whereas overall symptomatic improvement appeared to be good for all groups, endoscopic evaluation showed a direct correlation between initial extent of disease and post-operative healing. Normal cavities were found in 77% of patients without polypoid disease. Patients with middle meatal polyps completely reversed their mucosal disease in 58% of cases. Only 24% of patients with diffuse polypoid disease reverted to normal cavities during the follow up period. When these results were analyzed with regards to the prognostic factors evaluated, only extent of disease was found to be statistically significant and therefore a staging system based upon the initial extent of sinus disease was proposed (Table 4).

Fang prospectively evaluated the maxillary sinus mucosa in 71 patients with nasal polyposis and chronic rhino-sinusitis[11]. All patients underwent endoscopic sinus surgery utilizing the Messerklinger Technique. Dis-

Table 4. Kennedy Staging for Chronic Ethmoid Sinusitis (REF)[10]

Stages

I	Anatomic abnormalities All unilateral sinus disease Bilateral disease limited to ethmoid sinuses
II	Bilateral ethmoid disease with involvement of one dependant sinus
III	Bilateral ethmoid disease with involvement of two or more dependant sinuses on each side
IV	Diffuse sino-nasal polyposis

ease presence greater than 7 years, initial polyposis within the maxillary antrum, and mucocilliary clearance time >36 minutes (Saccharin test) were found to be negative prognostic indicators. Outcome was not significantly altered by the presence of allergy.

Levine evaluated 154 patients with polyposis and found that 88% of patients reported overall symptomatic improvement[12]. Ten percent of patients were unavailable for review. Topical nasal steroids were given if polypoid disease remained post-operatively. Ten percent of patients had persistent polyps post-surgery. Also, Levine found that 33% of patients with chronic rhinosinusitis also had polyps within the anterior ethmoid at the time of surgery.

Faugere et al evaluated a mixed group of patients with chronic rhinosinusitis and nasal polyposis[13]. They found a direct correlation between the length of follow up and incidence of recurrent polyposis. Thirty six percent of patients available for post-operative examination were found to have recurrent polyps. In addition, symptomatic improvement also declined over time so that only 40% of patients were free of disease at five years.

Sogg evaluated the results of non-endoscopic sinus surgery in patients with polyposis[14]. Outcome was measured in terms of recurrent polyps or nasal purulence although the exact method of obtaining results was not reported. In addition, medical therapy was not discussed. Patients with associated allergy had a worse outcome and 13% of these patients required revision surgery.

May evaluated 60 patients with polyposis and asthma or Samter's Triad 6–48 months following endoscopic sinus surgery and found that only 39% and 35% of patients respectively, showed symptomatic improvement[15]. Patients without these other factors improved in 65% of cases. Friedman also found little difference in outcome between patients with asthma and additional ASA sensitivity[16]. However, overall improvement was substantially better in Friedman's series (82%). In both series, patients

were not staged. In addition, post-operative care including medical therapy was not reported.

In addition to asthma being considered as a prognostic indicator in patients with sino-nasal polyposis, several authors have evaluated changes in asthma following sinus surgery. Asthma may be present in >25% of patients with nasal polyps[17]. English reviewed 205 patients with nasal polyps, asthma and aspirin sensitivity following sinus surgery[18]. He found that 40% of patients who required periodic bursts of oral steroids prior to surgery for asthma control were non-steroid dependant for at least 6 months after surgery. However, most patients requiring daily oral steroids remained steroid dependant following surgery. He also reported that 40% of patients developed some degree of bronchospasm during surgery despite pre-treatment with oral steroids. Intra-operative bronchodialators along with a boost in the steroid dose seemed to control the bronchospasm.

Lawson evaluated 36 patients with asthma in whom 29 also had polyps[19]. Thirty three percent of these patients reported subjective improvement in their asthma following surgery, 66% were unchanged, and 10% were worse. Medical therapy was not discussed.

Korchia et al performed pre and post-operative pulmonary function tests in patients with asthma who underwent sinus surgery for polyposis[20]. No improvement was found. Previous reports prior to the steroid era showed exacerbation of pulmonary symptoms following polypectomy[21,22]. Even though a definitive statement regarding asthma outcome following polypectomy and sinus surgery can not be made, most authors do report that stabilization of the overall sino-pulmonary mucosal lining with oral and inhaled steroids prior to surgery helps prevent intra-operative bronchospasm[23].

Finally, outcome measures related to improvement in frontal sinus obstruction resulting from frontal recess disease is important to review since it is within this key area that most otolaryngologists will have the most difficulty. The decision to dissect the frontal recess is based upon a careful review of the patients symptomatology, radiographic evaluation and pre-operative as well as intra-operative endoscopic exam. Patients with chronic frontal sinusitis resulting from polypoid obstruction within the frontal recess require removal of obstructing osteitic bone and polyps. However no attempt should be made to strip hyperplastic mucosa from within the frontal sinus ostium, skull base, or medial orbital wall. A record or photograph of the frontal ostium should be obtained for post-operative reference. Many patients with diffuse sino-nasal polyposis will have marked mucosal hyperplasia within the frontal sinus and this should remain undisturbed. Post-operative medical therapy including long-term culture directed antibiotics along with topical and oral corticosteroids should be given. Short term use of dexamethasone ophthalmic drops placed in the Moffet position may also be helpful. Dissecting the frontal recess markedly increases the need for aggressive endoscopic post-operative care if stenosis of the ostium is to be avoided.

Schaefer and Close reviewed 36 patients up to 26 months following endoscopic frontal sinusotomy for signs and symptoms of chronic frontal sinusitis[24]. Fifteen patients had frontal sinus polyps. All patients received topical nasal steroids for at least 6 months. Sixty five percent of patients reported symptomatic improvement. Prognostic indicators of poor outcome were not addressed.

COMPLICATIONS

The best way to prevent complications during surgery is to have a thorough knowledge of the anatomy of the paranasal sinuses as well as experience with the technique to be used. In addition, careful pre-operative endoscopic examination allows the surgeon to assess the degree of inflammation, extent of disease present, and presence of significant landmark distortion. In this way, the surgeon knows what will be encountered during surgery and allows complicated cases to be referred to specialty centers if necessary. Kennedy et al surveyed the otolaryngologists of the American Academy of Otolaryngology-Head and Neck Surgery regarding post-operative complications from ethmoidectomy[25]. Completed questionnaires were received from 56% of surgeons of which 77% (3043) performed ethmoidectomy. The overall major complication rate was 0.4%. The CSF leak rate was 0.1%.

Table 5. Pre-operative Anatomic Review

Slope and integrity of the skull base and medial orbital wall

Uncinate rotation and maxillary sinus development

Vertical height of the posterior ethmoid as influenced by the posterior medial roof of the maxillary sinus and skull base

The presence of Onodi Cells

The attachment of the sphenoid sinus septation to the skull base in relation to the optic canal and internal carotid artery

---

CT is invaluable for pre-operative planning. Anatomic variation, skull base erosion, or obstructing new bone growth can be detected. Reviewing the pre-operative CT before and during surgery may help prevent surgical complications (Table 5).

Synechia

The most common complication following endoscopic sinus surgery is post-operative scar formation within the ethmoid cavity. Scar bands lead to continued obstruction, reduced mucocilliary clearance, and treatment failure. Small areas of scar formation in critical locations such as within the frontal recess and at the natural ostium of the maxillary sinus can produce major disruptions in mucociliary flow patterns giving rise to areas of recirculation.

The incidence of scar formation can be reduced in several ways. First, every attempt should be made to preserve the mucosa along the medial orbital wall and skull base during surgery. The use of through cutting instruments during surgery makes mucosal preservation easier. Second, careful endoscopic debridement in the post-operative period is critical. Crusts, mucus blood, and granulation can be removed before scarring forms. Finally, culture-directed systemic antibiotics, topical nasal steroids, and oral steroids as necessary help control underlying infection and inflammation which leads to earlier mucosal healing and less scarring.

Bleeding

Excessive bleeding can occur during surgery or in the postoperative period. Operative bleeding hinders the surgeons view of key landmarks and therefore increases the possibility of more serious complications. A thorough history should be obtained prior to surgery with questions directed toward the possibility of an underlying bleeding disorder. Maximal medical therapy prior to surgery is mandatory if bleeding is to be minimized during surgery. The use of pre-operative oral steroids should be considered in order to stabilize mucosa and reduce polyposis when possible. In addition, proper intra-nasal local anesthetic and vasoconstrictive injections combined with sphenopalatine artery block markedly reduce bleeding.

Recently, microarthroscopic debridement of polyps during surgery has been found to reduce intra-operative bleeding (Figure 1). A cutting blade oscillating within a sheath aspirates and removes polyps with ease. The

Table 6. Complications of Sinus Surgery

Ocular	Cranial base	Hemorrhage	Other
Hematoma	CSF Leak	Internal carotid Artery	Synechia
Optic Nerve Injury	Brain Abscess	Sphenopalatine Injury	Toxic Shock Syndrome
Diplopia	Pneumocephalus	Ethmoid artery Injury	Olfactory Loss
Epiphora	Intra-cranial Injury		Cavernous Sinus Thrombosis

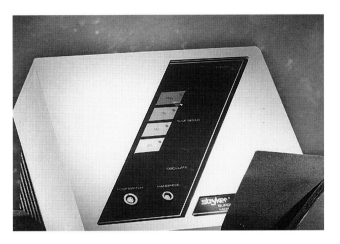

Figure 1. Microarthroscopy Debrider (The "Hummer") Stryker Instruments, Kalamazoo, MI

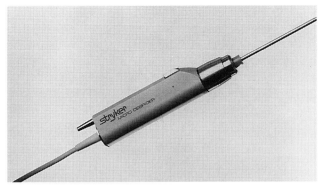

Figure 2. Stryker Microarthroscopy Debrider ("The Hummer")

"Hummer" works less well removing bone partitions. Not only is bleeding reduced, with this device mucosa is spared during the dissection. Mucosal preservation along the skull base and medial orbital wall improves postoperative care and facilitates healing.

Significant postoperative bleeding usually arises from branches of the sphenopalatine artery. In most cases bleeding can be controlled in the office using bipolar cautery or topical microfibrillar collagen*. Unipolar cautery is also effective; however there is a risk of optic nerve injury. A sphenopalatine injection through the greater palatine foramen may provide anesthesia and temporary slowing of the bleeding.

Fatal bleeding has occurred from injury to the internal carotid artery[26]. Absolutely no tissue should be removed from the sphenoid sinus without direct visualization. Kennedy found a 22% clinical dehiscence of the internal carotid artery in 188 specimens examined[27]. Internal carotid artery injury is difficult to control. The sphenoid sinus should immediately be packed and the patient prepared for angiography with possible balloon occlusion.

CSF Leak

Although the overall incidence of CSF leak resulting from endoscopic sinus surgery is low for experienced surgeons, it remains a significant complication from any sinus surgery. Patients with polyposis are at increased risk of CSF leak due to distorted anatomy, increased bleeding, and occasional skull base dehiscence. Dural injury can lead to meningitis, pneumocephalus, or brain abscess.

Intra-operative CSF leaks should be addressed during initial surgery. The skull base defect should be found and thoroughly examined. Surrounding disease should be re-

* Avitene, Medchem Products Inc. 232 West Cummings Park, Wobum, MA.

moved so that an adequate surface for grafting is obtained. A free mucosal graft from the opposite side of the septum can be used to close most defects[28].

Patients with post-operative CSF leaks may present with headache, meningeal signs, or intermittent watery rhinorrhea. CSF leaks can also be delayed in onset and be asymptomatic. A high degree of suspicion is necessary in some cases. Comprehensive nasal endoscopy should be performed in an attempt to identify the dural defect. Computed tomography of the skull base with fine cuts aids in identifying the site of injury (Fig. 2). Suspected fluid should be collected and analyzed for the presence of Beta-2 Transferrin[29]. When there is insufficient fluid for testing, Radionuclide CSF Imaging can be utilized[30]. If necessary, the defect can be localized using intra-thecal fluorescein and a blue filter attached to the endoscope. Most dural defects can be repaired intra-nasally using previously described techniques[28].

Orbital Injury

Blindness from sinus surgery results from direct trauma to the optic nerve or as a result of retro-orbital hematoma. Direct trauma to the optic nerve usually occurs in the sphenoid or when the most posterior ethmoid pneumatizes the sphenoid resulting in an Onodi Cell. Onodi cells are present in 12 to 42% of patients with a higher incidence in Asians[31]. These cells pneumatize around the optic nerve and therefore place the nerve in jeopardy during sinus surgery. Kainz and Stammberger found the bone covering the optic nerve to be dehiscent in 12% of specimens examined[32]. Onodi cells can be identified on preoperative CT. Direct injury to the optic nerve generally results in irreversible visual loss.

Visual loss from orbital hematoma usually occurs following injury to the lamina papyracea[33]. The orbit has a fixed volume and therefore small quantities of blood markedly raise intra-orbital pressure. Three cc's of blood produces 6mm of proptosis. Lymphedema and venous obstruction lead to inadequate perfusion and subsequent visual loss. Recognition of a hematoma is imperative if permanent visual loss is to be avoided. Proptosis, lid edema, ophthalmoplegia and decreased visual acuity should alert the surgeon to this complication. Nasal packing should be removed. If vision is intact, medical measures can be tried. These include gentle massage of the globe, cooling with ice, high dose systemic steroids, and diuretics. If these maneuvers do not result in a reversal of symptoms, then a lateral canthotomy with cantholysis should be performed or a formal orbital decompression.

Diplopia following endoscopic sinus surgery is rare and usually results from injury to the medial rectus[34]. The medial orbital wall in the posterior ethmoid is usually disrupted along with damage to the medial retinal muscle. Identification of the medial orbital wall early in the dissection is imperative if this complication is to be avoided.

Lacrimal Injury

Epiphora following endoscopic sinus surgery is rare; however inadvertent injury to the lacrimal system is more common. Bolger et al used intra-operative fluorescein injection into the lacrimal system during 24 randomized endoscopic sinus procedures in order to determine the incidence of intra-operative lacrimal duct injury[35]. They found a 15% incidence of lacrimal duct disruption. However, none of the patients with intra-operative lacrimal injury developed epiphora. Five of the injured patients were available for Jones testing nearly one year later. Two patients recannalized into the middle meatus and three patients continued to show fluorescein in the inferior meatus.

Occasionally only mucosa separates the lacrimal duct from the natural ostium of the maxillary sinus. Injury to the lacrimal system can be minimized by enlarging the maxillary antrostomy posteriorly and inferiorly thus avoiding the lacrimal system.

Rare Complications

Rare complications from sino-nasal surgery include olfactory loss and Toxic Shock Syndrome (TSS). Kimmelman analyzed 93 patients who were undergoing nasal surgery including polypectomy with the University of Pennsylvania Smell Identification Test[36]. Anosmia occurred in one patient following nasal septal reconstruction. The olfactory epithelium is assumed to be distributed over the superior nasal septum, cribriform plate, and superior turbinate based upon neuroepithelial studies. However, the exact distribution of the epithelium needs further investigation[37]. Occasionally polyps are seen medial and adjacent to the middle turbinate or attached to the superior nasal septum. Minimal resection of the superior turbinate along with mucosal sparing in these areas may help avoid post-operative anosmia.

TSS is characterized by multi-system organ failure in association with fever, rash, hypotension, and desquamation and is usually seen within 48 hours of surgery[38]. TSS is caused by specific toxin producing Staphloccocal organisms and was first described in menstruating women. Treatment includes rehydration and the administration of anti-Staphloccocal intravenous antibiotics. Pre-operative prophylactic antibiotics have not been shown to prevent TSS.

CONCLUSION

Surgical therapy in most cases is not curative. However, when combined with medical therapy, surgery is extremely effective in controlling polyposis, especially when patients are followed endoscopically. The surgical procedure which provides the greatest efficacy with the least collateral damage at this time is endoscopic sinus surgery. Since patients with polyposis usually present the most difficult surgical challenges, considerable endoscopic experience is required of the surgeon if major complications are to be avoided.

REFERENCES

1. Messerklinger, W. *Endoscopy of the Nose*. Urban and Schwarzenberg, Baltimore, 1978.
2. Zinreich J. Imaging of inflammatory sinus disease. Otolaryngology Clinics of North America, 26, 535–547, 1993.
3. Vleming M, de Vries N. Endoscopic paranasal sinus surgery: Results. American Journal of Rhinology, 4, 13–17, 1990.
4. Wigand E, Hosemann W. Results of endoscopic surgery of the paranasal sinuses and anterior skull base. Journal of Otolaryngology, 20, 385–389, 1991.
5. Gaskins R. A surgical staging system for chronic sinusitis. American Journal of Rhinology, 6, 5–12, 1992.
6. Stammberger H, Posawetz W. Functional endoscopic sinus surgery: Concept, indications and results of the Messerklinger technique. European Archives of Otorhinolaryngology, 247, 63–76, 1990.
7. Wigand M, Hosemann W. Microsurgical treatment of recurrent nasal polyposis. Rhinology Suppl., 8, 25–30, 1989.
8. Lund V, Mackay I. Outcome assessment of endoscopic sinus surgery. Journal of the Royal Society of Medicine, 87, 70–72, 1994.
9. Jankowski R, Goetz R, Moneret D, et al. Les insuffusances de l'ethmoidectomie dans la prise en charge therapeutique de la polypose. Ann. Oto-Laryng., 108, 298–306, 1991.
10. Kennedy D. Prognostic factors, outcomes, and staging in ethmoid sinus surgery. Laryngoscope, Suppl. 57, 1–18, 1992.
11. Fang S. Normalization of maxillary sinus mucosa after FESS. A prospective study of chronic sinusitis with nasal polyps. Rhinology, 32, 137–140, 1994.
12. Levine H. Functional endoscopic sinus surgery: Evaluation, surgery, and follow-up of 250 patients. Laryngoscope, 100, 79–84, 1990.

13. Faugere J, Mauruc B, Douce P, Gouteyron J. Indications et resultats a propos de 290 ethmoidectomies endonasales. Revue de laryngologie, 113, 191–195, 1992.

14. Sogg A. Long-term results of ethmoid surgery. Ann Otol Rhinol Laryngol, 98, 699–701, 1989.

15. May M, Levine H, Schaitkin B, Mester S. Results of surgery. In Levine H, May M. Endoscopic Sinus Surgery. New York, Thieme, pp. 176–192, 1993.

16. Friedman W, Katsantonis G. Intranasal and transantral ethmoidectomy: A 20-year experience. Laryngoscope, 100, 343–348, 1990.

17. Drake-Lee A. Medical treatment of nasal polyps. Rhinology, 32, 1–4, 1994.

18. English G. Nasal polypectomy and sinus surgery in patients with asthma and aspirin idiosyncrasy. Laryngoscope, 96, 374–380, 1986.

19. Lawson W. The intranasal ethmoidectomy: An experience with 1,077 procedures. Laryngoscope, 101, 367–371, 1991.

20. Korchia D, Thomassin J, Doris J, Badier M. [Asthma and polyposis. Efficacy and adverse effect of endonasal ethmoidectomy. Results of 70 patients]. Ann Otolaryngol Chir Cervicofac, 109, 359–363, 1992.

21. Vander Veer A. The asthma problem. NY Med J., 112, 392–399, 1920.

22. Francis C. Prognosis of operations for removal of nasal polyps in asthma. Practitioner, 123, 272–278, 1929.

23. English G. Nasal polyposis. In: English G, ed. Otolaryngology. New York, JB Lippincott Co. 1991; vol.2:chptr 19:1–19.

24. Schaefer S, Close L. Endoscopic management of frontal sinus disease. Laryngoscope, 100, 155–160, 1990

25. Kennedy D, Shaman P, Deems D, et al. Complications of ethmoidectomy: A survey of Fellows of the American Academy of Otolaryngology-Head and Neck Surgery. Otolaryngology Head and Neck Surgery, 111, 589–599, 1994.

26. Maniglia A. Fatal and other major complications of endoscopic sinus surgery. Laryngoscope, 101, 349–354, 1991.

27. Kennedy D, Zinreich J, Hassab M. The internal carotid artery as it relates to endonasal sphenoethmoidectomy. American Journal of Rhinology, 4, 7–12, 1990.

28. Maddox D, Kennedy D. Endoscopic management of cerebrospinal fluid leaks and cephaloceles. Laryngoscope, 100, 857–862, 1990.

29. Skedros D, Cass S, Hirsch B, Kelly R. Beta-2 Transferrin assay in clinical management of cerebrospinal fluid and perilymphatic fluid leaks. Journal of Otolaryngology, 22, 341–344, 1993.

30. Holmes R. Hoffman K. Central nervous system. In: Early P, Sodee D, ed. Principles and Practices of Nuclear Medicine. Philadelphia, Mosby. 1995; 549–578.

31. Yeoh K, Tan K. The optic nerve in the posterior ethmoid in Asians. Acta Otolaryngol, 112, 852–861, 1992.

32. Kainz J, Stammberger H. Danger areas of the posterior rhinobasis. Acta Otolaryngol, 112, 852–861, 1992.

33. Stankiewicz J. Blindness and intranasal ethmoidectomy: Prevention and management. Otolaryngology Head and Neck Surgery, 101, 320–329, 1989.

34. Eitzen J, Elsas F. Strabismus following endoscopic intranasal sinus surgery. J of Ped Opth and Strabismus, 228, 168–170, 1991.

35. Bolger W, Parsons D, Mair E, Kuhn F. Lacrimal drainage system injury in functional endoscopic sinus surgery. Archives of Otolaryngology Head and Neck Surgery, 118, 1179–1184, 1992.

36. Kimmelman C. The Risk to Olfaction from nasal surgery. Laryngoscope, 104, 981–088, 1994.

37. Paik S, Lehman M, Seiden A, Duncan H, Smith D. Human olfactory biopsy, the influence of age and receptor distribution. Archives of Otolaryngology, 118, 731–738, 1992.

38. Abram A, Bellian K, Giles W, Gross C. Toxic shock syndrome after functional endonasal sinus surgery: An all or none phenomenon? Laryngoscope, 104, 927–931, 1994.

Index